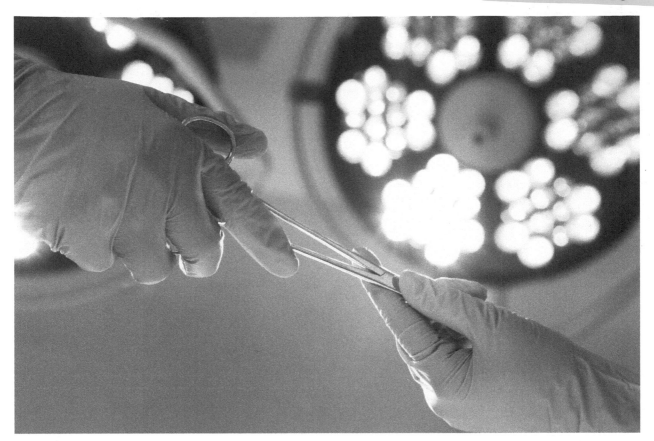

BMJ Clinical Review:

General Surgery

Edited by
Gopal K Mahadev & Eleftheria Kleidi

BPP
UNIVERSITY
SCHOOL OF HEALTH

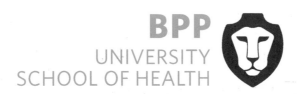

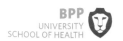

First edition August 2015

ISBN 9781 4727 3894 3
eISBN 9781 4727 4404 3
eISBN 9781 4727 4412 8

British Library Cataloguing-in-Publication Data
A catalogue record for this book is available from the British Library

Published by
BPP Learning Media Ltd
BPP House, Aldine Place
London W12 8AA

www.bpp.com/health

Printed in the United Kingdom by
Ashford Colour Press Ltd

Unit 600, Fareham Reach,
Fareham Road,
Gosport, Hampshire,
PO13 0FW

Your learning materials, published by BPP Learning Media Ltd, are printed on paper sourced from sustainable, managed forests.

The content of this publication contains articles from The BMJ which have been selected, collated and published by BPP Learning Media under a licence.

The contents of this book are intended as a guide and not professional advice. Although every effort has been made to ensure that the contents of this book are correct at the time of going to press, BPP Learning Media, the Editor and the Author make no warranty that the information in this book is accurate or complete and accept no liability for any loss or damage suffered by any person acting or refraining from acting as a result of the material in this book.

Every effort has been made to contact the copyright holders of any material reproduced within this publication. If any have been inadvertently overlooked, BPP Learning Media will be pleased to make the appropriate credits in any subsequent reprints or editions.

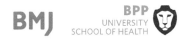

About the publisher

BPP Learning Media is dedicated to supporting aspiring professionals with top quality learning material. BPP Learning Media's commitment to success is shown by our record of quality, innovation and market leadership in paper-based and e-learning materials. BPP Learning Media's study materials are written by professionally-qualified specialists who know from personal experience the importance of top quality materials for success.

About The BMJ

The BMJ (formerly the British Medical Journal) in print has a long history and has been published without interruption since 1840. The BMJ's vision is to be the world's most influential and widely read medical journal. Our mission is to lead the debate on health and to engage, inform, and stimulate doctors, researchers, and other health professionals in ways that will improve outcomes for patients. We aim to help doctors to make better decisions. BMJ, the company, advances healthcare worldwide by sharing knowledge and expertise to improve experiences, outcomes and value.

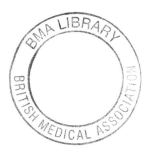

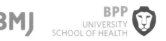

Contents

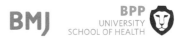

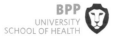

About the editors

Mr Gopal K Mahadev is a Consultant Surgeon with specialist interest in Breast Oncoplastic and General Surgery. He is member of Court of Examiners for MRCS with the Royal College of Surgeons of England & FRCS Intercollegiate Board and also involved in Quality Assurance of Assessments. He has worked as Senior Lecturer (Hon) in Medical Education and is a teacher, trainer, examiner and mentor for Medical Students, Surgical trainees as well as Consultants.

Mrs. Eleftheria Kleidi is a Specialty Registrar in Upper Gastrointestinal Surgery at Leighton Hospital, Crewe. She qualified from the Medical School of the University of Crete in 2004. After her foundation years, she started her training in general surgery in Athens and obtained her CCT in 2013. Since then, she has been specialising in UGI surgery and Bariatrics and was awarded the scholarship of the College of Surgeons of Greece for training in the UK. She completed her PhD in Bariatrics at the University of Athens in 2015.

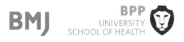

Introduction to General Surgery

Surgery continues to progress as new technology, techniques and knowledge are incorporated into the care of surgical patients. The creation of new books with updated and concentrated knowledge in the field has always been a necessity. As Theodore Billroth quoted, in the 19th century: *"It is a most gratifying sign of the rapid progress of our time that our best textbooks become antiquated so quickly"*.

General surgery is no longer an integrated specialty and is divided into a set of clearly defined subspecialties. However, the surgical challenges remain the same. These include the evolution of surgical practical performance, the efficient decision-making about patient management and the meticulous post-operative care. In this book, we have attempted to contribute to the advancement of the latter two challenges, by carefully selecting and compiling clinical reviews from the BMJ.

Clinical reviews from the BMJ provide a clear, up to date account of each topic including broad update of recent developments and their likely clinical applications in primary and secondary care. Its aim is to also stimulate readers to read further and therefore each article additionally indicates other sources of information. The clinical reviews provide a thorough, useful, readable and understandable knowledge on general surgery and surgical oncology. Updated principles and techniques are presented on the topics in various specialities. We expect this book to be used as an adjunct to the expansion of knowledge on surgical fields.

This book is designed to be equally useful to medical students, trainees in general surgery, Medical practitioners with an interest in expanding their knowledge in gastrointestinal pathologies and candidates for postgraduate exams from the concentrated and evidence-based knowledge encountered in this book. We do hope that you will find this book useful towards this direction.

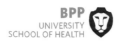

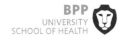

Treatment of breast infection

J Michael Dixon, professor of surgery and consultant surgeon[12],
Lucy R Khan, specialty registrar breast surgery[2]

[1]Breakthrough Research Unit, Edinburgh Breast Unit, Western General Hospital, Edinburgh EH4 2XU, UK

[2]Edinburgh Breast Unit

Correspondence to: J M Dixon jmd@ed.ac.uk

Cite this as: BMJ 2011;342:d396

DOI: 10.1136/bmj.d396

http://www.bmj.com/content/342/bmj.d396

A cohort study of American women reported that 10% of women who breast feed have mastitis,[1] and a recent Cochrane review reported the incidence to be as high as 33%.[2] Breast abscesses are seen less often, but when they do develop delays in referral to a specialist surgeon may occur. A recent survey in the United Kingdom found that many surgical units have no clear protocols for managing patients with breast infection who are referred to hospital.[3] Some surgeons aspirate breast abscesses under local anaesthesia, whereas others use general anaesthesia. The management of breast infection has evolved over the past two decades, with advances in both diagnosis and treatment. A new concept is bedside ultrasound, and this plays an important part in current management.

We review management of breast infection in the primary care setting and after hospital referral. The review is based on our current practice and the best quality evidence available. Few randomised controlled trials deal with this topic, and most breast specialists have adopted their own protocols for clinical management, loosely based on published algorithms, and largely dictated by their specific patient population and their clinical practice setting. This review provides a resource for those who see breast infection infrequently. Appropriate timely referral will help avoid unnecessary morbidity for patients.

What kinds of breast infection are there?

Infection can occur in the parenchyma of the breast or the skin overlying the breast (fig 1). Parenchymal breast infections can occur in lactating and non-lactating breasts. One cross sectional analysis of 89 patients with breast abscesses requiring surgical intervention found that 14% were lactational and 86% were non-lactational.[4]

Which micro-organisms are implicated?

An up to date retrospective case series shows that during lactation the most common organism responsible is *Staphylococcus aureus*,[6] including strains of meticillin resistant *S aureus* (MRSA), particularly if the infection was

SOURCES AND SELECTION CRITERIA

We conducted a Medline search using the key words "breast infection", "mastitis", and "breast abscess". This review focuses on parenchymal breast infection, with brief mention of infections of the skin overlying the breast. We do not include infection associated with implants. We selected articles that provided the best evidence available. Our experience from clinical practice is huge, and we have included many of the lessons learnt over the many years that we have managed patients with breast abscesses.

acquired in hospital.[1][7] Other organisms responsible include streptococci and *Staphylococcus epidermidis*. Organisms responsible for non-lactating breast infections include bacteria commonly associated with skin infections but also include enterococci and anaerobic bacteria such as *Bacteroides* spp and anaerobic streptococci.[8] Patients with recurrent breast abscesses have a higher incidence of mixed flora (20.5% in those with recurrence v 8.9% with a single episode), including anaerobic organisms (4.5% v 0%).[4]

Investigating and managing breast infection in lactating women

Who gets it and how do they present?

Lactating breast infection is most commonly seen within the first six weeks of breast feeding, although it can develop during weaning. The infection arises initially in a localised segment of the breast and can spread to the entire quadrant and then the whole of the breast if untreated.

A review of 946 cases of lactational mastitis in the United States found that women often gave a history of difficulty with breast feeding and many had experienced engorgement, poor milk drainage, or an excoriated nipple.[9] Population based studies have shown that risk factors for abscess formation include maternal age over 30 years, gestational age greater than 41 weeks, and a history of mastitis.[10][11] The examining doctor may see erythema, localised tenderness, localised engorgement, or swelling. Some women present with fever, malaise, and occasionally rigors.

SUMMARY POINTS

- Early prescription of appropriate antibiotics reduces the rate of breast abscess development
- Refer to hospital all patients whose infection does not settle rapidly after one course of appropriate antibiotics
- Use ultrasound routinely in patients referred with a suspected abscess to see whether pus is present
- Breast abscesses can usually be treated in the outpatients department by repeated aspiration or mini-incision and drainage under local anaesthesia
- Patients whose inflammatory changes do not settle after a course of antibiotics may have inflammatory breast cancer; in such cases perform imaging and image guided core biopsy if a localised suspicious abnormality is present
- Recurrent central infection is usually associated with periductal mastitis—a smoking related disease—and total duct excision is often needed

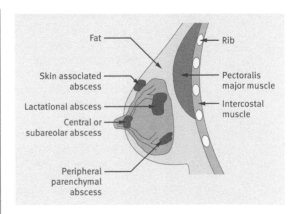

Fig 1 Diagram showing common sites and types of breast infection[5]

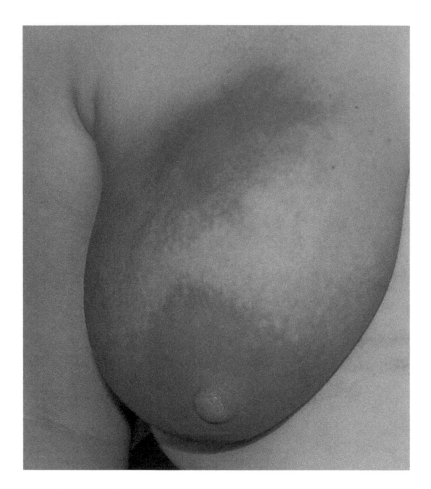

Fig 2 Lactating abscess at presentation with visible swelling and overlying erythema

A cohort study estimated that 2-10% of breastfeeding women get mastitis but only 0.4% develop an abscess.[1] A prospective study of 128 women reported that 5-10% of women with mastitis developed a breast abscess, possibly because of suboptimal management of their mastitis.[12]

How to treat mastitis

Guidelines from the World Health Organization and numerous reviews of the condition recommend treating lactating women with mastitis by prescribing appropriate oral antibiotics and encouraging milk flow from the engorged segment (by continuation of breast feeding or use of a breast pump). Such measures reduce the rate of abscess formation and thereby relieve symptoms.[2] A Cochrane review found only one reported randomised trial of antibiotic treatment versus breast emptying alone conducted among women with lactational mastitis that showed faster clearance (mean 2.1 v 4.2 days) of symptoms in women using antibiotics.[2] Oral antibiotics are usually sufficient, and only rarely do patients with sepsis require hospital admission and intravenous antibiotics. Lactating infection can be treated by flucloxacillin, co-amoxiclav, or a macrolide such as erythromycin or clarithromycin (in patients who are allergic to penicillin), given for at least 10 days. Tetracycline, ciprofloxacin, and chloramphenicol should not be used to treat lactating breast infection because these drugs can enter breast milk and harm the baby.

One report of using *Lactobacillus fermentum* and *Lactobacillus salivarius* as an alternative treatment has shown them to be as effective as antibiotics.[13] Further studies are needed before they can be used as an alternative to appropriate antibiotics.

There is an alarming trend towards believing that fungi are important in the aetiology of breast infection and deep breast pain associated with breast feeding, despite a lack of good quality evidence. The prescription of antifungals, such as fluconazole, is common despite the lack of good quality clinical evidence to support their use.[14]

A case series describes several patients with breast pain during breast feeding who did not have mastitis but Raynaud's disease of the nipple and who responded to nifedipine.[15] Prescription of anti-inflammatory drugs and the application of cold compresses or ice packs can help to alleviate pain. One small trial compared the effectiveness of chilled or room temperature cabbage leaves with ice packs and both produced identical symptom relief.[16]

We have found that it is not uncommon for patients to be referred late to hospital with established large volume abscesses (fig 2). Reasons for this include failure to refer infection that does not settle rapidly after one course of antibiotics; a lack of continuity of care in the community; use of inappropriate antibiotics; and delays as a result of using other treatment modalities, such as antifungal agents and cold compresses alone.

Investigating a suspected breast abscess

Ultrasound will establish the presence of pus and should be performed in any patient whose infection does not settle with one course of antibiotics, whether a breast abscess is suspected or not (fig 3). Even when clinical examination shows obvious signs of an abscess, ultrasound is useful because it may identify more than one collection of pus that might otherwise be missed.

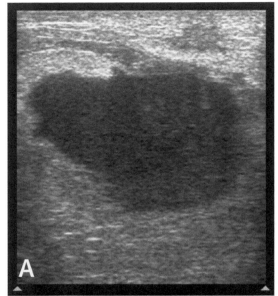

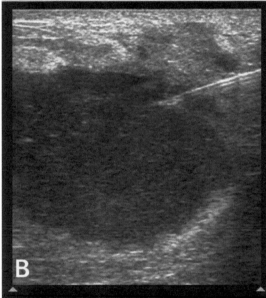

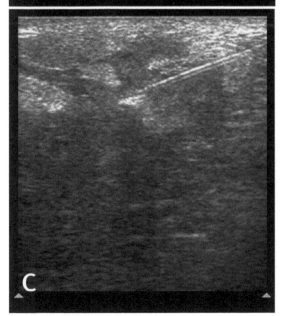

Fig 3 (A) Ultrasound of lactating breast abscess. (B) Lactating breast abscess; the needle is visible on the upper right immediately before aspiration. (C) Lactating breast abscess after aspiration; no more fluid is visible in the abscess, which has now collapsed

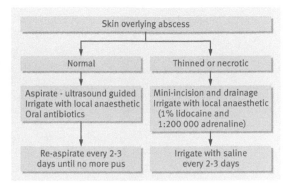

Fig 4 Breast abscess protocol

Draining an abscess

In our specialist practice we have developed and evaluated the following approach to the management of breast abscesses. We base our approach to draining the abscess on the appearance of the skin overlying the abscess (fig 4).

If the overlying skin is normal, we recommend aspiration of the abscess under ultrasound guidance using adequate local anaesthesia. A 21 gauge needle is introduced through the skin some distance away from the abscess and 1% lidocaine with 1:200 000 adrenaline is infiltrated into the skin and into the breast tissue under ultrasound image guidance. When reaching the abscess cavity (fig 3B), if the pus is thin enough it can be aspirated with the same needle. Once the pus has been aspirated the syringe is changed and the abscess cavity is irrigated with as much as 50 mL of 1% lidocaine and adrenaline. On ultrasound imaging the abscess cavity should be seen to expand and collapse as fluid is injected and aspirated to dryness (fig 3C).

If the pus is very thick and cannot be aspirated through a 21 gauge needle, then having waited for local anaesthetic to be effective, a larger gauge needle may be advanced through the skin and breast tissue into the cavity. The pus is diluted with local anaesthetic and adrenaline, after which this is aspirated. We find that using a combination of lidocaine and adrenaline in solution reduces pain and minimises bleeding and subsequent bruising. Irrigation is continued until all the pus is aspirated and the fluid used to irrigate comes back clear. The net effect of this procedure is to control pain by a combination of providing local anaesthesia and reducing the pressure within the abscess cavity by aspirating all the pus. We send a sample of pus to the microbiology department for culture and continue appropriate oral antibiotics and analgesia until the abscess resolves.

We review the patient every two to three days and repeat aspiration under ultrasound guidance if fluid is present in the abscess cavity. We continue with this approach until no further fluid is visible in the abscess cavity or the fluid aspirated does not contain pus. Few abscesses require more than two to three aspirations, although very large collections may require more. Characteristically, the fluid aspirated changes from pus to serous fluid and then to milk over a few days. Most abscesses in lactating breasts can be managed successfully in this manner.

If the skin overlying the abscess is compromised and is thin and shiny or necrotic we perform mini-incision and drainage (fig 5). Local anaesthetic is infiltrated into the skin overlying the abscess and left for a minimum of seven to eight minutes, and then a small stab incision with a number 15 blade is made into the abscess over the point of maximum fluctuation. If the point of maximum fluctuation is not clear, ultrasound can help to define the best site for incision. We excise any necrotic skin. Once the contents of the abscess cavity are drained, we irrigate the cavity thoroughly with local anaesthetic solution and repeat every two to three days until there is no evident leakage from the abscess, the wound closes, and no further pus is draining. Most patients whose abscess needs to be incised and drained can have the procedure performed under local anaesthesia in the outpatient clinic. Large incisions are not necessary to drain breast abscesses, and the cosmetic results of the small incisions needed are usually excellent. The placement of drains and insertion of packing have no role in the modern day management of breast abscesses.

If infection fails to regress with appropriate management, carry out further imaging combined with needle core biopsy of any suspicious abnormality to exclude an inflammatory cancer.

Breast feeding after breast infection

Although women are encouraged to continue breast feeding after treatment of mastitis or an abscess, it may be difficult to do so from the affected side. If the infant cannot relieve breast fullness during nursing, the woman may use hand expression or a breast pump to encourage and maintain milk flow until breast feeding can resume. Although most women are able to continue breast feeding even if they have excoriation of the nipple and pain, a few experience continuous and disabling pain (fig 6). If after discussion a woman chooses to stop breast feeding so that the breast infection can be controlled and the breast can heal, lactation can be suppressed using cabergoline.

Investigating and managing breast infection in non-lactating women

Who is at risk?

People at highest risk of developing an infection of breast tissue when not lactating are those who smoke and those with diabetes. A recent retrospective analysis found that patients with non-lactating skin associated abscesses who have diabetes or who smoke (or both) are likely to have recurrent episodes of breast infection.[17] Infections are categorised as central or subareolar infections and peripheral infections—each has different causes and treatments. Infections that occur in the skin of the breast are usually secondary to an underlying lesion such as a sebaceous cyst or hidradenitis suppurativa.

Types of infection

Central or subareolar infection

This is usually secondary to periductal mastitis, a condition in which the subareolar ducts are damaged and become infected, often by anaerobic bacteria.[8] Patients may present initially with subareolar inflammation (with or without an associated mass) or with an established abscess (fig 7A). Associated features include nipple retraction and a discharge from the nipple. Periductal mastitis predominantly affects young women, the average age being 32 years, and smoking is a major causative factor, with 90% of patients being smokers. Periductal mastitis and can also occur in men.[18] [19] Substances in cigarette smoke—such as lipid peroxidise, nicotine, and cotinine—concentrate in the breast and are found at much higher concentrations in subareolar ducts than in plasma. Either the toxic substances in cigarette smoke damage the ducts directly or local hypoxia causes subareolar duct damage and subsequent inflammation and infection.[18]

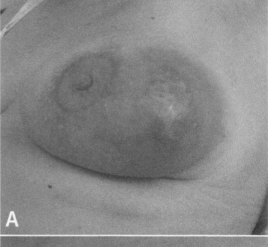

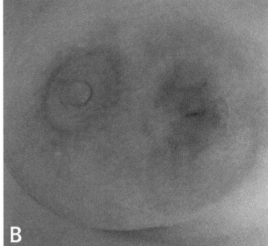

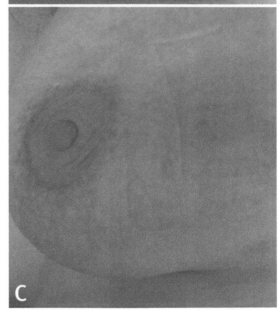

Fig 5 (A) Lactating breast abscess with thin overlying skin best treated by mini-incision and drainage under local anaesthesia. (B) Lactating breast abscess immediately after mini-incision and drainage. (C) One week after mini-incision and drainage

Patients with periductal mastitis can have bilateral disease, and some women present with bilateral fistulas and nipple changes on both sides. Smokers who have nipple piercing can develop persistent and troublesome infection. Breast abscesses can affect men as well as women.

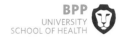

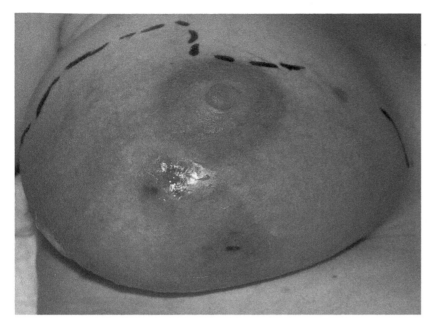

Fig 6 Extensive lactating breast infection with multiple abscesses. Patient had sepsis and was fatigued, and she decided to stop breast feeding

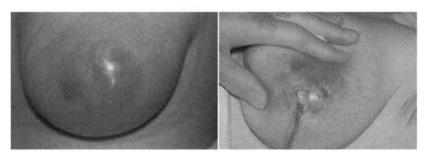

Fig 7 (A) Periareolar abscess with thin overlying skin. (B) Abscess during mini-incision and drainage

---

A PATIENT'S PERSPECTIVE

My problems with breast feeding started as soon as my baby was born with pain from sore, cracked, and bleeding nipples. During the first four weeks the pain increased until I developed extreme shooting pains, which would make my body writhe and jump in bed. I was unable to sleep and dreaded each feed. Then a hard lump developed in my breast. I thought it was a blocked duct and was advised to continue feeding. I sought out as much help and advice as possible from midwives, general practitioners, health visitors, breastfeeding councillors, and breastfeeding groups. The lump continued to grow until I could cup it in my hand. I was advised to try fluconazole but was not given antibiotics. In the end, I had to ask the fourth general practitioner I saw to make an emergency referral to the breast unit.

By the time I was seen, several weeks after the lump developed, I was desperate for somebody to do something. I was becoming depressed with the pain and at the thought of having to give up breast feeding, but I knew I could not continue on in agony. My 7×7 cm breast abscess had to be aspirated six times over two weeks and I took antibiotics for 10 days. It was extremely important to me that I was seen by the same person each time I attended. I have been able to continue breast feeding and my breast has now recovered completely.

Peripheral non-lactating infection

This is less common than central infection. Peripheral infection has been associated with diabetes, rheumatoid arthritis, steroid treatment, trauma, and granulomatous lobular mastitis but often there is no underlying cause. Occasionally, comedo ductal carcinoma in situ can become infected and present with inflammation or as an abscess; we therefore recommend that patients over 35 years with peripheral infection and no obvious cause undergo bilateral mammography once the infection has resolved.

Granulomatous lobular mastitis

One cause of peripheral infection is granulomatous lobular mastitis, a condition of unknown aetiology. It can present as a peripheral inflammatory mass that masquerades as cancer or as an area of infection with or without overlying skin ulceration. Although this condition mostly affects young parous women, who develop multiple and recurrent abscesses, it is seen in nulliparous women as well. It has been suggested that *Corynebacterium* spp play a part in this condition,[20] but antibiotics effective against these organisms rarely lead to resolution of disease and thus they are unlikely to have a major aetiological role.

Skin associated infection

Sebaceous cysts are common over the skin of the breast and these can become infected to form local abscesses. Cellulitis of the breast with or without abscess formation is common in patients who are overweight, have large breasts, or have had breast surgery or radiotherapy. It occurs in the lower half of the breast and also under the breast where sweat accumulates and intertrigo develops. Intertrigo may be a recurrent problem in women with large ptotic breasts. *Staphylococcus aureus* is the usual causative organism. Although antifungal creams are commonly prescribed, there is no evidence that fungi play an aetiological role in this condition.[21] Hidradenitis suppurativa commonly affects the axilla and groin and can also affect the skin of the lower half of the breast, resulting in recurrent episodes of infection and abscess formation.

Which antibiotic is best?

We recommend treating non-lactating and skin associated breast infections with amoxicillin and clavulanic acid or, if the patient is allergic to penicillin, a combination of erythromycin and metronidazole.

Managing abscesses

Non-lactating abscesses are managed in a similar way to lactating breast abscesses by aspiration or mini-incision and drainage (fig 7B) combined with appropriate oral antibiotics. Recurrence is common after resolution of central or subareolar non-lactating abscesses because the underlying pathology in the central ducts often persists. Patients with recurrent disease require definitive surgery in the form of total duct excision to remove the diseased ducts and stop the cycle of recurrent infection.

Recurrent episodes of periductal mastitis and infection can result in a mammary duct fistula. In such cases, excision of the fistula combined with total duct excision or laying open the fistula is usually effective. To reduce the risk of recurrence, all the ducts must be excised right up to the back of the nipple, leaving only nipple skin.[22] It is sometimes necessary to remove the nipple areolar complex in cases with recurrent infection. All patients who smoke should be advised of the risks of continued smoking and its association with recurrent breast infection and fistula formation.

Granulomatous lobular mastitis eventually resolves without active intervention so management is focused on treating abscesses appropriately.[23] Steroids have been used,[24] but we do not recommend them for this condition.

Managing skin related infections

For abscesses related to sebaceous cysts, incision under local anaesthesia with irrigation of the cavity and evacuation of the sebaceous material is usually effective. After resolution

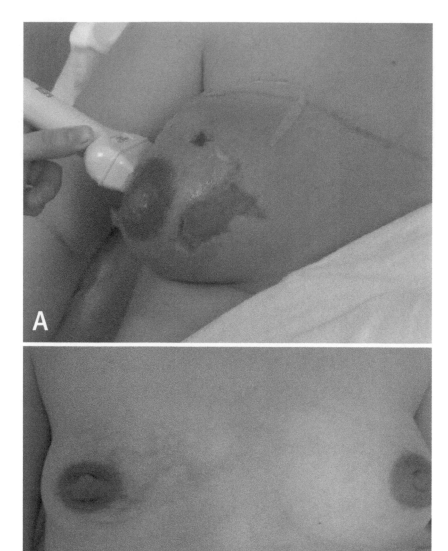

Fig 8 (A) Abscess where referral was greatly delayed.
(B) Same patient one year later showing major asymmetry as a result of tissue loss

of the abscess, the sebaceous cyst is usually sufficiently scarred that it does not require formal excision. If the sebaceous cyst persists, then consider excision of the cyst under local anaesthetic once all infection has resolved.

Abscesses related to hidradenitis are treated by mini-incision and drainage combined with appropriate antibiotics. Options for recurrent infection include treatment with retinoids in mild cases. Surgical excision of the affected area or skin grafting results in long term control in 20-50% of women.[25] Consider referring patients with severe hidradenitis to a dermatologist or plastic surgeon.

The primary management of recurrent infections and intertrigo affecting the lower half of the skin of the breast should aim to keep the area as clean and dry as possible. In our experience, it is important for patients to wash at least twice a day and avoid all creams (including antifungals) and talcum powder. Cotton bras or a cotton T shirt or vest worn inside the bra may help keep the area clean and dry.

Conclusion

The management of breast infection has changed and doctors in primary and secondary care should be aware of current protocols and management pathways. Breast infection is common and most cases resolve with antibiotics. Urgently refer any patient whose infection does not settle rapidly after one course of appropriate antibiotics to minimise the associated morbidity. Delay in referral or instituting inappropriate antibiotic treatment can have serious consequences, with loss of large volumes of breast tissue and substantial asymmetry (fig 8). Such a result has potential medicolegal consequences in modern medicine.

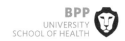

TIPS FOR NON-SPECIALISTS

- Prescribe appropriate antibiotics early to minimise subsequent abscess development
- In lactating infections, promote milk drainage by encouraging women to continue breast feeding
- Refer the patient urgently to a specialist breast surgeon if infection does not settle rapidly after one course of appropriate antibiotics
- Consider breast cancer in patients with an inflammatory lesion that persists despite appropriate management

ADDITIONAL EDUCATIONAL RESOURCES

Resources for healthcare professionals

- Dixon JM. Benign breast disease. In: Burnand KG, Young AE, Lucas J, eds. A new Airds companion to surgical studies. Elsevier, 2005:506-17
- Beers MH, Berkow R, eds. Breast disease. The Merck manual of diagnosis and therapy. 17th ed. Merck Research Laboratories, 1999
- Dixon JM. Breast infection. In: ABC of breast diseases. Blackwell Publishing, 2006:19-23

Resources for patients

- NHS Choices (www.nhs.uk/Conditions/Breast-abscess)— Information on breast abscesses including causes, symptoms, diagnosis, risks, and treatment; has links to other useful resources
- Patient UK (www.patient.co.uk/health/Mastitis-(Breast-Infection).htm)—Information on symptoms and treatment; allows patients to discuss their experiences

Contributors: LRK wrote the first draft. JMD helped finalise the manuscript and provided images.

Competing interests: All authors have completed the Unified Competing Interest form at www.icmje.org/coi_disclosure.pdf (available on request from the corresponding author) and declare: no support from any organisation for the submitted work; no financial relationships with any organisations that might have an interest in the submitted work in the previous three years; no other relationships or activities that could appear to have influenced the submitted work.

Provenance and peer review: Commissioned; externally peer reviewed.

Patient consent obtained.

1 ACOG. Committee opinion no 361: Breastfeeding: maternal and infant aspects. *Obstet Gynaecol* 2007;109:479-80.
2 Jahanfar S, Ng CJ, Teng CL. Antibiotics for mastitis in breastfeeding women. *Cochrane Database Syst Rev* 2009;1:CD005458.
3 Thrush S, Dixon JM. Treatment of loculated lactational breast abscess with a vacuum biopsy system. *Br J Surg* 2006;93:251.
4 Bharat A, Gao F, Aft RL, Gillanders WE, Eberlein TJ, Margenthaler JA. Predictors of primary breast abscesses and recurrence. *World J Surg* 2009;33:2582-6.
5 Hughes LE, Mansel RE, Webster DJT. Miscellaneous conditions. In: Hughes LE, Mansel RE, Webster DJT, eds. Benign disorders and diseases of the breast: current concepts and clinical management. Edward Arnold, 2000:230.
6 Moazzez A, Kelso RL, Towfigh S, Sohn H, Berne TV, Mason RJ. Breast abscess bacteriologic features in the era of community-acquired methicillin-resistant Staphylococcus aureus epidemics. *Arch Surg* 2007;142:881-4.
7 Schoenfeld EM, McKay MP. Mastitis and methicillin-resistant Staphylococcus aureus (MRSA): the calm before the storm? *J Emerg Med* 2010;38:e31-4.
8 Bundred NJ, Dixon JM, Lumsden AB, Radford D, Hood J, Miles RS, et al. Are the lesions of duct ectasia sterile? *Br J Surg* 1985;72:844-5.
9 Foxman B, D'Arcy H, Gillespie B, Bobo JK, Schwartz K. Lactation mastitis: occurrence and medical management among 946 breastfeeding women in the United States. *Am J Epidemiol* 2002;155:103-14.
10 Berens PD. Prenatal, intrapartum, and postpartum support of the lactating mother. *Pediatr Clin North Am* 2001;48:365-75.
11 Kvist LJ, Rydhstroem H. Factors related to breast abscess after delivery: a population-based study. *BJOG* 2005;112:1070-4.
12 Dener C, Inan A. Breast abscesses in lactating women. *World J Surg* 2003;27:130-3.
13 Arroyo R, Martin V, Maldonado A, Jimenez E, Fernandez L, Rodriguez JM. Treatment of infectious mastitis during lactation: antibiotics versus oral administration of lactobacilli isolated from breast milk. *Clin Infect Dis* 2010;50:1551-8.
14 Carmichael AR, Dixon JM. Is lactation mastitis and shooting breast pain experienced by women during lactation caused by Candida albicans? *Breast* 2002;11:88-90.
15 Anderson JE, Held N, Wright K. Raynaud's phenomenon of the nipple: a treatable cause of painful breastfeeding. *Pediatrics* 2004;113:360-4.
16 Roberts KL. A comparison of chilled cabbage leaves and chilled gelpaks in reducing breast engorgement. *J Hum Lact* 1995;11:17-20.
17 Rizzo M, Peng L, Frisch A, Jurado M, Umpierrez G. Breast abscesses in nonlactating women with diabetes: clinical features and outcome. *Am J Med Sci* 2009;338:123-6.
18 Dixon JM. Periductal mastitis and duct ectasia: an update. *Breast* 1998;7:128.
19 Bundred NJ, Dover MS, Aluwihare N, Faragher EB, Morrison JM. Smoking and periductal mastitis. *BMJ* 1993;307:772-3.
20 Paviour S, Musad S, Roberts S, Taylor G, Taylor S, Shore K, et al. Corynebacterium species isolated from patients with mastitis. *Clin Infect Dis* 2002;35:1434-40.
21 Janniger CK, Schwartz RA, Szepietowski JC, Reich A. Intertrigo and common secondary skin infections. *Am Fam Physician* 2005;72:833-8.
22 Dixon JM, Kohlhardt SR, Dillon P. Total duct excision. *Breast* 1998;7:216.
23 Galea MH, Robertson JF, Ellis IO, Elston CW, Blamey RW. Granulomatous lobular mastitis. *Aust N Z J Surg* 1989;59:547-50.
24 Wilson JP, Massoll N, Marshall J, Foss RM, Copeland EM, Grobmyer SR. Idiopathic granulomatous mastitis: in search of a therapeutic paradigm. *Am Surg* 2007;73:798-802.
25 Mansel RE, Webster DJT, Sweetland HM. Miscellaneous conditions. In: Mansel RE, Webster DJT, Sweetland HM, eds. Benign disorders and diseases of the breast: current concepts and clinical management. 3rd ed. Saunders, Elsevier, 2009:273-96.

Related links

bmj.com/archive
- Pharmacological prevention of migraine (2011;342: d583)
- Telehealthcare for long term conditions (2010;342:d120)
- Preventing exacerbations in chronic obstructive pulmonary disease (2010;342:c7207)
- Islet transplantation in type 1 diabetes (2010;342:d217)
- Diagnosis and management of hereditary haemochromatosis (2010;342:c7251)

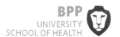

Ductal carcinoma in situ of the breast

Nicola L P Barnes, specialist registrar breast surgery[1], Jane L Ooi, consultant breast and oncoplastic surgeon[1], John R Yarnold, professor of clinical oncology[2], Nigel J Bundred, professor of surgical oncology[3]

[1]Breast Unit, Royal Bolton Hospital, Bolton BL4 0JR, UK

[2]Radiotherapy Unit, Institute of Cancer Research and Royal Marsden Hospital, London, UK

[3]Department of Surgical Oncology, South Manchester University Hospital, Manchester, UK

Correspondence to: N L P Barnes
nicolabarnes@doctors.org.uk

Cite this as: BMJ 2012;344:e797

DOI: 10.1136/bmj.e797

http://www.bmj.com/content/344/bmj.e797

Ductal carcinoma in situ (DCIS) is a preinvasive (also termed non-invasive) breast cancer, where proliferations of malignant ductal epithelial cells remain confined within intact breast ducts (fig 1). DCIS is a precursor lesion that has the potential to transform into an invasive cancer over a timescale that may be a few years or decades long. The development of its ability to invade and metastasise is as yet unquantifiable and is attributed to the accumulation of somatic mutations in premalignant cells. Treatment aims to prevent DCIS from progressing to invasive breast cancer.

DCIS was rarely diagnosed before the introduction of national screening programmes but is now common, accounting for 20% of screen detected cancers in the United Kingdom.[1] Treatment usually comprises surgery (mastectomy or wide local excision), with or without adjuvant radiotherapy. However, it is possible that a subset of these lesions would never progress to invasive breast cancer over the lifetime of the patient if left untreated, and in this (as yet undefined) population traditional management may represent overtreatment. Deciding on appropriate personalised treatment for individual patients diagnosed with DCIS is an ongoing challenge, because the optimum management remains controversial. We review relevant randomised controlled trials, meta-analyses, preclinical, and clinical studies to provide the reader with an overview of the evidence base underpinning current management of patients with DCIS and to highlight controversies and unanswered research questions.

How does DCIS develop?

The natural course of DCIS is poorly understood. It is categorised into low grade, intermediate grade, and high grade disease according to combinations of cell morphology, architecture, and the presence of necrosis. High grade DCIS has pleomorphic, irregularly spaced, large nuclei that vary in size and have irregular nuclear contours, coarse chromatin, prominent nucleoli, and frequent mitoses. Low grade DCIS has monomorphic, evenly spaced cells with rounded centrally placed nuclei, inconspicuous nucleoli, infrequent mitoses, and rarely necrosis of individual cells. Intermediate grade DCIS lies within these extremes—the nuclei are typically larger than in low grade DCIS and show moderate pleomorphism.[2] The developmental pathway of

SOURCES AND SELECTION CRITERIA

We searched Medline and PubMed for meta-analyses, randomised controlled trials, and original peer reviewed articles, using ductal carcinoma in situ, DCIS, preinvasive, non-invasive, treatment, radiotherapy, endocrine therapy, and psychosocial as main search terms. Only papers written in English were selected and we obtained the full text for each. We searched the Cochrane database for relevant reviews and www.Clinicaltrials.gov for current research.

low grade and intermediate grade DCIS is thought to differ from that of high grade disease. Low grade tumours show a loss in the 16q chromosome, whereas high grade disease more often shows 17q gain.[3] Atypical ductal hyperplasia is thought to be a precursor lesion of low grade DCIS and has a similar fivefold increased risk of subsequent invasive cancer. High grade DCIS has no obvious precursor lesion. Low grade DCIS, if it progresses, tends to develop into low grade invasive cancer, whereas high grade DCIS progresses to high grade invasive disease.

Risk factors for developing DCIS include a family history of breast cancer, nulliparity, older age at birth of first child, and positivity for BRCA1 and BRCA2.[4][5] Since the publication of the Women's Health Initiative and the Million Women Study,[6][7] the association between invasive breast cancer and combined oestrogen and progesterone hormone replacement therapy has been well documented. However, hormone replacement therapy did not significantly increase the risk of developing DCIS in these two studies. In the Women's Health Initiative study there were 47 cases of DCIS in the hormone replacement therapy group versus 37 cases in the control group (hazard ratio 1.18; weighted P=0.09).[6] The Million Women study did not report an association with DCIS. A large surveillance study published in 2009 found that atypical ductal hyperplasia (and by implication, low grade DCIS) has become less common since women stopped using hormone replacement therapy.[8] This suggests that, although hormone replacement therapy may not increase the risk of developing DCIS, it may promote the growth of pre-existing populations of oestrogen receptor positive DCIS progenitor cells.

When considering referral to a family history clinic, a case of DCIS in the family should count towards the indicators for genetic testing in the same way that an invasive cancer does. Non-screen detected DCIS is rare in the UK, and a diagnosis of DCIS in a first degree relative under screening age may also warrant consideration of family history risk assessment.

How might DCIS present?

More than 90% of cases of DCIS are detected at screening while asymptomatic. About 6% of all symptomatic breast cancers are preinvasive.[1] Some patients present with Paget's disease of the nipple (an eczematous-type nipple lesion that does not resolve with topical steroid treatment), nipple discharge (which is usually from a single duct and

SUMMARY POINTS

- Ductal carcinoma in situ (DCIS) is a preinvasive breast cancer—malignant cells are confined within an intact ductal basement membrane
- Most cases (90%) are asymptomatic and detected at screening, but it can present as Paget's disease of the nipple, nipple discharge, or a lump
- Treatment aims to prevent invasive disease
- Oestrogen receptor status tends to be preserved in recurrences or disease progression; this has implications for adjuvant treatment and reducing risk of recurrence
- The optimum treatment is unclear, and urgent clarification is needed
- Women with DCIS should have the option of entering high quality randomised controlled trials

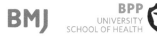

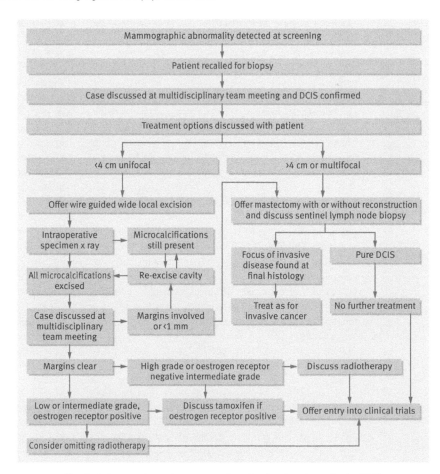

Fig 1 Difference between normal, ductal carcinoma in situ (DCIS), and invasive disease

either blood stained or clear), or a palpable mass. DCIS that presents with clinical signs is more likely to be extensive or to have an invasive component.

Men can also develop DCIS and tend to present with symptoms of blood stained nipple discharge or a retroareolar mass. The standard treatment for men is mastectomy with excision of the nipple-areola complex. DCIS accounts for about 5% of breast cancers in men,[9] but the proportion of men who would progress to invasive cancer if DCIS was not treated is unknown.

How is DCIS diagnosed and treated?

At screening mammography, malignant looking microcalcifications are the most common abnormality. Architectural distortion, ill defined masses, nodules, or ductal asymmetry can also indicate underlying DCIS. Figure 2 shows a flow chart of a typical screen detected treatment pathway. Women with an abnormal mammogram will be recalled for an image guided biopsy, under local anaesthetic, with either a 14 gauge core biopsy gun or vacuum assisted biopsy device. If the area of abnormality is extensive, multiple cores of different areas can be taken, to try to increase the chance of detecting a coexistent invasive tumour. Core biopsy and vacuum assisted biopsy are preferable to fine needle aspiration, which cannot discriminate between in situ and invasive cancer because it provides no information on the basement membrane. A recent meta-analysis showed that, compared with 14 gauge core biopsy, use of an 11 gauge vacuum assisted biopsy device halves the risk of missing a coexisting invasive cancer (P=0.006).[10] Other factors associated with missing associated invasive disease include having a high grade lesion (P<0.001), an imaging size greater than 20 mm (P≤0.001), a breast imaging reporting and data system (BI-RADS) score of 4 or 5 (P for trend=0.005), a mass visible at mammography (v calcification only, P<0.001), and a palpable abnormality (P<0.001).[10]

Fig 2 Typical screen detected treatment pathway for ductal carcinoma in situ (DCIS)

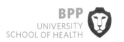

For symptomatic cases the diagnostic pathway will depend on presentation—core biopsy for a palpable lump, punch biopsy for Paget's disease of the nipple, and smear cytology to look for malignant cells for nipple discharge. Microdochectomy (removal of just the symptomatic breast duct(s)) or total duct excision will need to be performed if the only symptom is persistent clear or bloody discharge to exclude underlying DCIS (or invasive disease).

The breast surgeon and breast care nurse will then counsel the patient on the surgical options. One option is breast conserving surgery by means of wide local excision, usually using wire localisation (a wire inserted stereotactically, under mammographic guidance; more than one wire may be needed to bracket large areas). This allows the surgeon to excise the lesion accurately. The patient will be offered mastectomy if the area of DCIS is extensive or breast size in relation to lesion size does not allow for cosmetically or surgically acceptable wide local excision, and occasionally because of patient preference. National Institute for Health and Clinical Excellence (NICE) guidance suggests that sentinel lymph node biopsy (to stage the axilla) should be performed at the time of mastectomy for lesions greater than 4 cm because of the small incidence of occult invasive disease in extensive DCIS.[11] Axillary surgery is not indicated alongside wide local excision.

Women with extensive DCIS, if medically fit, are excellent candidates for immediate breast reconstruction. In the UK, about 35% of women with DCIS have a mastectomy and 72% have wide local excision.[1]

After wide local excision, the specimen is x rayed to ensure that all suspicious microcalcifications have been removed. After mastectomy, the histopathologist may request imaging of specimen slices to aid detection of the disease and its extent.

After surgery, the case will be discussed at a multidisciplinary team meeting (comprising radiologists, pathologists, oncologists and surgeons) to ensure that margins are clear histologically and radiologically. The optimum margin width is controversial, but a circumferential margin of at least 1 mm is generally accepted. If margins are close (<1 mm) or involved after wide local excision, cavity re-excision or mastectomy should be offered to achieve clear margins.

What other investigative tools are useful in diagnosis and treatment?

Ductoscopy is not used routinely in the management of DCIS and is currently mainly a research tool. However, direct visualisation of the ductal system is an appealing option for a disease that is located purely within the ducts and may be especially useful for cases of nipple discharge. Instillation of chemotherapy agents directly into the ducts is also a theoretical possibility,[12] and this feature may be exploited in the future.

There is increasing evidence that magnetic resonance imaging may have an important role in the clinical assessment of the extent of DCIS.[13] Several ongoing trials are looking at the use of magnetic resonance imaging in the diagnosis and treatment planning of DCIS. This technique may be able identify occult multifocal or contralateral disease in patients with DCIS, but there is still some concern that overestimation of the extent of disease may lead to wider than necessary margins or unnecessary mastectomy, in addition to identifying high numbers of contralateral lesions that turn out to be benign.

What adjuvant treatments can be used in DCIS?

No further treatment is needed after mastectomy for pure DCIS. However, after breast conserving surgery the optimum adjuvant treatment is uncertain. Large randomised controlled trials (RCTs) have looked at the use of radiotherapy and tamoxifen as adjuvant treatments for DCIS.

Radiotherapy

Four RCTs have looked at using adjuvant radiotherapy after breast conserving surgery for DCIS—EORTC 10853,[14] NSABP B-17,[15] UK/ANZ DCIS,[16] and SweDCIS,[17] with a subsequent Cochrane review.[18] All of the trials showed a significant reduction in DCIS and invasive recurrence after radiotherapy (all used 50 Gy, standard fractionation, and no tumour bed boost dose), and all have long term follow-up (8-10 years). Radiotherapy also significantly reduced ipsilateral recurrence from 15-20% to 5-9% at five years and from 24% to 12% at 10 years of follow-up.[14][15][16][17] On pooling the trial results in the Cochrane review, ipsilateral invasive recurrence was halved at 10 years across the trials (hazard ratio 0.50, 95% confidence interval 0.32 to 0.76; P=0.0001).[18] About 50% of the recurrences over all the trials were invasive cancer, and 50% further DCIS.

The Cochrane review looked at the subgroups of age above or below 50 years, presence or absence of comedo necrosis (areas of necrotic debris within the DCIS), and size greater than or less than 10 mm; all subgroups benefited from the addition of radiotherapy, with recurrence rates approximately halving. Older (>50 years) patients had greater benefit from radiotherapy than younger ones (0.35 (>50) v 0.67 (<50)).[18] None of these trials was prospectively designed for these subgroup analyses, so the results should be interpreted with caution. The NSABP B-17 trial recently published long term (>10 year follow-up) results, which showed that recurrence of an invasive tumour in the ipsilateral breast was associated with a slightly increased risk of death (1.75, 1.45 to 2.96; P<0.001), whereas recurrence of DCIS was not.[19] Twenty two of the 39 deaths were attributed to breast cancer.[19] Such an effect was not seen in the 10 year follow-up of the UK/ANZ DCIS trial, which showed no increased risk of death after wide local excision alone.[16]

In practice, the trial results show that nine women require treatment with radiotherapy to prevent one ipsilateral recurrence (50% of recurrences are further DCIS).[18] Clinicians can therefore advise patients that for every 100 women who opt for radiotherapy, five to 10 fewer invasive breast cancers develop. Most of the invasive cancers that do occur are detected at surveillance mammography and will probably be small, subclinical, of early stage, and cured by further treatment (mastectomy, endocrine therapy, or chemotherapy, or a combination thereof). Having a recurrence of any type will not strike most women as a trivial risk, but they will need to be carefully counselled about their risk-benefit profile, especially because patients randomised to radiotherapy in the UZ/ANZ DCIS trial had an increase in death from cardiovascular disease (P=0.008), although numbers were small.[16]

Tamoxifen

Two large RCTs have looked at using tamoxifen in addition to radiotherapy after breast conserving surgery. Neither trial tested oestrogen receptor (ER) status at the time of diagnosis, so trial entrants were both ER positive and negative. The NSABP B-24 trial found that the addition of tamoxifen to radiotherapy decreased subsequent invasive cancer from 7% to 4% at five years.[20] This effect was maximal

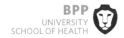
in younger women (<50) and at retrospective review was shown to be of benefit only in ER positive cases.[21] At long term review, the addition of tamoxifen to radiotherapy reduced recurrence of an invasive tumour in the ipsilateral breast (at median follow-up of 163 months) by 32% (0.68, 0.49 to 0.95; P=0.025).[19] The UK/ANZ DCIS trial showed that tamoxifen reduced recurrent ipsilateral DCIS (0.70, 0.51 to 0.86; P=0.003) and contralateral tumours (0.44, 0.25 to 0.77; P=0.005), but it did not show a significant effect on ipsilateral invasive disease (0.95, 0.66 to 1.38; P=0.8), at a median follow-up of 12.7 years.[16] However, the ER status of these patients was unknown. In this trial tamoxifen was more effective in low grade and intermediate grade tumours than in high grade ones; this is probably because low grade DCIS tends to be nearly 100% ER positive, with only 60% of high grade cases expressing ER.[22] The UK/ANZ DCIS trial authors suggested that the variation in findings between the two trials may have resulted from around 34% of women in the NSABP B-24 trial being under 50 years,[20] whereas more than 90% of women in the UK trial were over 50.[16] Tamoxifen had no significant effects on mortality in either trial.

The IBIS-II study and the NSABP B-35 trial are investigating the use of aromatase inhibitors as adjuvant treatment in DCIS. The MAP.3 trial, which looked at the aromatase inhibitor exemestane as preventive treatment in postmenopausal women, showed that exemestane reduced the number of further breast events in women who had undergone mastectomy for DCIS, although the numbers of events were small.[23]

What is the potential of DCIS to become invasive, and could we be overtreating it?

Pure DCIS poses no threat to life. The goal of treating DCIS is to prevent invasive cancer. The introduction of national breast screening programmes was partly based on the premise that the detection and treatment of DCIS would, after a lag phase, result in a decrease in the incidence of invasive breast cancer. However, such a decrease has not occurred,[24] and this has led to speculation that we may be overtreating women with low risk DCIS that may never progress to invasive disease or pose a threat to life. It has been suggested that DCIS should be reclassified as a "ductal intraepithelial neoplasia,"[25] to distance it from invasive disease. This has not been generally adopted. An investigator initiated clinical trial studying the effect of preoperative endocrine treatment in DCIS found marked morphological changes, decreased proliferation, and changes in protein expression in DCIS after neoadjuvant endocrine treatment. The authors suggested that selected cases of DCIS could be treated by endocrine therapy alone (if ER positive)[26] or even "watchful waiting" with no intervention at all.[24]

This hypothesis is backed up by the previously discussed study on atypical ductal hyperplasia, which showed that this disease (and by implication, low grade DCIS) has become less common since women stopped using hormone replacement therapy.[8] Low grade DCIS is highly oestrogen dependent and unlikely to progress to invasive disease once the oestrogenic drive is removed, either postmenopausally or by the use of aromatase inhibitors. Postmenopausal women comprise the bulk of the screening population, and the recent MAP.3 trial suggests that exemestane reduces the development of DCIS in a prevention setting.[23] It is ER positive cases of low risk DCIS that, in theory, may not need surgical treatment. However, accurate and confident definition of these "low

risk" groups, if they exist, is still elusive and the existing evidence shows that overall invasive recurrence rates are as high as 10-20% after surgery alone at 15 years.[16] [19]

ER negative DCIS has a higher recurrence rate and is not affected by endocrine treatment, so effective local control is essential. There tends to be receptor preservation between DCIS and its subsequent recurrence. ER negative DCIS tends to recur as ER negative DCIS or ER negative invasive disease. This has implications when considering adjuvant treatment and reducing the risk of recurrence. If ER negative DCIS recurs as invasive cancer it invariably needs chemotherapy.

Genotyping might help identify high risk and low risk patients, as it does for invasive disease. Genomic Health has recently released the Oncotype DX Breast Cancer Assay for DCIS—an assay of 21 cancer related genes—which they state can estimate the likelihood of local recurrence (DCIS or invasive carcinoma) at 10 years (www.oncotypedx.com/en-US/Breast/HealthcareProfessional/DCIS.aspx). Its clinical applicability will become apparent only with time.

Which women are at risk of recurrence after treatment for DCIS?

After a diagnosis of DCIS, NICE guidance suggests that patients should be offered annual mammography for five years (or until they reach screening age) and then return to the national screening programme.[11]

After mastectomy the risk of recurrence is low, at about 1%, although ipsilateral recurrences are mostly invasive disease. This is probably because follow-up imaging is not routinely performed on the ipsilateral side after mastectomy, so any skin flap or chest wall disease is seen only when it becomes palpable, at which point it is likely to be invasive.

The overall risk after wide local excision alone with no attention to margin status is higher, at about 25%.[15] [27] Recurrences are split equally between further DCIS and invasive disease. The woman's individual risk of recurrence—most importantly invasive recurrence and subsequent risk of death—should guide any offers of adjuvant treatments after breast conserving surgery.

Key risk factors for recurrence have been identified in the main RCTs in DCIS. The most important and modifiable risk factor is involved margins at breast conserving surgery and failure to remove all suspicious microcalcifications. Younger age at diagnosis (<40 years), high grade disease, and the presence of comedo necrosis are also important[15] [20] [27] [28] [29] (box). The University of Southern California/Van Nuys prognostic index is an American scoring system that brings together some of these risk factors. It was designed to achieve a less than 20% recurrence rate at 12 years (fig 3).[30] It has not yet been independently validated, however, and its effect on a UK screening population, where most tumours are small (<2 cm), is limited. It has not been shown to be prognostic for this screen detected population,[31] so its use is not encouraged in these patients.[31]

RISK FACTORS FOR RECURRENCE OF DUCTAL CARCINOMA IN SITU
• Involved or close (<1 mm) excision margins after breast conserving surgery
• High grade or poorly differentiated disease
• Comedo necrosis
• Younger age at diagnosis (<40 years)
• Oestrogen receptor negative disease
• Symptomatic presentation

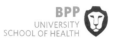

Breast cancer stem cells could contribute to recurrence of DCIS. These cells can self renew, proliferate, and avoid apoptosis. Aberrant activation of cell signalling pathways involved in stem cell self renewal (such as the Notch protein) might contribute to the recurrence of DCIS by allowing the cells to survive and proliferate.[32] These pathways are also under investigation as potential therapeutic targets.

What is the psychosocial impact of a diagnosis of DCIS?

The perceived risk of recurrence after treatment for DCIS is often higher than the actual risk. A study of 487 women with DCIS, treated with both mastectomy and breast conserving surgery, showed that 39% of women thought they had at least a moderate (25-30%) likelihood of developing invasive cancer in the next five years and 28% thought there was a moderate likelihood of DCIS spreading to other parts of their body.[33] A recent descriptive qualitative study highlighted that women can find it especially difficult to accept the perceived paradox between having a "precancerous" condition and the extensive surgery that is sometimes needed. Women more easily accepted the need for wide local excision than for mastectomy.[34] In the same study, some of the women did not like the term "precancerous"—they found it unhelpful and thought that it lessened the importance of the diagnosis. Women also found the need to continually justify having their treatment to themselves and others and found it difficult to explain their diagnosis.[34] This is an area where the support, counselling, and information provided by breast care nurses is invaluable.

The potential of audit data to inform future practice

The Sloane project is a prospective UK based audit on screen detected DCIS, lobular carcinoma in situ, atypical ductal hyperplasia, and atypical lobular hyperplasia. The main aim of the project is to record the current management of non-invasive breast disease and atypical hyperplasia in the UK by collecting information on the radiological and pathological features of cases, surgical and adjuvant treatment, and recurrences. It will hopefully help to answer questions about the diagnosis, treatment, and clinical outcomes of these diseases. It is the largest audit of its kind, and currently 10 732 cases have been submitted by participating UK breast screening units. Although the addition of new

---

TIPS FOR NON-SPECIALISTS

- Refer patients with persistent eczematous changes of the nipple to a breast clinic for exclusion of Paget's disease of the nipple
- Stress to the patient that a diagnosis of pure ductal carcinoma in situ (DCIS) has no direct impact on mortality
- Medically fit women who need a mastectomy for DCIS are often excellent candidates for immediate reconstruction, which should be offered to all appropriate patients
- Women may be confused about their optimum treatment. Explain treatment options and up to date research findings carefully, taking time to ensure that the patient understands
- Inclusion in ongoing clinical trials should be offered to all suitable patients

---

ONGOING RESEARCH

- IBIS-II trial: Investigating the benefit of tamoxifen versus the aromatase inhibitor anastrozole (or placebo) in postmenopausal women after breast conserving surgery for ductal carcinoma in situ (DCIS) (in active follow-up)
- ICICLE trial: Trying to identify genes that increase the risk of developing DCIS in addition to which women with DCIS are at risk of developing invasive disease if left untreated
- NSABP B-35 trial: Comparing anastrozole with tamoxifen for postmenopausal women with DCIS after lumpectomy and radiotherapy (in active follow-up)
- NSABP B-43 trial: Comparing trastuzumab (Herceptin) with radiotherapy or radiotherapy alone for women with HER2 positive DCIS treated by lumpectomy (still recruiting)
- The Memorial Sloan-Kettering Cancer Centre (USA) is conducting a trial of breast magnetic resonance imaging as a preoperative tool for DCIS
- The National Cancer Institute in France is evaluating the diagnostic performance of magnetic resonance imaging with or without biopsy to optimise the resection of DCIS
- The Mayo Clinic (USA) is looking at molecular breast imaging in patients with suspected DCIS
- The National Cancer Institute/University of Pennsylvania is undertaking a phase I/II study of vaccines made from the patient's white blood cells mixed with peptides (which may help the body mount an effective immune response against tumour cells) in patients with DCIS

ADDITIONAL EDUCATIONAL RESOURCES

Resources for healthcare professionals
- The Sloane Project (www.sloaneproject.co.uk)—UK wide prospective audit of screen detected non-invasive and atypical hyperplasia of the breast
- National Institute for Health State of the Science Conference on Diagnosis and Management of DCIS report 2009 (www.consensus.nih.gov)—Summary statement from the meeting
- 2009 National Institutes for Health state-of-the-science meeting on ductal carcinoma in situ: management and diagnosis. *J Natl Cancer Inst Monogr* 2010;41:111-222
- Goodwin A, Parker S, Ghersi D, Wilcken N. Post-operative radiotherapy for ductal carcinoma in situ of the breast. *Cochrane Database Syst Rev* 2009;21:CD000563

Resources for patients
- National Breast and Ovarian Cancer Centre. Understanding ductal carcinoma in situ (DCIS) and deciding about treatment (www.psych.usyd.edu.au/cemped/docs/dcisgw.pdf)—A communication aid booklet for women with DCIS
- Health Talk On Line (www.healthtalkonline.org)—Large database of patient interviews, where real patients talk about their experiences in dealing with a wide range of health topics including DCIS
- MacMillan Cancer Support (www.macmillan.org.uk)—Comprehensive website of cancer information and support
- Cancer Prevention Institute of California (www.dcis.info)—Information on DCIS

Score	1	2	3
Size (mm)	≤15	16-40	>40
Margin (mm)	≥10	1-9	<1
Class	Grade 1/2 no necrosis	Grade 1/2 no necrosis	Grade 3
Age (years)	>60	40-60	<40

Scores for each category are added up to give an overall score from 3 to 12, which is then referenced to a recurrence prediction and management suggestion table

Score	Treatment
4-6	Wide local excision
7: margins ≥3 mm	Wide local excision
7: margins <3 mm	Wide local excision and radiotherapy
8: margins ≥3 mm	Wide local excision and radiotherapy
8: margins <3 mm	Mastectomy
9: margins ≥5 mm	Wide local excision and radiotherapy
9: margins <5 mm	Mastectomy
10-12	Mastectomy

Fig 3 Van Nuys prognostic index

QUESTIONS FOR FUTURE RESEARCH

- How can we identify women with "low risk" disease who do not need treatment and those at "high risk" who need maximal treatment?
- Can genotyping of ductal carcinoma in situ (DCIS) help predict risk of progression to invasive disease or recurrence after initial treatment?
- Will magnetic resonance imaging aid diagnosis and follow-up of patients with DCIS?
- Can ductoscopy be used in the diagnosis and treatment of DCIS?

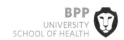

cases is anticipated to end in April 2012, the collection of data on future events for cases already in the audit will hopefully continue into the foreseeable future.

What does the future hold?

There is no agreed practice in the UK or elsewhere for the use of radiotherapy or tamoxifen after breast conserving surgery for DCIS, so there is no clear standard of care. Two very different approaches could potentially be considered—evidence suggests that all women benefit from radiotherapy after breast conserving surgery, yet some experts suggest that we should be considering (at the most extreme) "watchful waiting." Current practice seems to be somewhere in the middle, with patients being offered surgery, and to a variable and unstandardised extent, radiotherapy and tamoxifen. We urgently need to be able to distinguish between "low risk" women who could be safely treated with surgical excision alone, hormonal therapy alone, or possibly "watchful waiting" and "high risk" patients who need all available adjuvant treatment. This can be achieved only with a randomised controlled trial of active treatment versus active monitoring, stratified according to DCIS grade. Women with DCIS should therefore have the option of entering into high quality randomised controlled trials that will help to determine optimum treatment.

We thank the Sloane Project management team for up to date information on the Sloane Project numbers. JRY acknowledges NHS funding to the NIHR Biomedical Research Centre. NJB acknowledges funding from the NIHR Programme and Cancer Research UK.

Contributors: NLPB planned and drafted the article, JLO and JRY revised the article, and NJB planned and revised the article. NLPB is guarantor.

Funding: None received.

Competing interests: All authors have completed the ICMJE uniform disclosure form at www.icmje.org/coi_disclosure.pdf (available on request from the corresponding author) and declare: no support from any organisation for the submitted work; no financial relationships with any organisations that might have an interest in the submitted work in the previous three years; no other relationships or activities that could appear to have influenced the submitted work.

Provenance and peer review: Not commissioned; externally peer reviewed.

1   NHS cancer screening programmes. All breast cancer report. An analysis of all symptomatic and screen detected breast cancers diagnosed in 2006. NHS breast screening programme Oct 2009.
2   NHS Breast Screening Programme. Pathology reporting of breast disease. National Pathology Co-ordinating Group. Publication no 58, 2005.
3   Hwang ES, DeVries S, Chew KL, Moore DH 2nd, Kerlikowske K, Thor A, et al. Patterns of chromosomal alterations in breast ductal carcinoma in situ. Clin Cancer Res2004;10:5160-7.
4   Claus EB, Stowe M, Carter D. Breast carcinoma in situ: risk factors and screening patterns. J Natl Cancer Inst 2001;93:1811-7.
5   Claus EB, Petruzella S, Matloff E, Carter D. Prevalence of BRCA1 and BRCA2 mutations in women diagnosed with ductal carcinoma in situ. JAMA2005;293:964-9.
6   Chlebowski RT, Hendrix SL, Langer RD, Stefanick ML, Gass M, Lane D, et al; WHI Investigators. Influence of estrogen plus progestin on breast cancer and mammography in healthy postmenopausal women: the Women's Health Initiative Randomized Trial. JAMA2003;289:3243-53.
7   Beral V; Million Women Study Collaborators. Breast cancer and hormone-replacement therapy in the Million Women Study. Lancet2003;362:419-27.
8   Menes TS, Kerlikowske K, Jaffer S, Seger D, Miglioretti DL. Rates of atypical ductal hyperplasia have declined with less use of postmenopausal hormone treatment: findings from the Breast Cancer Surveillance Consortium. Cancer Epidemiol Biomarkers Prev2009;18:2822-8.
9   Pappo I, Wasserman I, Halevy A. Ductal carcinoma in situ of the breast in men: a review. Clin Breast Cancer2005;6:310-4.
10 Brennan ME, Turner RM, Ciatto S, Marinovich ML, French JR, Macaskill P, et al. Ductal carcinoma in situ at core-needle biopsy: meta-analysis of underestimation and predictors of invasive breast cancer. Radiology2011;260:119-28.
11 National Institute for Health and Clinical Excellence. Early and locally advanced breast cancer diagnosis and treatment. CG80. 2009. www.nice.org.uk/CG80.
12 Tang S, Twelves D, Isacke C, Gui G. Mammary ductoscopy in the current management of breast disease. Surg Endosc 2010;25:1712-22.
13 Lehman CD. Magnetic resonance imaging in the evaluation of ductal carcinoma in situ. J Natl Cancer Monogr2010;2010:150-1.
14 Bijker N, Meijnen P, Peterse JL, Bogaerts J, Van Hoorebeeck I, Julien JP, et al. Breast-conserving treatment with or without radiotherapy in ductal carcinoma in situ: ten-year results of EORTC randomized phase III trial 10853. J Clin Oncol2006;243:381-7.
15 Fisher ER, Dignam J, Tan-Chiu E, Costantino J, Fisher B, Paik S, et al. Pathologic findings from the National Surgical Adjuvant Breast Project (NSABP) eight year update of protocol B17: intraductal carcinoma. Cancer1999;86:429-38.
16 Cuzick J, Sestaka I, Pinder SE, Ellis IO, Forsyth S, Bundred NJ, et al. Effect of tamoxifen and radiotherapy in women with locally excised ductal carcinoma in situ: long-term results from the UK/ANZ DCIS trial. Lancet Oncol2010;12:21-9.
17 Emdin SO, Granstrand B, Ringberg A, Sandelin K, Arnesson LG, Nordgren H, et al. SweDCIS: radiotherapy after sector resection for ductal carcinoma in situ of the breast. Results of a randomised trial in a population offered mammography screening. Acta Oncol2006;45:536-43.
18 Goodwin A, Parker S, Ghersi D, Wilcken N. Post-operative radiotherapy for ductal carcinoma in situ of the breast. Cochrane Database Syst Rev2009;21:CD000563.
19 Wapnir IL, Dignam JJ, Fisher B, Mamounas EP, Anderson JJ, Julien TB, et al. Long-term outcomes of invasive ipsilateral breast tumor recurrences after lumpectomy in NSABP B-17 and B-24 randomized clinical trials for DCIS. J Natl Cancer Inst2011;103:478-88.
20 Fisher B, Dignam J, Wolmark N,Wickerman DC, Fisher ER, Mamounas EP, et al. Tamoxifen in the treatment of intraductal breast cancer: national surgical adjuvant breast and bowel project B-24 randomised controlled trial. Lancet1999;353:1993-2000.
21 Allred DC, Bryant J, Land S, Paik S, Fisher E, Julien T, et al. Estrogen receptor expression as a predictive marker of the effectiveness of tamoxifen in the treatment of intraductal breast cancer: findings of the NSABP protocol B-24 [abstract]. Breast Cancer Res Treat2002;76(suppl 1):S36.
22 Barnes NL, Boland GP, Davenport A, Knox WF, Bundred NJ. Relationship between hormone receptor status and tumour size, grade and comedo necrosis in ductal carcinoma in situ. Br J Surg2005;92:429-34.
23 Goss PE, Ingle JN, Alés-Martínez JE, Cheung AM, Chlebowski RT, Wactanski-Wende J, et al; NCIC CTG MAP.3 Study Investigators. Exemestane for breast-cancer prevention in postmenopausal women. N Engl J Med2011;364:2381-91.
24 Ozanne EM, Shieh Y, Barnes J, Bouzan C, Hwang ES, Esserman LJ. Characterizing the impact of 25 years of DCIS treatment. Breast Cancer Res Treat2011;129:165-73.
25 Graff S. Ductal carcinoma in situ: should the name be changed? J Natl Cancer Inst2010;102:6-8.
26 Chen YY, DeVries S, Anderson J, Lessing J, Swain R, Cin K, et al. Pathologic and biologic response to preoperative endocrine therapy in patients with ER-positive ductal carcinoma in situ. BMC Cancer2009;9:285.
27 Jullen J, Bijker N, Fentiman I, Peterse JL, Delledonne V, Rouanet P, et al. Radiotherapy in breast-conserving treatment for ductal carcinoma in situ: first results of the EORTC randomized phase III trial 10853. Lancet2000;355:528-33.
28 Bijker N, Peterse JL, Duchateaul, Julien JP, Fentiman IS, Duval C, et al. Risk factors for recurrence and metastasis after breast conserving therapy for ductal carcinoma in situ: analysis of EORTC trial. J Clin Oncol2001;19:2263-71.
29 Houghton J, George WD, Cuzick J, Duggan C, Fentiman IS, Spittle M. Radiotherapy and tamoxifen in women with completely excised ductal carcinoma in situ of the breast in the UK, Australia, and New Zealand: randomised controlled trial. Lancet2003;362:95-102.
30 Silverstein MJ, Lagios MD. Choosing treatment for patients with DCIS: fine tuning the University of Southern California/Van-Nuys prognostic index. J Natl Cancer Inst Monogr2010;41:193-6.
31 Boland GP, Chan KC, Knox WF, Roberts SA, Bundred NJ. Value of the Van Nuys prognostic index in prediction of recurrence o ductal carcinoma in situ after breast-conserving surgery. Br J Surg2003;90:426-32.
32 Harrison H, Farnie G, Howell SJ, Rock RE, Stylianou S, Brennan KR, et al. Regulation of breast cancer stem cell activity by signaling through the Notch4 receptor. Cancer Res2010;70:709-18.
33 Partridge A, Adloff K, Blood E, Dees EC, Kaelin C, Golshan M, et al. Risk perceptions and psychosocial outcomes of women with ductal carcinoma in situ: longitudinal results from a cohort study. J Natl Cancer Inst2008;100:243-51.
34 Kennedy F, Harcourt D, Rumsey N. The shifting nature of women's experiences and perceptions of ductal carcinoma in situ. Journal of Advanced Nursing2012;68:856-67.

Related links

bmj.com
- Managing retinal vein occlusion (2012;344:e499)
- New recreational drugs and the primary care approach to patients who use them (2012;344:e288)
- Diagnosis and management of Raynaud's phenomenon (2012;344:e289)
- Improving healthcare access for people with visual impairment and blindness (2012;344:e542)

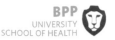

Management of women at high risk of breast cancer

Anne C Armstrong, consultant medical oncologist[1],
Gareth D Evans, professor of medical genetics and cancer epidemiology[23]

[1]Department of Oncology, Christie Hospital Manchester, Manchester, UK

[2]Manchester Centre for Genomic Medicine, Manchester Academic Health Science Centre, University of Manchester, Manchester, UK

[3]Department of Genetic Medicine, St Mary's Hospital, Central Manchester Foundation Trust, Manchester, UK

Correspondence to: A C Armstrong anne.armstrong@christie.nhs.uk

Cite this as: BMJ 2014;348:g2756

DOI: 10.1136/bmj.g2756

http://www.bmj.com/content/348/bmj.g2756

Breast cancer is the commonest malignancy diagnosed in women worldwide and accounts for over 30% of all cancers diagnosed in women in the United Kingdom.[1] The average lifetime risk of developing breast cancer for women in the United Kingdom and United States is estimated to be 12%,[1] although this may be an overestimate, as it is not clear what age this assumes a woman lives to and whether full adjustment has been made for those who die young from other causes. It is also unclear whether multiple breast cancers in a single woman are counted as several women with breast cancer.

The risk of breast cancer is multifactorial and is an interaction between environmental, lifestyle, hormonal, and genetic factors.[2] [3] Some women have a particularly high risk of breast cancer owing to their family history, or, less commonly, after supradiaphragmatic radiotherapy for Hodgkin's lymphoma. This review discusses how to identify women who are at high risk of breast cancer as a result of their family history or irradiation and outlines the management options for such women, including surveillance and risk reducing strategies. A further group of women diagnosed on the basis of a breast biopsy as having atypical ductal or lobular hyperplasia are also at increased risk of breast cancer; these women are not discussed further in this review.

When should a woman be considered at high risk of breast cancer?

A risk assessment for breast cancer is complex and no consistent definition or threshold for high risk has been established. Within UK practice, high risk, as defined by the National Institute for Health and Care Excellence,[4] is a lifetime risk of 30% or greater, which equates to a more than 8% risk of breast cancer at age 40-50 years. The high risk threshold used in the United Kingdom is similar to that in other European countries, although in North America the threshold for screening using magnetic resonance imaging is a lifetime risk of 20-25%.[5] NICE guidelines have algorithms for identifying high risk women, which include two close (first or second degree) relatives with breast cancer with an average age of less than 50, three with breast cancer aged less than 60, or four with breast cancer at any age. These are "catch all" criteria, which will not make all women who meet these criteria fit the lifetime or 10 year risk criterion. Another high risk criterion includes women with a family history of both breast and ovarian cancer, which specifically highlights the possibility of a BRCA1/2 mutation given the increased risk of both cancers associated with mutations in these genes.

In most women with breast cancer the cause is unknown. Those with breast cancer can be considered at high risk if they meet the criteria mentioned above, including their own breast cancer. Each close relative with a diagnosis of breast cancer increases a woman's risk of developing breast cancer, especially with a diagnosis at a young age (<50 years). Such families may have a genetic predisposition to the development of breast cancer, with about 5% of all breast cancers being attributable to inherited mutations in specific genes such as BRCA1, BRCA2, and TP53. In any individual the genetic risk factors will be modified by other risk factors.

In women of Ashkenazi Jewish descent a family history of breast cancer poses a higher risk than in women of non-Jewish descent because of the high prevalence and penetrance of BRCA1 and BRCA2 mutations (2.5%).[6] In this population any breast cancer is associated with a 10% carrier rate of BRCA1/2, with higher rates for women with a diagnosis at a younger age. Furthermore, three specific "founder" mutations (two in BRCA1 and one in BRCA2) have been identified within this population, making genetic testing based on only these mutations a much more sensitive and specific test.

It is also clear that women who received supradiaphragmatic radiotherapy at a young age as treatment for Hodgkin's lymphoma have a high risk of breast cancer, which 20-40 years after treatment is nearly as high as that of carriers of BRCA1/2.[7] The peak risk is around age 14 years, which may be attributable to the accumulation of radiation damage in dividing cells during breast development.

Which genes are implicated in a high risk of breast cancer?

Several genes are associated with a high risk of breast cancer. Of the known high risk genes, mutations in BRCA1 and BRCA2 are the most common and account for about 20% of the familial component. Germline mutations in other high risk genes such as TP53, PTEN, and STK11 are less common and identified in less than 1% of families with breast cancer (table 1).[8]

SOURCES AND SELECTION CRITERIA

We searched PubMed using search terms such as "breast cancer risk" and "hereditary breast cancer." Studies included were those written in English, and included case-control studies, randomised control trials, and meta-analyses. We also consulted relevant national and international guidelines, including those of the National Institute for Health and Care Excellence, and we were part of the NICE Guideline Development Group where all relevant evidence was identified and summarised.

SUMMARY POINTS

- The risk of breast cancer is multifactorial, but some women will have a high risk because of a genetic predisposition or, rarely, as a consequence of radiotherapy at a young age
- Women with a family history suggestive of a genetic predisposition to cancer should be referred to local genetics services for formal assessment
- Annual magnetic resonance imaging and mammography (unless a carrier of the TP53 gene) in high risk women identifies more breast cancers than does mammography alone
- Risk reducing bilateral salpingo-oophorectomy and risk reducing mastectomy reduces the risk of breast cancer by 50% and 90-95%, respectively, in carriers of BRCA1 and BRCA2 mutations
- Chemoprevention with drugs such as tamoxifen for five years reduces the risk of breast cancer by about 30% and can be a useful alternative to risk reducing surgery

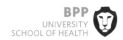
Table 1 Breast cancer associated cancer predisposition syndromes and associated risk of breast cancer[9]

Disease gene	Location	Tumours	Tumour age (years)	Risk (%)	Birth incidence of mutations	Life expectancy
CHEK2	22q	Breast cancer	>25	20	1 in 200	?Normal
ATM	11q	Breast cancer	>25	20	1 in 200	?Normal
BRIP		Breast cancer	>25	20	1 in 1000	?Normal
PALB2		Breast cancer	>25	30-40	<1 in 1000	?Normal
NF1	17q	Neurofibroma, glioma, breast cancer	1st year, 1st year, >25	100, 12, 17	1 in 2600	54-72 years
PTEN Cowden	10q	Breast cancer, thyroid	>25, 30	60, 10	1 in 200 000-250 000	Reduced in women
PJS STK11	19p	Gastrointestinal malignancy, breast	20, >25	60, 40	1 in 25 000	58 years
LFSTP53	17p	Sarcoma, breast cancer (women), gliomas	1st year, >16, 1st year	80, 95, 20	1 in 30 000	Severely reduced
CDH1	16q	Gastric, breast (women)	>16, >35	70-80, 20-40	Rare	Reduced
BRCA2	13q	Breast/ovary (women), prostate (men), pancreas	>18, >30, >30	40-90, 20, 5	1 in 800	68 years
BRCA1	17q	Breast (women), ovary	>18, >20	60-90, 40-60	1 in 1000	62 years

Carriers of mutations in BRCA1 and BRCA2 have a high lifetime risk of breast cancer (around 65-85% with BRCA1 and 40-85% with BRCA2)[10 11 12] as well as a high risk of ovarian cancer (40-60% with BRCA1 and 10-30% with BRCA2). BRCA2 mutations also confer an excess risk of prostate cancer, pancreatic cancer, and melanoma. The frequencies of BRCA1/BRCA2 mutations in breast cancer populations unselected for family history or age of diagnosis are, however, low and account for about 2-3% of breast cancers overall,[13] but they are about 10% in founder populations such as Ashkenazi Jewish.

Most breast cancers that arise in carriers of the BRCA1 mutation are "triple negative"—that is, the cancers lack receptors for oestrogen, progesterone, and human epidermal growth factor receptor 2 (Her2).[13] The immune phenotye of cancers associated with BRCA2 mutations reflect that of sporadic cancers, with most cancers expressing receptors for oestrogen and progesterone with only 16% triple negative.[14]

When and how should a family history be taken?
Although 2004 guidelines from NICE did not advocate taking a family history proactively, much has changed in terms of extra available surveillance and preventive options for those women with at least moderate risk.[15] Moderate risk as defined by NICE is a lifetime risk of 17-29% or a 10 year risk at age 40 of 3-7.9%. When risk is being assessed in primary or secondary care, at least a two generation family history, including paternal relatives, should be taken from women seeking advice. A family history of breast cancer should also be sought in women aged more than 30 starting combined oral contraception and women aged more than 50 starting combined hormone replacement therapy. Women meeting at least moderate risk criteria (for instance a mother or sister with breast cancer at age <40 or two close relatives at any age) should be offered a referral to secondary care (the local family history clinic or breast clinic) but for women with a known family gene mutation, direct referral to genetic services is appropriate (table 2). In the United Kingdom, family history clinics are available in most localities, with over 100 countrywide, but models may differ in other countries. None the less, much management of familial breast cancer does take place in secondary care around the world, with surveillance organised by local breast surgeons and gynaecologists.

When referred to a secondary care clinic, women will have a preclinic questionnaire administered to assess eligibility or a family history elicited directly. Other non-genetic risk factors such as pregnancy history and age at menarche and menopause are also taken. The woman's risk is assessed usually by use of a risk algorithm such as Tyrer-Cuzick[16] or BOADICEA.[17] If a woman is in the high risk category (lifetime risk .30%) or she or her affected relative has a

Table 2 Referral criteria for family history and genetics clinics*[4]

Referral to family history clinics/secondary care	Referral to genetics clinics/tertiary care
One first degree relative with breast cancer at age <40 years	Triple negative breast cancer at age <40 years
One first degree male relative with breast cancer at any age	Two first or second degree relatives with breast cancer at age <50 years
Two first or second degree relatives with breast cancer at any age	Three first or second degree relatives at age <60 years with breast cancer
Two close relatives with breast cancer at any age and a close relative with ovarian cancer	Four first degree relatives with breast cancer at any age
Three first or second degree relatives with breast cancer at any age	Ovarian or male breast cancer at any age and on same side of family and any of: one first or second degree relative aged <50 years; two first or second degree relatives aged <60 years; another ovarian cancer at any age
Three first or second degree relatives with breast cancer at any age	Any breast cancer and Jewish ancestry

*For bilateral breast cancer each breast cancer counts as one relative.

Table 3 Screening for women at high risk of breast cancer*[4]

Age (years)	Annual mammographic surveillance	Annual breast magnetic resonance imaging
,29	No surveillance	TP53 carrier†
30-39	Known or suspected BRCA1/BRCA2 mutation	Known or suspected BRCA1/BRCA2/TP53 mutation
40-49	Known or suspected BRCA1/BRCA2 mutation	Known or suspected BRCA1/BRCA2/TP53 mutation
50-59	Known or suspected BRCA1/BRCA2 mutation	Known TP53 mutation
60-69	Known or suspected BRCA1/BRCA2 mutation	Known TP53 mutation

*For guidance on surveillance for women at moderate risk of breast cancer see National Institute for Health and Care Excellence guidelines.[4]

†Mammographic surveillance is not recommended for TP53 carriers owing to risk of ionising radiation in this patient group.

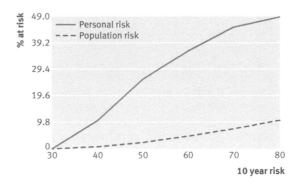

Woman aged 30 years
Age at menarch, 12 years
Age at first birth, 26 years
Person is premenopausal
Height, 5 ft 4 in (1.63 m)
Weight 9 stone (57.2 kg)
Never used hormone replacement therapy
Risk after 10 years, 10.26%
10 year population risk, 0.523%
Lifetime risk, 48.82%
Lifetime population risk, 10.21%
Probability of being a carrier of BRCA1 gene, 20.97%
Probability of being a carrier of BRCA2 gene, 22.55%

Tyrer-Cuzick readout of a woman (arrowed) at high risk of breast cancer. The woman is eligible without genetic testing for annual screening by magnetic resonance imaging aged 30-50 and for genetic testing. Her affected mother and aunt, if alive, can be offered genetic testing for BRCA1/2 as they qualify on all algorithms (Manchester score 30 is well above the 15 threshold for 10%). If they are not alive the proband and her sister could have genetic testing as they have a >10% chance of a BRCA1/2 mutation. The sister, now aged 35, could be offered tamoxifen for five years

10% or more chance of carrying a BRCA1/2 mutation she will be offered referral to a tertiary care genetics service. Extra surveillance will be offered as appropriate (table 3). An assessment will also be made of others in the family who may benefit from screening or genetic testing. Use of a risk algorithm to assess the 10% threshold can be made in family history clinics using a simple scoring system such as the Manchester score[18] or a computer algorithm such as BOADICEA.[17] Women from founder populations such as Ashkenazi Jewish (carrier frequency 2.5%) and Icelandic (0.5%) can be considered for BRCA1/2 testing with much less significant family histories. Several algorithms may be used in tertiary care. The figure shows an example of a risk output from Tyer-Cuzick version 6. Fully comprehensive algorithms such as Tyrer-Cuzick incorporate family history with other known risk factors such as age at menarche and menopause and at first full term pregnancy, overweight or obesity, and breast biopsy information. Newer risk factors such as mammographic density are being incorporated. Efforts are under way internationally to target screening, and preventive measures by proper risk stratification and accurate risk assessments are vital to this aim.

Counselling
Counselling includes advising women about their risk of breast cancer and what they can do about it, as well as the possibility of genetic testing. Although many genes and genetic factors have been identified, currently there is really only good utility in offering testing for women with high risk genes and in particular mutations in BRCA1 and BRCA2. Testing will usually start with the woman who has breast or ovarian cancer to develop a definitive test for that family. Women undergoing testing need to be aware of the likelihood of testing positive for a mutation that causes disease as well as for a variant of uncertain significance (about 5% of BRCA1/2 tests find missense mutations, most of which are thought to be harmless).

The decision to undergo presymptomatic testing for a known BRCA1/2 mutation can involve complex emotions and bring back memories of a relative's diagnosis, treatment, and death. Many women do not choose to have testing, and those that do may leave this for many years, particularly if they are a young adult when first eligible. As such most genetics centres see women at least twice before taking a predictive sample. Women who are considering being tested for a known family mutation or being considered for testing where no living relative is available will need a full discussion of their risks for breast and ovarian cancer, how these can be managed, and any effects on life or health insurance dependent on where they live.

How are high risk women followed up?
Surveillance
Breast screening aims to diagnose cancer earlier to allow timely therapeutic intervention that may consequently be more effective than if left to later. In all women, breast screening with mammography is predicted to reduce breast cancer mortality,[19] although controversy remains about the absolute benefit of screening as well as the impact of overdiagnosis and overtreatment of screen detected low grade and in situ breast cancers. In the United Kingdom, women are offered screening from age 47-50 within the NHS breast screening programme. Many similar screening programmes exist across Europe and worldwide.

Mammographic screening of younger women is generally less effective than of older women because of increased breast density. Digital mammography is more accurate than film mammography in younger women with dense breasts and is therefore recommended for the high risk population. There are, however, concerns about exposing young women to regular doses of ionising radiation. One study modelled the risk of radiation induced cancers against reductions in mortality from mammographic screening in carriers of the BRCA mutation and suggested no net benefit of

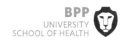
mammographic screening in women aged less than 30.[20] NICE advocate no mammography in women aged less than 30 with a familial risk.[2] Breast magnetic resonance imaging, with no exposure to radiation, has a sensitivity of about 80% and identifies more cancers in high risk women than does mammography (sensitivity 30-40%).[21][22] Magnetic resonance imaging is less specific, leading to additional imaging and biopsies. In high risk women, surveillance with both magnetic resonance imaging and mammography is better than either test alone.[22][23]

National[2] and international guidelines recommend enhanced screening for women with a very high risk of familial breast cancer who have not had risk reducing mastectomies (table 3). This includes annual surveillance with magnetic resonance imaging from age 30-49 years for women who have a known BRCA1, BRCA2, or TP53 mutation or are at a more than 30% probability of such and, for BRCA1/2, annual mammography from the age of 40 to 69. UK guidelines also recommend the use of annual mammography and magnetic resonance imaging in women who have received supradiaphragmatic radiotherapy when less than 36, starting eight years after treatment.[24]

Breast cancer surveillance is non-invasive, has few adverse long term effects, and does not interfere with child bearing. The risk of false positive results can lead to additional investigations, including imaging and biopsies, and some women find magnetic resonance imaging unacceptably claustrophobic. Furthermore, magnetic resonance imaging does not prevent breast cancer and there is no evidence as yet that breast screening reduces the risk of breast cancer deaths in high risk women.

When is prophylactic surgery or chemoprevention considered?

Risk reducing mastectomies

Women with high risk of breast cancer may decide to undergo surgery to reduce their risk. Bilateral risk reducing mastectomies remove most but not all breast tissue. Case-control studies in patients with BRCA1/2 mutations found than surgery reduced the risk of breast cancer by 90-95%.[25] Although randomised trials comparing the efficacy of bilateral risk reducing mastectomy with regular surveillance would be an ethical challenge, prospective observational studies have been published, with one study of more than 2000 years of patient observation finding 57 breast cancer cases in the surveillance group compared with none in the surgical group.[26] Overall survival benefits from bilateral risk reducing mastectomy alone have yet to be shown, but one study reported that any form of risk reducing surgery in women with BRCA1 or BRCA2 mutations improved survival,[27] and in two recent studies contralateral mastectomy has been shown to improve survival in women with BRCA1/2 mutations.[28][29]

Bilateral risk reducing mastectomy is a major undertaking for women, who need time to discuss their options and the risks of each procedure, including the potential for ongoing interventions such as surgical revisions and nipple tattooing. There is a small (about 2-5%) possibility of finding an occult malignancy during risk reducing mastectomy, despite preoperative screening investigations.[26] Several studies have evaluated the psychological impact of bilateral risk reducing mastectomies, which in general (but not universally) show good levels of satisfaction and reduced anxiety after the procedure.[30][31]

Bilateral risk reducing salpingo-oophorectomy

Women who have inherited mutations of BRCA1 and BRCA2 may also undergo risk reducing bilateral salpingo-oophorectomy. This reduces the risk of ovarian and breast cancer; a meta-analysis of all case series of the procedure suggesting that bilateral salpingo-oophorectomy performed before natural menopause reduces the risk of breast cancer by up to 50%.[32] This is thought to be due to the reduction in circulating oestrogen. The benefits of risk reducing bilateral salpingo-oophorectomy may be greater in carriers of the BRCA2 mutation compared with BRCA1 mutation, which is likely to relate to the greater frequency of oestrogen receptor positive breast cancer in carriers of the BRCA2 mutation. Nevertheless, ongoing breast surveillance is still recommended in these women and there are some prospective case series that suggest the incidence of breast cancer after risk reducing bilateral salpingo-oophorectomy is still high.[33]

The ideal age for risk reducing bilateral salpingo-oophorectomy remains uncertain, but studies suggesting an earlier age of onset of cancers in carriers of the BRCA1 mutation support earlier intervention compared with carriers of the BRCA2 mutation. A surgical menopause can result in acute symptoms and long term risks of oestrogen deficiency. Although the use of hormone replacement therapy after natural menopause has been in decline since the association between breast cancer and hormone replacement therapy use in the Million Womens Study,[34] the use of hormone replacement therapy for women with BRCA1 and BRCA2 mutations until the age of an expected menopause seems to be safe[35] and is advised.[4] Risk reducing bilateral salpingo-oophorectomy at ages 38-40 for carriers of the BRCA1 mutation and at ages 40-45 for carriers of the BRCA2 mutation would seem to be a reasonable balance.

Chemoprevention

In women with a diagnosis of (an oestrogen receptor positive) cancer, selective oestrogen receptor modulators, such as tamoxifen and raloxifene, and aromatase inhibitors reduce the risk of recurrence of that cancer as well as the risk of a contralateral primary breast cancer. Such drugs have therefore been investigated as preventive agents as an alternative to risk reducing surgery in women with a high risk of breast cancer. Tamoxifen has efficacy in premenopausal and postmenopasual women, whereas aromatase inhibitors are only effective in postmenopausal women. Raloxifene only has efficacy data in postmenopausal women.

A meta-analysis of randomised trials of selective oestrogen receptor modulators for breast cancer prevention, with data on 83 000 women, showed a 38% reduction in incidence of oestrogen receptor positive (but not oestrogen receptor negative) breast cancer with five years of treatment.[36] The absolute benefit of treatment depended on the absolute risk of breast cancer, but overall this equated to a need to treat 42 women to prevent one cancer. Similar to the benefit of adjuvant endocrine treatment for breast cancer, the benefits of chemoprevention extend beyond the five years that the drug is taken, with evidence of risk reduction extending to at least five years after completion.

Other studies have investigated the use of the aromatase inhibitors, exemestane and anastrozole, as chemopreventive agents. The recently published IBIS-II study, in which 3864 postmenopausal women were randomly assigned to anastrazole 1 mg daily or to placebo, showed an enhanced risk reduction with anastrazole treatment for five years compared with the risk reduction seen in the studies using selective oestrogen receptor modulators. After five years of follow-up 40 women in the anastrazole arm had developed

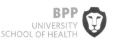

QUESTIONS FOR FUTURE RESEARCH

- Does surveillance with magnetic resonance imaging improve overall survival in patients at high risk of breast cancer?
- What are the differences in clinical and psychological outcomes in women who chose to have or chose not to have risk reducing surgery?
- Is chemoprevention effective in carriers of BRCA1/2 mutations and in women who received supradiaphragmatic radiotherapy at a young age?
- Are aromatase inhibitors more effective than tamoxifen at reducing the risk of breast cancer in women at high risk?

TIPS FOR NON-SPECIALISTS

- Breast cancer in general is a multifactorial disease and only about 5% of breast cancers are due to inherited mutations in high risk genes such as BRCA1/2 and TP53
- Genetic testing for high risk genes is performed only after suitable counselling in family history clinics and with informed consent

ADDITIONAL EDUCATIONAL RESOURCES

Healthcare professionals

- National Institute for Health and Care Excellence. Familial breast cancer: classification and care of people at risk of familial breast cancer and management of breast cancer and related risks in people with a family history of breast cancer. (Clinical guideline 164.) NICE, 2013—current UK guidance on the management of patients at high risk of breast cancer due to their family history
- Hilgart JS, Coles B, Iredale R. Cancer genetic risk assessment for individuals at risk of familial breast cancer. *Cochrane Database Syst Rev* 2012;2:CD003721—assesses the impact of risk assessment services on this group of patients
- National Cancer Institute Cancer Topics (www.cancer.gov/cancertopics/pdq/genetics/breast-and-ovarian/HealthProfessional)—information about breast cancer genetics, other risk factors, and breast cancer prevention

Patients

- Breast Cancer Care (www.breastcancercare.org.uk/breast-cancer-information/breast-awareness/am-i-risk/family-history-assessment)
- Cancer Research UK (www.cancerresearchuk.org/cancer-help/type/breast-cancer/about/risks/definite-breast-cancer-risks)

breast cancer compared with 85 in the placebo arm (hazard ratio 0.47, 95% confidence interval 0.32 to 0.68).[37] Selective oestrogen receptor modulators and aromatase inhibitors have yet to be compared head to head in the same study.

No study has as yet shown an overall survival advantage from any chemopreventive strategy. Furthermore, from the available evidence the drugs prevent the incidence of oestrogen receptor positive but not oestrogen receptor negative cancers and may not be as effective in BRCA1 carriers where triple negative cancers predominate. Chemoprevention can be associated with potentially serious adverse events—for example, tamoxifen causes a small excess risk of venous thrombosis (around 4-7 events per 1000 women over five years) and endometrial malignancy (around 4 excess cases per 1000, with most of the excess risk in postmenopausal women).[38] Aromatase inhibitors (which are not currently approved for chemoprevention by NICE) cause loss of bone mineral density and an increased risk of osteoporosis. All women starting treatment with an aromatase inhibitor should have baseline bone mineral density monitoring according to national guidelines.[39]

The uptake of chemoprevention worldwide is low despite favourable national guidance by NICE (for tamoxifen and raloxifene), the American Society of Clinical Oncology, and other institutions. Possible explanations for this include concerns about side effects of the drugs and a lack of awareness among women and healthcare providers.[40] For women at high risk of an oestrogen receptor positive breast

cancer, these drugs can be a useful option if they wish to avoid or delay risk reducing surgery. The drugs are, however, less effective than risk reducing surgery and have the potential for serious adverse events. The potential benefits and risks of these drugs require careful counselling and quantifying, which may best be performed within secondary or tertiary care settings. Decision aids are being developed to help women make a decision regarding treatment with these drugs.

Competing interests: We have read and understood the BMJ Group policy on declaration of interests and declare the following interests: AA was an expert member of the NICE Familial Breast Cancer Guideline Development Group (2013 update). GE was the chair of the same group. GE and AA are coauthors of a manuscript in preparation.

Provenance and peer review: Commissioned; externally peer reviewed.

1 Cancer Research UK. Breast cancer incidence statistics. 2012. www.cancerresearchuk.org/cancer-info/cancerstats/types/breast/incidence/#risk.
2 Parkin DM, Boyd L, Walker LC. The fraction of cancer attributable to lifestyle and environmental factors in the UK in 2010. Summary and conclusions. *Br J Cancer* 2011;105(S2):S77-81.
3 Turkoz FP, Solak M, Petekkaya I, Keskin O, Kertmen N, Sarici F, et al. Association between common risk factors and molecular subtypes in breast cancer patients. *Breast* 2013;22:344-50.
4 National Institute for Health and Care Excellence. Familial breast cancer: classification and care of people at risk of familial breast cancer and management of breast cancer and related risks in people with a family history of breast cancer. (Clinical guideline 164.) 2013. http://guidance.nice.org.uk/CG164.
5 Saslow D, Boetes C, Burke W, Harms S, Leach MO, Lehman CD, et al. American Cancer Society guidelines for breast screening with MRI as an adjunct to mammography. *CA Cancer J Clin* 2007;57:75-89.
6 Rubinstein WS. Hereditary breast cancer in Jews. *Fam Cancer* 2004;3:249-57.
7 Swerdlow AJ, Cooke R, Bates A, Cunningham D, Falk SJ, Gilson D, et al. Breast cancer risk after supradiaphragmatic radiotherapy for Hodgkin's lymphoma in England and Wales: a national cohort study. *J Clin Oncol* 2012;30:2745-52.
8 Lalloo F, Evans DG. Familial breast cancer. *Clin Genet* 2012;82:105-14.
9 Evans DG, Ingham RL. Reduced life expectancy seen in hereditary diseases which predispose to early-onset tumors. *Appl Clin Genet* 2013;6:53-61.
10 Antoniou A, Pharoah PD, Narod S, Risch HA, Eyfjord JE, Hopper JL, et al. Average risks of breast and ovarian cancer associated with BRCA1 or BRCA2 mutations detected in case series unselected for family history: a combined analysis of 22 studies. *Am J Hum Genet* 2002;72:1117-30.
11 Chen S, Parmigiani G. Meta-analysis of BRCA1 and BRCA2 penetrance. *J Clin Oncol* 2007;25:1329-33.
12 Evans DG, Shenton A, Woodward E, Lalloo F, Howell A, Maher ER. Penetrance estimates for BRCA1 and BRCA2 based on genetic testing in a clinical cancer genetics service setting: risks of breast/ovarian cancer quoted should reflect the cancer burden in the family. *BMC Cancer* 2008;8:155.
13 Papelard H, de Bock GH, van Eijk R, Vliet Vlieland TP, Cornelisse CJ, Devilee P, et al. Prevalence of BRCA1 in a hospital-based population of Dutch breast cancer patients. *Br J Cancer* 2000;83:719-24.
14 Mavaddat N, Barrowdale D, Andrulis IL, Domchek SM, Eccles D, Nevanlinna H, et al. Pathology of breast and ovarian cancers among BRCA1 and BRCA2 mutation carriers: results from the Consortium of Investigators of Modifiers of BRCA1/2 (CIMBA). *Cancer Epidemiol Biomarkers Prev* 2012;21:134-47.
15 Harris H, Nippert I, Julian-Reynier C, Schmidtke J, van Asperen C, Gadzicki D, et al. Familial breast cancer: is it time to move from a reactive to a proactive role? *Fam Cancer* 2011;10:501-3.
16 Tyrer J, Duffy SW, Cuzick J. A breast cancer prediction model incorporating familial and personal risk factors. *Stat Med* 2005;23:1111-30.
17 Antoniou AC, Hardy R, Walker L, Evans DG, Shenton A, Eeles R, et al. Predicting the likelihood of carrying a BRCA1 or BRCA2 mutation: validation of BOADICEA, BRCAPRO, IBIS, Myriad and the Manchester scoring system using data from UK genetics clinics. *J Med Genet* 2008;45:425-31.
18 Evans DG, Lalloo F, Cramer A, Jones E, Knox F, Amir E, et al. Addition of pathology and biomarker information significantly improves the performance of the Manchester scoring system for BRCA1 and BRCA2 testing. *J Med Genet* 2009;46:811-7.
19 Independent UK Panel on Breast Cancer Screening. The benefits and harms of breast cancer screening: an independent review. *Lancet* 2012;380:1778-86.
20 Berrington de Gonzalez A, Berg CD, Visvanathan K, Robson M. Estimated risk of radiation-induced breast cancer from mammographic screening for young BRCA mutation carriers. *J Natl Cancer Inst* 2009;101:205-9.

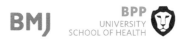

21 Kriege M, Brekelmans CT, Boetes C, Besnard PE, Zonderland HM, Obdeijn IM, et al. Efficacy of MRI and mammography for breast-cancer screening in women with a familial or genetic predisposition. *N Engl J Med* 2004;351:427-37.

22 Leach MO, Boggis CR, Dixon AK, Easton DF, Eeles RA, Evans DG, et al. MARIBS study group. Screening with magnetic resonance imaging and mammography of a UK population at high familial risk of breast cancer: a prospective multicentre cohort study (MARIBS). *Lancet* 2005;365:1769-78.

23 Warner E, Messersmith H, Causer P, Eisen A, Shumak R, Plewes D. Systematic review: using magnetic resonance imaging to screen women at high risk for breast cancer. *Ann Intern Med* 2008;148:671-9.

24 Ralleigh G, Given-Wilson R. Breast cancer risk and possible screening strategies for young women following supradiaphragmatic irradiation for Hodgkin's disease. *Clin Radiol* 2004;59:647-50.

25 Rebbeck TR, Friebel T, Lynch HT, Neuhausen SL, van't Veer L, Garber JE, et al. Bilateral prophylactic mastectomy reduces breast cancer in BRCA1 and BRCA2 mutation carriers: the PROSE Study Group. *J Clin Oncol* 2004;22:1055-62.

26 Heemskerk-Gerritsen BA, Menke-Pluijmers MB, Jager A, Tilanus-Linthorst MM, Koppert LB, Obdeijn IM, et al. Substantial breast cancer risk reduction and potential survival benefit after bilateral mastectomy when compared with surveillance in healthy BRCA1 and BRCA2 mutation carriers: a prospective analysis. *Ann Oncol* 2013;24:2029-35.

27 Ingham SL, Sperrin M, Baildam A, Ross GL, Clayton R, Lallo F, et al. Risk-reducing surgery increases survival in BRCA1/2 mutation carriers unaffected at time of family referral. *Breast Cancer Res Treat* 2013;142:611-8.

28 Evans DG, Ingham SL, Baildam A, Ross GL, Lalloo F, Buchan I, et al. Contralateral mastectomy improves survival in women with BRCA1/2-associated breast cancer. *Breast Cancer Res Treat* 2013;140:135-42.

29 Metcalfe K, Gershman S, Ghadirian P, Lynch HT, Snyder C, Tung N, et al. Contralateral mastectomy and survival after breast cancer in carriers of BRCA1 and DRCA2 mutations: retrospective analysis. *BMJ* 2014;348:g226.

30 Hallowell N, Baylock B, Heiniger L, Butow PN, Patel D, Meiser B, et al. Looking different, feeling different women's reactions to risk-reducing breast and ovarian surgery. *Fam Cancer* 2012;11:215-24.

31 Montgomery LL, Tran KN, Heelan MC, Van Zee KJ, Massie MJ, Payne DK, et al. Issues of regret in women with contralateral prophylactic mastectomies. *Ann Surg Oncol* 1999;6:546-52.

32 Rebbeck TR, Kauff ND, Domchek SM. Meta-analysis of risk reduction estimates associated with risk-reducing salpingo-oophorectomy in BRCA1 or BRCA2 mutation carriers. *J Natl Cancer Inst* 2009;101:80-7.

33 Fakkert IE, Mourits MJ, Jansen L, van der Kolk DM, Meijer K, et al. Breast cancer incidence after risk-reducing salpingo-oophorectomy in BRCA1 and BRCA2 mutation carriers. *Cancer Prev Res (Phila)* 2012;5:1291-7.

34 Beral V; Million Women Study Collaborators. Breast cancer and hormone-replacement therapy in the Million Women Study. *Lancet* 2003;362:419-27.

35 Rebbeck TR, Friebel T, Wagner T, Lynch HT, Garber JE, Daly MB, et al. Effect of short-term hormone replacement therapy on breast cancer risk reduction after bilateral prophylactic oophorectomy in BRCA1 and BRCA2 mutation carriers: the PROSE Study Group. *J Clin Oncol* 2005;23:7804-10.

36 Cuzick J, Sestak I, Bonanni B, Costantino JP, Cummings S, et al. Selective oestrogen receptor modulators in prevention of breast cancer: an updated meta-analysis of individual participant data. *Lancet* 2013;381:1827-34.

37 Cuzick J, Sestak I, Forbes JF, Dowsett M, Knox J, Cawthorn S, et al. Anastrozole for prevention of breast cancer in high-risk postmenopausal women (IBIS-II): an international, double-blind, randomised placebo-controlled trial. *Lancet* 2013;383:1041-8.

38 Moyer VA. Medications for risk reduction of primary breast cancer in women: US Preventative Services Task Force recommendation statement. *Ann Intern Med* 2013;159:698-708.

39 Reid DM, Doughty J, Eastell R, Heys SD, Howell A, et al. Guidance for the management of breast cancer treatment-induced bone loss: a consensus position statement from a UK Expert Group. *Cancer Treat Rev* 2008;34(Suppl 1):S3-18.

40 Waters EA, McNeel TS, Stevens WM, Freedman AN. Use of tamoxifen and raloxifene for breast cancer chemoprevention in 2010. *Breast Cancer Res Treat* 2012;134:875-80.

Related links

bmj.com

Previous articles in this series

- Gallstones (BMJ 2014;348: g2669)
- First seizures in adults (BMJ 2014;348:g2470)
- Obsessive-compulsive disorder (BMJ 2014;348:g2183)
- Modern management of splenic trauma (BMJ 2014;348:g1864)
- Fungal nail infection: diagnosis and management (BMJ 2014;348:g1800)

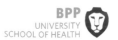

Post-mastectomy breast reconstruction

Paul T R Thiruchelvam, specialist registrar breast and general surgery[1],
Fiona McNeill, consultant oncoplastic and reconstructive breast surgeon[2],
Navid Jallali, consultant plastic and reconstructive surgeon[1],
Paul Harris, consultant plastic and reconstructive breast surgeon[2],
Katy Hogben, consultant oncoplastic and reconstructive breast surgeon[1]

[1]Imperial College NHS Trust, Charing Cross Hospital, London W6 8RF, UK

[2]Royal Marsden Hospital, London, UK

Correspondence to:
P T R Thiruchelvam
paul.thiruchelvam@imperial.ac.uk

Cite this as: BMJ 2013;347:f5903

DOI: 10.1136/bmj.f5903

http://www.bmj.com/content/347/bmj.f5903

Breast cancer is the most common cancer in women, with almost 1.38 million new cases a year worldwide; it accounts for 23% of all cancers and 14% of deaths from cancer.[1] However, mortality from breast cancer is declining—increasing numbers of women are long term survivors (>5 years) (currently 549 000 in the United Kingdom).[2][3] Surgery remains a mainstay of treatment, either breast conservation or mastectomy, but any breast surgery can greatly alter breast aesthetics and body image.

Breast reconstruction restores breast symmetry after a mastectomy by creating a breast mound, similar in size, shape, contour, and "out of bra position" to the contralateral breast. In England and Wales in 2002, about 10% of women had immediate breast reconstruction; by 2009 this had risen to 21%.[4] Post-mastectomy breast reconstruction is associated with improved body image, quality of life, self confidence, and wellbeing.[5]

In this review, we outline the indications for breast reconstruction along with the timing and techniques available to patients after mastectomy.

What is post-mastectomy breast reconstruction?

Breast reconstruction is a surgical procedure that restores shape to the breast after mastectomy. Although it will not re-create the exact look and feel of a natural breast, it aims to create a breast mound contour similar to that before mastectomy.

When, and to whom, should breast reconstruction be offered?

In 2009 the National Institute for Health and Clinical Excellence (NICE) revised guidance on improving breast cancer outcomes. It recommended discussing immediate reconstruction with all patients having a mastectomy and offering it unless serious comorbidity or the need for adjuvant therapy precludes this option. It also recommended offering and discussing all appropriate breast reconstruction options with patients, irrespective of whether they are available locally.[6] Fifty three per cent of women having surgery for breast cancer will undergo mastectomy (box 1).[7][8]

SUMMARY POINTS

- Breast reconstruction should be discussed with all women who undergo mastectomy
- The type of mastectomy undertaken directly influences the reconstructive outcome and aesthetics
- All reconstructive options should be discussed with the patient regardless of local expertise and appropriate referral made to specialist centres if necessary
- If radiotherapy is needed, delayed reconstruction minimises the risk of complications and improves aesthetic outcomes
- Follow-up studies show that women have a high level of satisfaction with the reconstructive option they chose, although those who opted for no reconstruction also report a high level of satisfaction

SOURCES AND SELECTION CRITERIA

We searched Medline, Embase, and the Cochrane collaboration for articles using the keywords "breast reconstruction". Wherever possible we used evidence from randomised controlled trials, systematic reviews, and meta-analyses from the past five years to provide an up to date review. We also consulted the Association of Breast Surgeons (ABS) guidelines (2009), ABS and British Association of Plastic Reconstructive and Aesthetic Surgeons guidelines (2012), and the fourth annual report of the National Mastectomy and Breast Reconstruction Audit (NMBRA) 2011.

BOX 1 INDICATIONS FOR MASTECTOMY

- Large tumour size to breast volume ratio
- Breast conserving surgery did not work
- Multicentric disease (multiple foci in more than one quadrant)
- Large in situ tumour
- Patient choice
- Recurrence in a previously conserved breast
- Patient not suitable for radiotherapy—for example, patient has already received mantle radiotherapy for Hodgkin's disease

In the UK and United States, bilateral mastectomy is increasingly being used for risk reduction in *BRCA* carriers, for those with a high risk of developing breast cancer (lifetime risk of 30%), or as a planned management strategy for unilateral cancer (fig 1).[9][10][11][12][13][14][15] In general, bilateral mastectomy is associated with a higher rate of breast reconstruction. A recent Cochrane review showed that bilateral prophylactic (risk reduction) mastectomy reduced the incidence of, and death from, breast cancer, but it highlighted that more rigorous prospective studies are needed to assess absolute risk reduction.[16] The review also found that although contralateral prophylactic (risk reduction) mastectomy decreases the incidence of cancer in the contralateral breast, it is unclear whether, and for whom, this practice improves survival.[16]

How is a mastectomy performed?

When performing a mastectomy, the anatomical (oncological) plane between breast tissue and subcutaneous fat needs to be identified. It is, however, impossible to remove all breast tissue because the oncological plane is not uniform throughout the breast. A standard (simple) mastectomy removes the breast skin envelope, but a skin sparing mastectomy preserves the breast skin envelope (with or without the nipple) along with the inframammary crease. Skin sparing mastectomy is the technique of choice for immediate breast reconstruction because it gives a more favourable aesthetic outcome, although it is associated with a 10-22% risk of skin flap necrosis.[17] The incidence of local

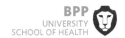

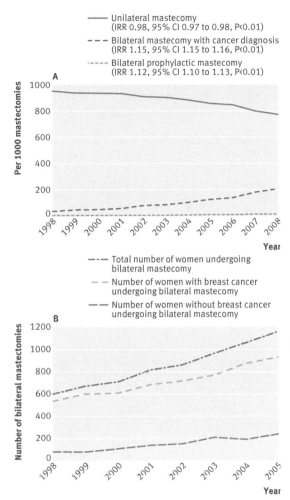

— Unilateral mastecomy
(IRR 0.98, 95% CI 0.97 to 0.98, P<0.01)
- - - Bilateral mastecomy with cancer diagnosis
(IRR 1.15, 95% CI 1.15 to 1.16, P<0.01)
····· Bilateral prophylactic mastecomy
(IRR 1.12, 95% CI 1.10 to 1.13, P<0.01)

—·— Total number of women undergoing
bilateral mastecomy
— — Number of women with breast cancer
undergoing bilateral mastecomy
—— Number of women without breast cancer
undergoing bilateral mastecomy

Fig 1 (A) Mastectomy rates in the United States, 1998-2008.[15]
(B) Bilateral mastectomy rates in the United Kingdom, 2002-09.[13]
CI=confidence interval; IRR=incidence rate ratio

recurrence is similar to that seen for simple mastectomy (2.9% at 10 years in a recent retrospective review).[18] In patients with large breasts and excess skin a controlled reduction in the skin envelope can be achieved.

Preservation of the native nipple-areola complex (NAC) is the ultimate extension of breast envelope preservation.[19] A questionnaire study of women in a single unit compared nipple sparing mastectomy and reconstruction (n=310) with simple mastectomy and reconstruction (n=143, including NAC reconstruction).[20] Body image was more positive and satisfaction with the final appearance of the nipple was higher in the NAC sparing group.[20]

However the nipple is affected in 5-31% of invasive or in situ breast cancers.[21] Two large retrospective case series found that tumour size (particularly >4 cm) and distance of the tumour from the NAC were independent predictors of nipple involvement.[22][23] One large single institution retrospective case series review of nipple sparing mastectomies found a nipple necrosis rate of 20% (partial 19%; total 2%); risk factors included hypertension, diabetes, obesity, smoking, and larger breast size (although this last factor was not significant).[24] Other complications include nipple malposition or asymmetry and reduced sensation in the preserved nipple. A novel technique called "nipple delay" seeks to reduce the risk of nipple necrosis in women at high risk of nipple loss and is performed seven to 21 days before mastectomy.[25] During the procedure, a skin flap is elevated in the plane of a

therapeutic mastectomy beneath the nipple-areola complex and surrounding mastectomy skin.

When should breast reconstruction be performed?
Breast reconstruction can be performed at the time of mastectomy (immediate/primary) or at any later date (delayed/secondary). Patients who are uncertain about reconstruction are best advised to consider delayed reconstruction. The main advantage of immediate reconstruction is preservation of the native breast skin envelope and inframammary fold, which enables a more natural and symmetrical outcome. However, immediate reconstruction can delay adjuvant therapy if postoperative complications arise.

Delayed reconstruction is best for patients who want to focus on the cancer treatment or need more time to consider the various breast reconstruction options. Delayed breast reconstruction is technically more challenging because the native skin envelope is removed at the time of standard mastectomy. Extra skin must therefore be recruited from skin expansion (where an expander implant is used to stretch the skin) or from a donor site. This can result in a less natural and symmetrical appearance and longer scars.

The UK National Mastectomy and Breast Reconstruction Audit (NMBRA) prospectively evaluated complications and patient reported outcomes in a cohort of patients from more than 200 centres between January 2008 and March 2009.[26] Nearly 17 000 women underwent mastectomy—21% had immediate and 11% had delayed reconstruction (table). Outcome questionnaires were completed at baseline, three months, and 18 months (fig 2). The audit found that patients who chose delayed reconstruction had better satisfaction scores after reconstruction, possibly because they had lived with a flat chest wall before reconstruction.[26]

Immediate breast reconstruction is associated with a higher complication rate than delayed reconstruction.[27][28] The latest Cochrane review found no clear evidence to support immediate reconstruction over delayed reconstruction.[29] Further research is needed to provide reliable evidence for patients to make more informed decisions about the best type and most appropriate timing of breast reconstruction.

What options are available for breast reconstruction?
Various techniques are available for breast reconstruction. The process can take 12-24 months and multiple surgical procedures may be needed to achieve the optimal outcome. Aesthetic outcomes are unpredictable and the reconstructed breast can be insensate. The reconstruction technique used depends on individual requirements, determined by patient choice, advice of the reconstructive surgeon, comorbidities (body habitus, smoking, diabetes), potential loss of high end function (with the latissimus dorsi or transverse rectus abdominus myocutaneous (TRAM) flap), cancer biology, and anticipated post-mastectomy therapy, particularly the need for radiotherapy. Options for reconstruction include silicone tissue expander/implants, autologous tissue flaps, or a combination of the two (box 2).

Implant with or without acellular dermal matrices
Implant based reconstruction accounts for 61% and 37% of reconstructions in the US and UK, respectively.[26][30] It enables formation of a breast mound without the donor site scaring and morbidity associated with autologous reconstruction. Reconstruction can be a one stage or two stage procedure. An implant is placed in a pocket created under the pectoral muscle with a port (remote or integrated) to enable volume

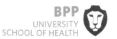

Experience of care at 3 months
9 out of 10 women felt that they had received the right amount of information about their procedure (mastectomy ± reconstruction)
Most women were satisfied with the information on their surgical procedure (how it was performed, recovery, and possible complications)
The national satisfaction score was 72 (scale from 0 (low satisfaction) to 100 (high satisfaction))
90% of women rated their care as excellent after mastectomy and reconstruction

National patient reported outcomes at 18 months after surgery
Mastectomy only
83% of women were satisfied with how they looked in the mirror with clothes, 42% of women were satisfied with how they looked in the mirror unclothed
75% reported feeling confident in a social setting
10% reported tenderness in the breast area
Women having an immediate reconstruction
90% of women were satisfied with how they looked in the mirror with clothes, 59% of women were satisfied with how they looked in the mirror unclothed
85% reported feeling confident in a social setting
7% reported tenderness in the breast area
Women having a delayed reconstruction
93% of women were satisfied with how they looked in the mirror with clothes, 76% of women were satisfied with how they looked in the mirror unclothed
92% reported feeling confident in a social setting
4% reported tenderness in the breast area

Fig 2 National mastectomy and breast reconstruction audit 2011. Assessment of care at three months after surgery; patient reported outcomes 18 months after surgery[26]

Type of primary reconstruction in women in the National Mastectomy and Breast Reconstruction Audit[24]		
Type of surgery	Immediate reconstruction (n (%))	Delayed reconstruction (n (%))
Implant or expander only	1246 (37)	281 (16)
Pedicle flap + implant or expander	735 (22)	438 (25)
Pedicle flap (autologous)	932 (27)	446 (26)
Free flap	476 (14)	566 (33)
Total	3389	1731

expansion. To achieve complete submuscular coverage, a portion of the serratus muscle can be raised laterally and sutured to the pectoralis muscle. The expansion process begins two to three weeks postoperatively, resulting in gentle stretching of the overlying skin and soft tissue until the desired volume is achieved. The tissue expander is replaced three to six months later with a definitive fixed volume implant. A one stage procedure (using a fixed

volume implant) avoids a second operation, but a two stage procedure enables adjustments to be made if necessary. Box 3 lists the associated complications.

Tissue coverage of the inferior pole of the implant may also be provided by a de-epithelialised inferior pole dermal sling (using tissue from the lower pole of the patient's breast) or an acellular dermal matrix. Acellular dermal matrices are collagen sheets derived from human, bovine, and porcine tissues, which become incorporated into the host tissue over time (figs 3 and 4). These grafts have several benefits—shorter operative time; no need to recruit serratus anterior muscle (decreases chest wall morbidity); fewer postoperative expansions needed to achieve the desired volume; and the inframammary and lateral mammary folds can be redefined.[31][32] Although expensive, these matrices enable larger initial volume implants to be used and result in lower rates of capsular contracture.[32][33] Higher incidences of seroma, infection, and partial mastectomy flap necrosis have been reported, however.[34]

Closure of the breast implant manufacturer Poly Implant Prothèse, because of the use of unapproved silicone filler, led to the re-establishment of the UK breast implant registry by the Medicines and Healthcare Products Regulatory Agency in June 2013.[35] The registry was initially established in 1993, but was closed in 2005 because too few women wished to take part in the scheme. The Poly Implant Prothèse implant episode highlighted areas where UK and European medical device regulation requires strengthening.

Autologous tissue reconstruction
Autologous breast reconstruction uses the patient's own tissue. It can be performed using pedicled flaps or free tissue transfers (free flaps). Pedicled flaps, such as the latissimus dorsi flap, maintain the existing blood supply to the transferred tissue so avoid microsurgery. Free (perforator)

BOX 2 ADVANTAGES AND DISADVANTAGES OF BREAST RECONSTRUCTION TECHNIQUES

Implant based

Advantages
- Less invasive
- Less operative time with shorter recovery time
- No donor site morbidity

Disadvantages
- Requires numerous tissue expansions postoperatively
- Does not feel "natural"
- Difficult to match ptosis in large breast
- May require implant exchange
- Implant infection and removal

Autologous

Advantages
- Does not degrade
- More natural appearance and feel

Disadvantages
- Flap failure (partial or complete) and fat necrosis
- Donor site morbidity
- Long operative time
- Large scar (usually in the abdomen after a deep inferior epigastric perforator flap reconstruction)

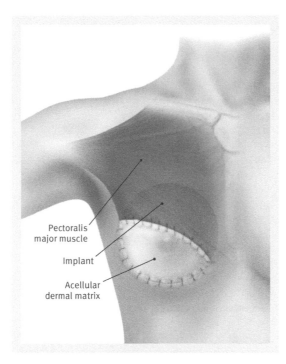

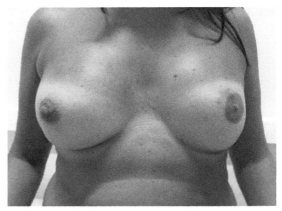

Fig 4 Woman with left sided breast cancer treated with left skin sparing mastectomy and reconstruction with acellular dermal matrix and implant, left nipple reconstruction, and areola tattoo. She subsequently underwent risk reducing skin and nipple sparing (envelope) mastectomy of the right breast, together with reconstruction with acellular dermal matrix and implant. Picture courtesy of Katy Hogben, consultant oncoplastic breast surgeon, Charing Cross Hospital, London

Fig 3 Illustration showing the usual placement of an acellular dermal matrix in an implant based reconstruction. Reproduced, with permission, from LifeCell

flaps, however, are raised on a pedicle (including a known artery and vein), divided, transferred to the recipient site and then anastomosed to the vessels in the chest or axilla (internal mammary or axillary vessels, respectively).

The major advantage of autologous reconstruction is that revision surgery is less likely because the transferred tissue adjusts to changes in body weight.[36] [37] Several patient reported outcome studies suggest that autologous tissue provides a more consistent and durable reconstruction, with higher long term satisfaction, compared with implant based reconstructions.[36] [38] However, in one retrospective review, patients with an expander or implant based reconstruction had the highest satisfaction scores (compared with latissimus dorsi flaps and TRAM flaps), despite having higher reoperation rates and lower aesthetic scores.[39]

Pedicled flaps include latissimus dorsi and TRAM flaps. Refinements in microsurgical techniques have led to the advent of perforator flaps, such as the deep inferior epigastric perforator (DIEP; fig 5) flap, superior inferior epigastric artery flap, and transverse upper gracilis flap (fig 6). Autologous breast reconstruction is technically challenging, with a longer operative time and hospital stay than implant based reconstructions. Patients with a history of obesity, diabetes, autoimmune disease, and smoking may not be suitable owing to increased perioperative morbidity.[40]

Non-abdominal based autologous breast reconstruction
Latissimus dorsi flap reconstruction involves the pedicled transfer of the latissimus dorsi with its overlying fat and skin. This is one of the most commonly used flaps for breast reconstruction in the UK.[26] This flap can be used on its own to reconstruct a small to moderately sized breast defect or it can be used in conjunction with an implant to provide increased volume. If used alone, an extended autologous latissimus dorsi flap can incorporate a larger volume of muscle and fat to increase the bulk of the flap. The NMBRA showed that the pedicled latissimus dorsi flap is extremely robust, with a reported failure rate of 1%, but it is

associated with a high rate of donor site seroma formation (50-80%).[26] [41] Patients may also experience shoulder pain, back pain, tightness when stretching the arm, and difficulty in carrying or lifting heavy objects (box 3).[26]

The transverse upper gracilis flap is an autologous free flap that is suitable for women with small or medium sized breasts, who may not be suitable for an abdominal based autologous reconstruction, or may not accept scars on the abdomen, back, or gluteal regions. The flap consists mainly of adipose tissue and is harvested from the inner thigh. This flap is smaller than the DIEP and TRAM free flaps, and it provides a thinner fat pad, so for larger volumes two flaps may be needed.

The superior gluteal artery perforator flap is the second choice if the abdominal donor site is unavailable. Its major drawback is that it leaves a scar on the buttock and the consistency of the fat does not match the breast as closely as abdominal fat.[42] [43] [44]

BOX 3 COMPLICATIONS AFTER BREAST RECONSTRUCTION

Implant based reconstructions
- Implant infection or rotation
- Extrusion or rupture of implant
- Capsular formation
- Seroma or haematoma
- Implant rippling (wrinkling or creasing)
- Inframammmary fold problem and bottoming out (inferior displacement of the implant)
- Skin flap necrosis
- Siliconoma or gel bleed

Autologous reconstructions (deep inferior epigastric perforator, transverse rectus abdominus myocutaneous, or latissimus dorsi flap)
- Flap failure (partial or total)
- Fat necrosis
- Abdominal bulge or hernia (seen with the deep inferior epigastric perforator flap)
- Seroma
- Haematoma
- Donor site morbidity
- Shoulder or back pain (seen with the latissimus dorsi flap)

Abdominal based autologous breast reconstruction

The abdomen is the main choice for autologous reconstruction because a large enough volume of tissue is usually available. Furthermore, the fat has a similar consistency to breast tissue and closely matches its feel. Several abdominal based flaps are available but the two most common variants are the TRAM and DIEP flaps. For the TRAM flap, skin, subcutaneous fat, and rectus abdominus muscle are harvested from below the umbilicus, either as a pedicled or free flap. The major drawback is that the loss of the rectus abdominus muscle can result in an abdominal bulge and increases the risk of hernia formation. The pedicled TRAM is the most common autologous reconstruction performed in the US.[45] Both pedicled and free TRAM flaps are associated with an increased risk of abdominal hernia, umbilical necrosis, and partial or complete flap necrosis.[46]

The DIEP flap is an evolution and refinement of the TRAM flap—it preserves the entire rectus abdominus muscle and sheath, allowing transfer of skin and subcutaneous fat only. Retrospective reviews have shown that despite being more complex, this procedure results in significantly lower donor site morbidity, shorter hospital stay, decreased postoperative pain, and better recovery of sensation than a traditional TRAM flap. It is also more cost effective.[47 48] In our units, the default option is to carry out a DIEP flap, reverting to a muscle sparing TRAM option if the perforators are poor.

What secondary procedures might be necessary after breast reconstruction?

NAC reconstruction

Patient reported outcome studies have found that NAC reconstruction significantly improves patient satisfaction with breast reconstruction.[49 50 51] The ideal nipple reconstruction should be symmetrical in shape, site, size, texture, and pigmentation. The procedure is often delayed until three to four months after reconstruction of the breast mound. Loss of projection of the reconstructed nipple remains a problem and can require revision. The nipple can be reconstructed using several techniques including the use of local flaps (subdermal and pedicle based), grafting from distant sites, nipple sharing, and nipple banking. Nipple sharing is performed after a unilateral breast reconstruction, once the breast mound is complete. Half of the contralateral nipple is harvested and then grafted on to a patch of de-epithelialised skin on the reconstructed breast. Nipple banking is performed at mastectomy. The areola is harvested as a full thickness graft combined with the nipple and temporarily transferred to the prearranged banking site, usually the groin, abdomen, or buttocks. Frozen sections are often taken from the base of each nipple, intraoperatively, to determine malignant involvement. Three months after reconstruction, the "banked" nipple is replanted on to the new breast mound. The areola is commonly reconstructed with intradermal tattooing. This procedure is undertaken in an outpatient clinic setting (20-30 minutes) and may require local anaesthetic. Tattoos fade with time, and further tattooing procedures might be needed.

Lipomodelling

This procedure is performed under general anaesthesia and involves the transfer of autologous fat by blunt needle aspiration from a donor site (usually abdomen, hips, and inner thigh) to the breast. It improves breast shape, symmetry, and volume after breast conserving surgery or

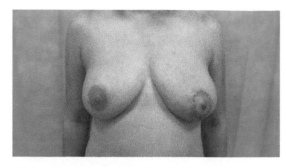

Fig 5 Immediate breast reconstruction after right mastectomy using a deep inferior epigastric perforator flap. Nipple reconstruction and tattooing of the areola were carried out separately. The patient then underwent a symmetrising left breast mastopexy. Courtesy of Navid Jallali, consultant plastic surgeon, Charing Cross Hospital, London

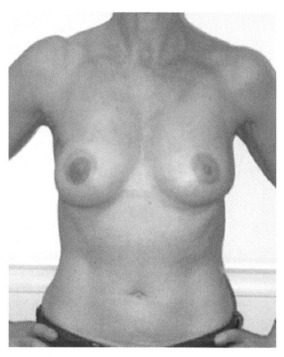

Fig 6 Breast reconstruction after right skin sparing mastectomy and immediate reconstruction using a double transverse upper gracilis flap. The patient subsequently underwent right nipple reconstruction and areola tattooing. Courtesy of Paul Harris, consultant plastic surgeon, Royal Marsden Hospital, London

a breast mound reconstruction. Several procedures may be needed to obtain an optimal outcome because fat reabsorption results in a loss of 10-30% of volume after injection.[52 53] Complications include liponecrosis, infection, calcification (potentially affecting radiological follow-up), and formation of an unspecified palpable mass.[52] Furthermore, care must be taken not to sacrifice autologous donor sites, such as the abdomen, for future use.

Symmetrisation procedures

Once the mastectomy site has been reconstructed, the next step may involve creating a symmetrical contralateral breast. Contralateral mastopexy (breast lift), reduction mammoplasty (breast reduction), or augmentation may be performed at the same time as the reconstruction or delayed.

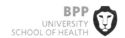

ADDITIONAL EDUCATIONAL RESOURCES

Resources for healthcare professionals

- Association of Breast Surgery (www.associationofbreastsurgery.org.uk)—Information about different types of breast reconstruction surgery, including how to find a surgeon
- British Association of Plastic, Reconstructive and Aesthetic Surgeons (www.bapras.org.uk)— Provides details about specific plastic surgery procedures and techniques involved in breast reconstruction

Resources for patients

- American Society of Plastic Surgeons (www.plasticsurgery.org/Reconstructive-Procedures/ Breast-Reconstruction.html)—Provides information on breast reconstructive techniques, costing preparation for surgery, and postoperative recovery
- Cancer Research UK (www.cancerresearchuk.org/cancer-help/type/breast-cancer/treatment/ surgery/reconstruction/about-breast-reconstruction)—Cancer charity, providing a detailed overview on breast cancer management, including including breast reconstruction
- Breast Cancer Care (www.breastcancercare.org.uk/breast-cancerinformation/treating-breast-cancer/surgery/reconstruction)—Information and support for everyone affected by breast cancer; patients discuss their reasons for deciding whether to have breast reconstruction after surgery
- Macmillan Cancer Support (www.macmillan.org.uk/Cancerinformation/Cancertreatment/ Treatmenttypes/Surgery/Breastreconstruction/Breastreconstruction.aspx)—Practical, medical, and financial support; helps patients understand what breast reconstruction is and the possible benefits and difficulties they might experience

A PATIENT'S PERSPECTIVE: DEEP INFERIOR EPIGASTRIC PERFORATOR FLAP RECONSTRUCTION

I was diagnosed with invasive ductal carcinoma in May 2011, aged 49 years. I underwent six courses of chemotherapy and hoped that a lumpectomy and lymph node removal would clear the cancer. Unfortunately it didn't work, so I had to have a mastectomy. I was sent to discuss the operation with my surgeon.

As well as being petrified at having a diagnosis of cancer, the thought of losing a breast was devastating, and I felt that my whole world had ended. Since the age of 17, I had been a model, so glamour and having the "perfect body" had been my life.

On meeting my surgeon he instantly put me at ease, and his professionalism and kindness reassured me. He explained the main options of breast reconstruction, and after discussing these options I felt happy that the deep inferior epigastric perforator technique was the right one for me. I mainly chose this option because my own tissues would be used, resulting in a natural look and feel.

I recovered from the surgery faster than I had imagined. My breast felt quite comfortable, but sitting, standing straight, and rising from a chair or bed was painful because of the tissue that had been taken from my abdomen. After a week it became easier to move about, and after two weeks I was moving around as normal. I was over the moon about how natural the breast reconstruction looked and felt, even down to still having a mole in the same place.

It is now 18 months since I had the surgery and my breast is complete, with a nipple and tattoo areolar—it looks amazing. The symmetry looks perfectly natural, as does the shape, although I have no sensation in the breast tissue. However, it looks and feels natural to my husband.

My pelvis has a very faint scar line, and although it is quite long I hardly notice it. I love the fact that at 50 I have a flat tummy. My belly button also has a faint scar around it, but again it is barely noticeable.

On the whole, for something that I feared so much, the whole experience was nowhere near as traumatic as I originally thought, mainly because of the kindness and expertise of the surgical team.

A PATIENT'S PERSPECTIVE: IMPLANT BASED RECONSTRUCTION

When I noticed a lump on my left breast I went to see my general practitioner, who referred me to Charing Cross Hospital for a scan and a biopsy. I assumed it was just a routine check and thought "I'm only 27, no one can get breast cancer at that age." After a long week of waiting for my results the day finally came. All I can remember is the doctor saying "I'm afraid it's bad news—you have breast cancer." After that, I can't remember anything, it was like someone has cut the sound off. I was diagnosed with a grade 2 invasive ductal cancer. For the next few days I couldn't stop crying. I couldn't eat or sleep—my world was falling apart, and I thought that everything was over. All I could think was "I am going to die." After a few stressful days I was back at the hospital. This is when everything changed, owing to the professionalism of the doctors, nurses, and everyone else at the hospital who helped me understand what my options were and how I could fight this horrible disease. I had decided that the best option was to have chemotherapy to shrink the tumour, then a mastectomy to remove any chance of the tumour coming back.

Again, I have so much praise for the hospital staff who helped me all the time, answered my questions, and gave me all the information that I needed. I had done a lot of research on the internet and knew what to expect during the treatment. I was ready to fight back.

Two days after I turned 28 I started my chemotherapy. After the first session my body reacted well to the treatment—I was really happy. I had a total of six sessions during which I lost all my hair—this was the worst side effect. But at the end of the treatment the tumour had shrunk. The day I was waiting for was coming—I was going to get the tumour out of my body. I had a mastectomy and a reconstruction with an implant. It hasn't been easy, but I recovered well. I had to go back to the hospital every other week so that the surgeon could check on how the wound was healing and also inflate my expander implant.

I was really happy with the way everything was going, the tumour was gone, my breast was near enough as it was before, and my hair had started to grow back. But I was always checking my right breast and always had the feeling that I could feel lumps, so I decided to have a risk reducing mastectomy with immediate expander implants in the other breast too.

I have had my expander implants changed to fixed volume ones, followed by a nipple reconstruction and a tattoo. It's been three years since everything started, it was very hard at times, but happily I have now finished all the surgery. I am very pleased with the results of my surgery and treatment. A big thank you to my surgical team, who have helped me get through this.

THE ROLE OF THE BREAST CARE NURSE IN BREAST RECONSTRUCTION

The breast care nurse is part of the multidisciplinary team and plays a pivotal role in ensuring that the reconstructive options are presented to the patient in a consistent way. Many women will need time to consider their options; look at photographs; and talk to partners, friends, or family before making a decision. Breast care nurses add a human element to the information given at consultations because we can spend more time with patients and listen to their concerns. We are able to make the information more meaningful for each patient, thereby helping to manage expectations of cosmetic outcome.

As a point of contact, breast care nurses provide confidence and support in the postoperative period when patients may feel more vulnerable, begin to experience doubts about their decisions, and lose confidence in the eventual outcome. Reconstructive surgery is a process, not a single procedure; recovery can be long and the outcome is not always as expected immediately. We can provide support outside of set clinic times, be on the end of a phone to discuss worries, and enable patients to manage their emotional and physical recovery. Being able to quickly manage concerns about complications such as infection or wound problems maintains the confidence and trust that a woman has in her surgical team and may ultimately affect her perception of the cosmetic outcome. Nikki Snuggs, Breast Care Nurse, Royal Marsden Hospital, London

What happens if the patient needs radiotherapy?

Radiotherapy after immediate reconstruction can have a detrimental effect on long term aesthetic outcomes owing to tissue fibrosis, oedema, and microvascular changes.[54 55 56 57 58 59 60 61] The effects are worse for implant based techniques, with capsular contracture, loss of shape and volume, pain, and higher revision rates.[58 62] Radiotherapy also affects autologous tissue flaps, resulting in flap contracture and loss of volume.[63 64] Randomised trials are currently assessing the impact of radiotherapy on implant and autologous techniques.

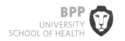

Before surgery it can be difficult to determine the need for post-mastectomy reconstruction and radiotherapy. Some units recommend against immediate reconstruction if radiotherapy is planned. Post-radiotherapy reconstruction is particularly challenging, owing to the poor quality of the irradiated tissue, and usually requires an autologous technique. If a patient who has opted for autologous reconstruction needs radiotherapy, a delayed procedure may therefore be recommended.

Does chemotherapy affect breast reconstruction?

Retrospective reviews have shown that chemotherapy given before (neo-adjuvant) or after (adjuvant) mastectomy does not significantly affect the long term outcome of breast reconstruction.[65] [66] A retrospective review (n=665) found that patients receiving neo-adjuvant chemotherapy were less likely to undergo immediate reconstruction and more likely to undergo delayed reconstruction than those receiving adjuvant chemotherapy.[67]

Evidence about whether immediate breast reconstruction delays adjuvant chemotherapy (systemic cancer directed treatment given after completion of definitive surgery and before recurrence) is conflicting; most of the studies were single institution ones, with small cohorts.[66] [68] [69] [70] [71] [72] One large (n=3643) multicentre cohort study found that immediate breast reconstruction was associated with a modest, but significant, delay in starting treatment, particularly in patients with a high body mass index (>35).[73] Both the Danish Breast Cancer Cooperative Group and the British Columbia Cancer Agency found no difference in overall survival between patients given chemotherapy early (less than three weeks) or later (up to 12 weeks postoperatively).[74] [75] However, delays of more than three months after surgery are associated with reduced disease-free survival and overall survival.

Informed consent and managing expectations in breast reconstruction

The weeks after a diagnosis of breast cancer are psychologically challenging. Women must be allowed to take part in the decision making process, particularly when considering the risk and benefits of the reconstructive options available. An option for no reconstruction must be included. Appropriate management of the patient's expectations for breast reconstruction should include what she will expect at the different postoperative stages, highlighting that reconstruction will not restore the original breast, and a reconstructed breast will not look or feel the same. Exploring the patient's expectations allows the surgeon to recognise those patients who have unrealistic expectations and deal with this problem preoperatively through individualised patient education. This may avoid the disappointment of having an outcome that is not what the woman had envisioned. A small single centre study found that patients who took an active part in the decisions about their treatment were more satisfied with the results of treatment, with more positive outcomes.[76]

Contributors: All authors contributed equally in the preparation of this article. PT is guarantor.

Funding: No special funding received.

Competing interests: We have read and understood the BMJ Group policy on declaration of interests and declare the following interests: None.

Provenance and peer review: Not commissioned; externally peer reviewed.

1   Jemal A, Bray F, Center MM, Ferlay J, Ward E, Forman D. Global cancer statistics. *CA Cancer J Clin*2011;61:69-90.

2   Maddams J, Brewster D, Gavin A, Steward J, Elliott J, Utley M, et al. Cancer prevalence in the United Kingdom: estimates for 2008. *Br J Cancer*2009;101:541-7.

3   Maddams J, Utley M, Moller H. Projections of cancer prevalence in the United Kingdom, 2010-2040. *Br J Cancer*2012;107:1195-202.

4   Jeevan R, Cromwell D, Browne J, van der Meulen J, Caddy CM, Pereira J, et al. Second annual report of the national mastectomy and breast reconstruction audit 2009. NHS Information Centre, 2009. www.rcseng. ac.uk/surgeons/research/surgical-research/docs/national-mastectomy-and-breast-reconstruction-audit-second-report-2009.

5   Lee C, Sunu C, Pignone M. Patient-reported outcomes of breast reconstruction after mastectomy: a systematic review. *J Am Coll Surg*2009;209:123-33.

6   National Institute for Health and Care Excellence. Early and locally advanced breast cancer diagnosis and treatment, 2009. www.nice.org. uk/nicemedia/pdf/cg80niceguideline.pdf.

7   Jeevan R, Browne J, van der Meulen J, Caddy CM, Pereira J, Sheppard C. First Annual Report of the National Mastectomy and Breast Reconstruction Audit 2008. NHS Information Centre, 2008. www.rcseng.ac.uk/surgeons/research/surgical-research/docs/national-mastectomy-and-breast-reconstruction-audit-first-report.

8   Bates T, Kearins O, Monypenny I, Lagord C, Lawrence G. Clinical outcome data for symptomatic breast cancer: the breast cancer clinical outcome measures (BCCOM) project. *Br J Cancer*2009;101:395-402.

9   Mahmood U, Hanlon AL, Koshy M, Buras R, Chumsri S, Tkaczuk KH, et al. Increasing national mastectomy rates for the treatment of early stage breast cancer. *Ann Surg Oncol*2013;20:1436-43.

10   Tuttle TM, Habermann EB, Grund EH, Morris TJ, Virnig BA. Increasing use of contralateral prophylactic mastectomy for breast cancer patients: a trend toward more aggressive surgical treatment. *J Clin Oncol*2007;25:5203-9.

11   Metcalfe KA, Lubinski J, Ghadirian P, Lynch H, Kim-Sing C, Friedman E, et al. Predictors of contralateral prophylactic mastectomy in women with a BRCA1 or BRCA2 mutation: the Hereditary Breast Cancer Clinical Study Group. *J Clin Oncol*2008;26:1093-7.

12   National Institute for Health and Care Excellence. Familial breast cancer. Classification and care of people at risk of familial breast cancer and management of breast cancer and related risks in people with a family history of breast cancer. 2013. www.nice.org.uk/nicemedia/live/14188/64202/64202.pdf.

13   Neuburger J, Macneill F, Jeevan R, van der Meulen JH, Cromwell DA. Trends in the use of bilateral mastectomy in England from 2002 to 2011: retrospective analysis of hospital episode statistics. *BMJ Open*2013;3:e003179.

14   Habermann EB, Abbott A, Parsons HM, Virnig BA, Al-Refaie WB, Tuttle TM. Are mastectomy rates really increasing in the United States? *J Clin Oncol*2010;28:3437-41.

15   Albornoz C, Cemal Y, Mehrara B, Disa J, Pusic AL, McCarthy C, et al. The impact of bilateral mastectomy on reconstructive rate and method in the United States: a population based analysis. *Plast Reconstr Surg*2012;130(SS-1):3441.

16   Lostumbo L, Carbine NE, Wallace J. Prophylactic mastectomy for the prevention of breast cancer. *Cochrane Database Syst Rev*2004;11:CD002748.

17   Carlson GW. Technical advances in skin sparing mastectomy. *Int J Surg Oncol*2011;2011:396901.

18   Romics L Jr, Chew BK, Weiler-Mithoff E, Doughty JC, Brown IM, Stallard S, et al. Ten-year follow-up of skin-sparing mastectomy followed by immediate breast reconstruction. *Br J Surg*2012;99:799-806.

19   Nahabedian MY, Tsangaris TN. Breast reconstruction following subcutaneous mastectomy for cancer: a critical appraisal of the nipple-areola complex. *Plast Reconstr Surg*2006;117:1083-90.

20   Didier F, Radice D, Gandini S, Bedolis R, Rotmensz N, Maldifassi A, et al. Does nipple preservation in mastectomy improve satisfaction with cosmetic results, psychological adjustment, body image and sexuality? *Breast Cancer Res Treat*2009;118:623-33.

21   Rusby JE, Smith BL, Gui GP. Nipple-sparing mastectomy. *Br J Surg*2010;97:305-16.

22   Loewen MJ, Jennings JA, Sherman SR, Slaikeu J, Ebrom PA, Davis AT, et al. Mammographic distance as a predictor of nipple-areola complex involvement in breast cancer. *Am J Surg*2008;195:391-4; discussion 94-5.

23   Lambert PA, Kolm P, Perry RR. Parameters that predict nipple involvement in breast cancer. *J Am Coll Surg*2000;191:354-9.

24   Gould DJ, Hunt KK, Liu J, Kuerer HM, Crosby MA, Babiera G, et al. Impact of surgical techniques, biomaterials, and patient variables on rate of nipple necrosis after nipple-sparing mastectomy. *Plast Reconstr Surg*2013;132:330e-8e.

25   Jensen JA, Lin JH, Kapoor N, Giuliano AE. Surgical delay of the nipple-areolar complex: a powerful technique to maximize nipple viability following nipple-sparing mastectomy. *Ann Surg Oncol*2012;19:3171-6.

26   National Mastectomy and Breast Reconstruction Audit Report 2011, 2011. www.rcseng.ac.uk/surgeons/research/surgical-research/docs/national-mastectomy-and-breast-reconstruction-audit-fourth-report-2011.

27   Alderman AK, Wilkins EG, Kim HM, Lowery JC. Complications in postmastectomy breast reconstruction: two-year results of the Michigan Breast Reconstruction Outcome Study. *Plast Reconstr Surg*2002;109:2265-74.

28   Sullivan SR, Fletcher DR, Isom CD, Isik FF. True incidence of all complications following immediate and delayed breast reconstruction. *Plast Reconstr Surg*2008;122:19-28.

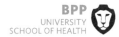

29 D'Souza N, Darmanin G, Fedorowicz Z. Immediate versus delayed reconstruction following surgery for breast cancer. *Cochrane Database Syst Rev* 2011;7:CD008674.

30 Albornoz CR, Bach PB, Pusic AL, McCarthy CM, Mehrara BJ, Disa JJ, et al. The influence of sociodemographic factors and hospital characteristics on the method of breast reconstruction, including microsurgery: a US population-based study. *Plast Reconstr Surg* 2012;129:1071-9.

31 Salzberg CA, Dunavant C, Nocera N. Immediate breast reconstruction using porcine acellular dermal matrix (Strattice): long-term outcomes and complications. *J Plast Reconstr Aesthet Surg* 2013;66:323-8.

32 Salzberg CA, Ashikari AY, Koch RM, Chabner-Thompson E. An 8-year experience of direct-to-implant immediate breast reconstruction using human acellular dermal matrix (AlloDerm). *Plast Reconstr Surg* 2011;127:514-24.

33 Schmitz M, Bertram M, Kneser U, Keller AK, Horch RE. Experimental total wrapping of breast implants with acellular dermal matrix: A preventive tool against capsular contracture in breast surgery? *J Plast Reconstr Aesthet Surg* 2013;33:675-80.

34 Sbitany H, Serletti JM. Acellular dermis-assisted prosthetic breast reconstruction: a systematic and critical review of efficacy and associated morbidity. *Plast Reconstr Surg* 2011;128:1162-9.

35 Health Do. Progress report after one year on the MHRA and DH response to the recommendations of the Howe review into Poly Implant Prothèse (PIP) breast implants. 2013. www.mhra.gov.uk/home/groups/comms-po/documents/news/con286825.pdf.

36 Yueh JH, Slavin SA, Adesiyun T, Nyame TT, Gautam S, Morris DJ, et al. Patient satisfaction in postmastectomy breast reconstruction: a comparative evaluation of DIEP, TRAM, latissimus flap, and implant techniques. *Plast Reconstr Surg* 2010;125:1585-95.

37 Fischer JP, Nelson JA, Cleveland E, Sieber B, Rohrbach JI, Serletti JM, et al. Breast reconstruction modality outcome study: a comparison of expander/implants and free flaps in select patients. *Plast Reconstr Surg* 2013;131:928-34.

38 Hu ES, Pusic AL, Waljee JF, Kuhn L, Hawley ST, Wilkins E, et al. Patient-reported aesthetic satisfaction with breast reconstruction during the long-term survivorship period. *Plast Reconstr Surg* 2009;124:1-8.

39 Spear SL, Newman MK, Bedford MS, Schwartz KA, Cohen M, Schwartz JS. A retrospective analysis of outcomes using three common methods for immediate breast reconstruction. *Plast Reconstr Surg* 2008;122:340-7.

40 Spear SL, Ducic I, Cuoco F, Taylor N. Effect of obesity on flap and donor-site complications in pedicled TRAM flap breast reconstruction. *Plast Reconstr Surg* 2007;119:788-95.

41 Clough KB, Louis-Sylvestre C, Fitoussi A, Couturaud B, Nos C. Donor site sequelae after autologous breast reconstruction with an extended latissimus dorsi flap. *Plast Reconstr Surg* 2002;109:1904-11.

42 Gagnon AR, Blondeel N. Superior gluteal artery perforator flap. *Semin Plast Surg* 2006;20:79-88.

43 Blondeel PN, Van Landuyt K, Hamdi M, Monstrey SJ. Soft tissue reconstruction with the superior gluteal artery perforator flap. *Clin Plast Surg* 2003;30:371-82.

44 LoTempio MM, Allen RJ. Breast reconstruction with SGAP and IGAP flaps. *Plast Reconstr Surg* 2010;126:393-401.

45 Gart MS, Smetona JT, Hanwright PJ, Fine NA, Bethke KP, Khan SA, et al. Autologous options for postmastectomy breast reconstruction: a comparison of outcomes based on the American College of Surgeons National Surgical Quality Improvement Program. *J Am Coll Surg* 2012;216:229-38.

46 Garvey PB, Buchel EW, Pockaj BA, Casey WJ, 3rd, Gray RJ, Hernandez JL, et al. DIEP and pedicled TRAM flaps: a comparison of outcomes. *Plast Reconstr Surg* 2006;117:1711-9; discussion 20-1.

47 Nahabedian MY, Momen B, Galdino G, Manson PN. Breast reconstruction with the free TRAM or DIEP flap: patient selection, choice of flap, and outcome. *Plast Reconstr Surg* 2002;110:466-75; discussion 76-7.

48 Chen CM, Halvorson EG, Disa JJ, McCarthy C, Hu QY, Pusic AL, et al. Immediate postoperative complications in DIEP versus free/muscle-sparing TRAM flaps. *Plast Reconstr Surg* 2007;120:1477-82.

49 Buck DW, 2nd, Shenaq D, Heyer K, Kato C, Kim JY. Patient-subjective cosmetic outcomes following the varying stages of tissue expander breast reconstruction: the importance of completion. *Breast* 2010;19:521-6.

50 Momoh AO, Colakoglu S, de Blacam C, Yueh JH, Lin SJ, Tobias AM, et al. The impact of nipple reconstruction on patient satisfaction in breast reconstruction. *Ann Plast Surg* 2012;69:389-93.

51 Goh SC, Martin NA, Pandya AN, Cutress RI. Patient satisfaction following nipple-areolar complex reconstruction and tattooing. *J Plast Reconstr Aesthet Surg* 2011;64:360-3.

52 Petit JY, Lohsiriwat V, Clough KB, Sarfati I, Ihrai T, Rietjens M, et al. The oncologic outcome and immediate surgical complications of lipofilling in breast cancer patients: a multicenter study—Milan-Paris-Lyon experience of 646 lipofilling procedures. *Plast Reconstr Surg* 2011;128:341-6.

53 Illouz YG, Sterodimas A. Autologous fat transplantation to the breast: a personal technique with 25 years of experience. *Aesthetic Plast Surg* 2009;33:706-15.

54 Prabhu R, Godette K, Carlson G, Losken A, Gabram S, Fasola C, et al. The impact of skin-sparing mastectomy with immediate reconstruction in patients with stage III breast cancer treated with neoadjuvant chemotherapy and postmastectomy radiation. *Int J Radiat Oncol Biol Phys* 2012;82:e587-93.

55 Tallet AV, Salem N, Moutardier V, Ananian P, Braud AC, Zalta R, et al. Radiotherapy and immediate two-stage breast reconstruction with a tissue expander and implant: complications and esthetic results. *Int J Radiat Oncol Biol Phys* 2003;57:136-42.

56 Cowen D, Gross E, Rouannet P, Teissier E, Ellis S, Resbeut M, et al. Immediate post-mastectomy breast reconstruction followed by radiotherapy: risk factors for complications. *Breast Cancer Res Treat* 2010;121:627-34.

57 Christensen BO, Overgaard J, Kettner LO, Damsgaard TE. Long-term evaluation of postmastectomy breast reconstruction. *Acta Oncol* 2011;50:1053-61.

58 Behranwala KA, Dua RS, Ross GM, Ward A, A'Hern R, Gui GP. The influence of radiotherapy on capsule formation and aesthetic outcome after immediate breast reconstruction using biodimensional anatomical expander implants. *J Plast Reconstr Aesthet Surg* 2006;59:1043-51.

59 Bentzen SM, Overgaard M, Thames HD, Christensen JJ, Overgaard J. Early and late normal-tissue injury after postmastectomy radiotherapy alone or combined with chemotherapy. *Int J Radiat Biol* 1989;56:711-5.

60 Borger JH, Kemperman H, Smitt HS, Hart A, van Dongen J, Lebesque J, et al. Dose and volume effects on fibrosis after breast conservation therapy. *Int J Radiat Oncol Biol Phys* 1994;30:1073-81.

61 Collette S, Collette L, Budiharto T, Horiot JC, Poortmans PM, Struikmans H, et al. Predictors of the risk of fibrosis at 10 years after breast conserving therapy for early breast cancer: a study based on the EORTC trial 22881-10882 "boost versus no boost." *Eur J Cancer* 2008;44:2587-99.

62 Kronowitz SJ, Robb GL. Radiation therapy and breast reconstruction: a critical review of the literature. *Plast Reconstr Surg* 2009;124:395-408.

63 Spear SL, Ducic I, Low M, Cuoco F. The effect of radiation on pedicled TRAM flap breast reconstruction: outcomes and implications. *Plast Reconstr Surg* 2005;115:84-95.

64 Thomson HJ, Potter S, Greenwood RJ, Bahl A, Barker J, Cawthorn SJ, et al. A prospective longitudinal study of cosmetic outcome in immediate latissimus dorsi breast reconstruction and the influence of radiotherapy. *Ann Surg Oncol* 2008;15:1081-91.

65 Monrigal E, Dauplat J, Gimbergues P, Le Bouedec G, Peyronie M, Achard JL, et al. Mastectomy with immediate breast reconstruction after neoadjuvant chemotherapy and radiation therapy. A new option for patients with operable invasive breast cancer. Results of a 20 years single institution study. *Eur J Surg Oncol* 2011;37:864-70.

66 Warren Peled A, Itakura K, Foster RD, Hamolsky D, Tanaka J, Ewing C, et al. Impact of chemotherapy on postoperative complications after mastectomy and immediate breast reconstruction. *Arch Surg* 2010;145:880-5.

67 Hu YY, Weeks CM, In H, Dodgion CM, Golshan M, Chun YS, et al. Impact of neoadjuvant chemotherapy on breast reconstruction. *Cancer* 2011;117:2833-41.

68 Wilson CR, Brown IM, Weiller-Mithoff E, George WD, Doughty JC. Immediate breast reconstruction does not lead to a delay in the delivery of adjuvant chemotherapy. *Eur J Surg Oncol* 2004;30:624-7.

69 Hamahata A, Kubo K, Takei H, Saitou T, Hayashi Y, Matsumoto H, et al. Impact of immediate breast reconstruction on postoperative adjuvant chemotherapy: a single center study. *Breast Cancer* 2013; published online 12 Jun.

70 Taylor CW, Kumar S. The effect of immediate breast reconstruction on adjuvant chemotherapy. *Breast* 2005;14:18-21.

71 Allweis TM, Boisvert ME, Otero SE, Perry DJ, Dubin NH, Priebat DA. Immediate reconstruction after mastectomy for breast cancer does not prolong the time to starting adjuvant chemotherapy. *Am J Surg* 2002;183:218-21.

72 Lee J, Lee SK, Kim S, Koo MY, Choi MY, Bae SY, et al. Does immediate breast reconstruction after mastectomy affect the initiation of adjuvant chemotherapy? *J Breast Cancer* 2011;14:322-7.

73 Alderman AK, Collins ED, Schott A, Hughes ME, Ottesen RA, Theriault RL, et al. The impact of breast reconstruction on the delivery of chemotherapy. *Cancer* 2010;116:1791-800.

74 Lohrisch C, Paltiel C, Gelmon K, Speers C, Taylor S, Barnett J, et al. Impact on survival of time from definitive surgery to initiation of adjuvant chemotherapy for early-stage breast cancer. *J Clin Oncol* 2006;24:4888-94.

75 Cold S, During M, Ewertz M, Knoop A, Moller S. Does timing of adjuvant chemotherapy influence the prognosis after early breast cancer? Results of the Danish Breast Cancer Cooperative Group (DBCG). *Br J Cancer* 2005;93:627-32.

76 Pusic AL, Klassen AF, Snell L, Cano SJ, McCarthy C, Scott A, et al. Measuring and managing patient expectations for breast reconstruction: impact on quality of life and patient satisfaction. *Expert Rev Pharmacoecon Outcomes Res* 2012;12:149-58.

Related links

bmj.com/archive
Previous articles in this series
• Identifying brain tumours in children and young adults (*BMJ* 2013;347:f5844)
• Gout (*BMJ* 2013;347:f5648)
• Testicular germ cell tumours (*BMJ* 2013;347:f5526)
• Managing cows' milk allergy in children (*BMJ* 2013;347:f5424)
• Personality disorder (*BMJ* 2013;347:f5276)

bmj.com
• Get Cleveland Clinic CME credits for this article

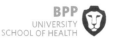

Dyspepsia

Alexander C Ford, senior lecturer and honorary consultant gastroenterologist[12],
Paul Moayyedi, chief of gastroenterology[3]

[1]Leeds Gastroenterology Institute, St James's University Hospital, Leeds, UK

[2]Leeds Institute of Biomedical and Clinical Sciences, Leeds University, Leeds, UK

[3]Gastroenterology Division, McMaster University, Health Sciences Center, Hamilton, ON, Canada

Correspondence to: AC Ford
alexf12399@yahoo.com

Cite this as: BMJ 2013;347:f5059

DOI: 10.1136/bmj.f5059

http://www.bmj.com/content/347/bmj.f5059

Definitions of the term dyspepsia vary but generally describe pain or discomfort in the epigastric region. People with dyspepsia have a normal life expectancy,[1] but symptoms impair quality of life,[2 3] and affect productivity.[4] Dyspepsia is estimated to cost the United Kingdom more than £1bn (€1.16bn; $1.55bn) annually,[5] so it is important to manage the condition appropriately. We summarise recent systematic reviews, meta-analyses, and randomised controlled trials to provide the general reader with an update on how to deal with this disorder effectively.

What is dyspepsia and who gets it?

Dyspepsia is a symptomatic diagnosis. A variety of definitions have been proposed, but a reasonable working definition for the primary care doctor is epigastric pain or discomfort for at least three months, in a patient who does not report predominant heartburn or regurgitation (although these symptoms can be part of the overall symptom complex). Gastro-oesophageal reflux disease (GORD) becomes the more likely diagnosis if symptoms of heartburn or regurgitation predominate, although this is one of the main areas of contention surrounding the definition of dyspepsia. The condition is common worldwide, with 20-40% of the world's population affected,[6] depending on the definition used. Epidemiological surveys show no consistent association with sex, age, socioeconomic status, smoking, or alcohol use.[3 7]

Dyspepsia is more common in people who take non-steroidal anti-inflammatory drugs (NSAIDs) and drugs such as calcium antagonists, bisphosphonates, nitrates, and theophyllines. It is also more common in people infected with Helicobacter pylori.[7] A population based study also found an association between anxiety and dyspepsia symptoms,[8] and certain genetic polymorphisms are more prevalent in those with the condition.[9] There is a strong overlap between irritable bowel syndrome, gastro-oesophageal reflux symptoms, and dyspepsia,[10 11] suggesting that common genetic or environmental factors are involved in the development of these disorders.

What causes dyspepsia?

Several diseases can cause symptoms of dyspepsia. A systematic review identified nine studies (5389 participants) that performed endoscopy in a general population sample with dyspepsia.[12] Overall, there was a 13% prevalence of erosive oesophagitis and 8% prevalence of peptic ulcer disease, with gastric or oesophageal cancer occurring in less than 0.3% of endoscopies. Oesophagitis was more prevalent in Western populations than in Asian ones (25% v 3%), whereas the opposite was true for peptic ulcer disease (3% v 11%). Overall, 70-80% of people with dyspepsia had no clinically significant findings at endoscopy. Such patients are classed as having functional dyspepsia. The Rome III criteria for functional dyspepsia divide it into two separate syndromes. In epigastric pain syndrome, patients report intermittent pain or burning localised to the epigastric region. Patients with postprandial distress syndrome have bothersome postprandial fullness after an ordinary sized meal or early satiation that prevents a meal being finished.[13]

The pathophysiology of dyspepsia depends on the underlying disease. Peptic ulcer disease is usually caused by H pylori infection, with a few cases being associated with NSAIDs. GORD is caused by a combination of failure of the gastro-oesophageal junction to prevent acid reflux and impaired clearance of acid from the oesophagus. Although technically distinct from dyspepsia, it may present with dyspeptic-type symptoms, rather than heartburn or regurgitation.[14] Acid reflux may be severe enough to damage the oesophageal mucosa, in which case erosive oesophagitis will be visible at endoscopy.

Around 70-80% of patients with epigastric pain will have functional dyspepsia, and the causes of this disorder are poorly understood. Gastroduodenal dysmotility, and sensitivity to both distension and acid,[15] have all been proposed as possible causes. As well as peripheral mechanisms, there are changes in brain activity,[16 17] suggesting that central processing is also abnormal. Functional dyspepsia has therefore been described as multifactorial, which is probably why any individual treatment is effective only in a small proportion of patients.

The causes of the central nervous system abnormalities, dysmotility, and hypersensitivity seen in functional dyspepsia are poorly understood. Several hypotheses have

---

SOURCES AND SELECTION CRITERIA

We searched Medline, Embase, the Cochrane Database of Systematic Reviews, and Clinical Evidence online using the search term "dyspepsia", as well as recent conference proceedings. We limited studies to those conducted in adults and focused on systematic reviews, meta-analyses, and high quality randomised controlled trials published during the past five years whenever possible.

SUMMARY POINTS

- Dyspepsia is common—about a fifth of people are affected at some point in their lives
- The condition is chronic, with a relapsing and remitting nature
- There is no evidence that dyspepsia adversely affects survival
- In most patients, no cause for dyspepsia is detected at endoscopy
- Gastro-oesophageal cancer is extremely rare in patients with dyspepsia who have no alarm symptoms
- Most treatments are safe and well tolerated, but there is little evidence that they have any long term effect on the natural course of the disorder

---

UPPER GASTROINTESTINAL ALARM SYMPTOMS (TAKEN FROM NATIONAL INSTITUTE FOR HEALTH AND CARE (FORMERLY CLINICAL) EXCELLENCE REFERRAL GUIDELINES FOR SUSPECTED CANCER[23])

- Age ≥55 years with new onset dyspepsia
- Chronic gastrointestinal bleeding
- Dysphagia
- Progressive unintentional weight loss
- Persistent vomiting
- Iron deficiency anaemia
- Epigastric mass
- Suspicious barium meal result

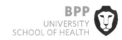

been proposed, including a subtle increase in inflammatory mediators in the upper gastrointestinal tract.[18] An observation that has garnered the most attention recently is the presence of eosinophils in the duodenum.[19] This has led to the hypothesis that the resulting increase in immune activation and inflammation may cause neuromodulation that gives rise to dysmotility, hypersensitivity, and central nervous system changes. The cause of this immune activation is uncertain, but it is most likely to be an infective process. The obvious candidate would be *H pylori* infection, but other infections can give rise to immune activation of the upper gastrointestinal tract. In support of this, it has been observed that dyspepsia is more common after an episode of acute gastroenteritis.[20]

How can the cause of dyspepsia be established?

Symptoms do not reliably distinguish between organic and functional disease,[21] and even alarm features (box), such as weight loss, are not particularly helpful.[22] Despite this, in the UK the presence of any of these alarm features is an indication for urgent specialist referral for endoscopy, to exclude upper gastrointestinal cancer.[23] Otherwise, endoscopy is not mandated in the management of dyspepsia, although it is the only way to accurately establish the underlying cause, including functional dyspepsia, which is a diagnosis of exclusion made in the absence of organic findings. However, no country can afford to perform endoscopy in all patients, and most guidelines recommend managing people under the age of 55 years with dyspepsia but no alarm features by testing for *H pylori* non-invasively with the urea breath test or stool antigen. Patients with positive results should be treated with eradication therapy and those with negative results given acid suppression therapy.[24] Gastric scintigraphy may help confirm delayed gastric emptying, particularly in patients with postprandial distress-type symptoms, to direct treatment, although the correlation between gastric emptying rates and symptoms is poor.[25]

What are the treatment options?

Uninvestigated dyspepsia in primary care or the community

An individual patient data meta-analysis of randomised controlled trials found that—although prompt endoscopy was superior to testing patients with uninvestigated dyspepsia for *H pylori*, and treating with eradication therapy if positive, in terms of symptom control at 12 months—it was not cost effective.[26] However, it is unclear whether a test and treat approach is preferable to empirical acid suppression first line, because a second individual patient data meta-analysis found no significant difference in symptoms or costs between the two.[27] Current guidelines state that either option can be used.[28] If the prevalence of *H pylori* in the population is known, it makes sense to use an acid suppression strategy first if prevalence is low (<10%) and an *H pylori* test and treat strategy if the prevalence is higher.[24] If these strategies are unsuccessful, other options (discussed below) can be considered, or the patient can be referred to secondary care for advice and further investigation if appropriate.

A six month primary care based Dutch trial compared two management strategies for uninvestigated dyspepsia based around empirical acid suppression.[29] One strategy used a step-up approach, starting with antacids, with treatment escalated to H2 antihistamines and then proton pump inhibitors (PPIs) if symptoms remained uncontrolled. The second used a step-down approach, with the drugs given in the reverse order and de-escalated if symptoms improved. Treatment success (adequate relief of symptoms) was similar at six months (72% with step-up v 70% with step-

down), but costs were significantly lower with the step-up approach. This, together with the small treatment effect in favour of step-up, meant that it came out top in a cost effectiveness analysis.

Another group of primary care patients who may benefit from *H pylori* test and treat are those who do not consult with dyspepsia very often but who require PPIs long term. A trial screened long term PPI users for *H pylori* and randomised those who were positive to eradication therapy or placebo.[30] Eradication therapy significantly reduced symptom scores, PPI prescriptions, consultations for dyspepsia, and dyspepsia related costs. The costs of detection and treatment were less than the money saved after two years of follow-up. Sensitivity analysis showed that the prevalence of *H pylori* would need to be less than 12% before this was no longer cost saving.

It has been estimated that 5% of dyspepsia in the community is attributable to *H pylori*,[7] so population screening and treatment for this organism could theoretically reduce dyspepsia related costs. Results from follow-up studies of people recruited to two large randomised controlled trials of population based screening (and eradication therapy or placebo if *H pylori* positive) in the UK suggest this might be the case, with significantly lower costs and fewer consultations after seven to 10 years.[31 32] However, these studies did not follow up all recruited people successfully, so currently there is insufficient evidence to institute population screening and treatment in the UK.

Peptic ulcer disease

The causal role of *H pylori* in peptic ulcer disease is well established, and patients with *H pylori* positive disease should receive eradication therapy. A Cochrane review found that the number needed to treat (NNT) with eradication therapy to prevent one duodenal ulcer relapse (26 placebo controlled trials) was 2 and for gastric ulcer (nine trials) the number was 3.[33] Although there was significant heterogeneity between studies in both analyses, all but one trial showed a significant benefit with eradication therapy. PPI triple therapy (a PPI plus two antibiotics (clarithromycin with amoxicillin or metronidazole)) should be used in areas like the UK where clarithromycin resistance is less than 10%, with bismuth quadruple therapy (bismuth plus a PPI and two antibiotics) being given where resistance is higher.[34] Most cases of *H pylori* negative peptic ulcer disease are caused by NSAIDs, and trials show that PPIs are superior to H2 antihistamines for ulcer healing in this situation.[35 36] *H pylori* negative, NSAID negative peptic ulcer disease is rare and probably requires long term PPI treatment.

Functional dyspepsia

Diet and lifestyle

Food diaries from a small study of 29 patients suggest that people with functional dyspepsia eat fewer meals and consume less energy and fat than healthy controls,[37] but whether this is a cause or a consequence of symptoms is unclear. Although the prevalence of undiagnosed coeliac disease is higher in people with symptoms of irritable bowel syndrome,[38] this is not the case in dyspepsia.[39] It is also unclear whether non-coeliac gluten sensitivity is involved in symptom generation in some patients with functional dyspepsia. Doctors often advise people with dyspepsia to lose weight, avoid fatty food and alcohol, or stop smoking, but there is little evidence that these measures improve symptoms.[40] As a result, drugs are the mainstay of treatment.

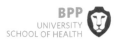

Acid suppression therapy
Antacids neutralise gastric acid, the production of which is controlled by gastrin, histamine, and acetylcholine receptors. Once stimulated, these receptors activate proton pumps in the parietal cell. H2 antihistamines and PPIs reduce acid production by blocking H2 receptors or the proton pump, respectively. Because PPIs act on the proton pump itself, these drugs lead to more profound acid suppression than H2 antihistamines or antacids.

A Cochrane review has studied the efficacy of acid suppressants in functional dyspepsia.[41] One placebo controlled trial of antacids showed no benefit. Twelve randomised controlled trials of H2 antihistamines versus placebo found that these drugs were effective for the treatment of functional dyspepsia (NNT=7). However, there was significant heterogeneity between studies, which was not explained by sensitivity analysis, and evidence of funnel plot asymmetry, suggesting publication bias or other small study effects. Their efficacy may therefore have been overestimated. Ten trials studied PPIs. Again, there was a significant benefit over placebo, although this was modest (NNT=10). There was significant heterogeneity between studies, with no obvious explanation, but no funnel plot asymmetry. A subgroup analysis conducted according to predominant symptom showed that PPIs were most beneficial in patients with reflux-type symptoms and more effective than placebo in patients with epigastric pain. However, they were no more effective than placebo in those with dysmotility-like functional dyspepsia.[42]

Most trials used PPIs for four to eight weeks. This seems a reasonable duration, especially as concerns have been raised recently about the safety of long term PPI use. Observational studies suggest that hip fracture, community acquired pneumonia, and *Clostridium difficile* infection are more common in PPI users,[43][44] although all these associations were extremely modest, and direct causation cannot be assumed from studies such as these.

H pylori eradication therapy
The benefit of eradication therapy is less pronounced in functional dyspepsia than in peptic ulcer disease, but treatment is still more effective than placebo. In a Cochrane review of 21 placebo controlled trials the NNT for improvement in symptoms after eradicating *H pylori* was 14, with no heterogeneity between studies and no evidence of funnel plot asymmetry.[45]

Prokinetic drugs
Prokinetics enhance gastrointestinal motility. Examples include 5-hydroxytryptamine-4 (5-HT4) receptor agonists, such as cispride and mosapride, and the dopamine antagonists metoclopramide and domperidone. A Cochrane review identified 24 placebo controlled trials of prokinetics in functional dyspepsia.[41] Most used cisapride, which has been withdrawn owing to concerns over cardiac safety, with only one trial studying mosapride or domperidone, and no randomised controlled trials of metoclopramide. Overall, these drugs seemed to be highly effective (NNT=6). However, there was significant heterogeneity between studies, which was not explained by sensitivity analysis, and funnel plot asymmetry, which suggests that their apparent efficacy may be due to publication bias. In addition, when only high quality trials were included in the analysis the benefit was no longer apparent.[46]

Antidepressants and psychological therapies
Patients with functional dyspepsia, as with most other functional gastrointestinal disorders, have higher rates of anxiety, depression, and other psychological conditions than healthy people.[47] Antidepressants seem to be of benefit in irritable bowel syndrome,[48] and three trials have recently been conducted in functional dyspepsia. In a Chinese study, a low dose of the tricyclic antidepressant imipramine was significantly more effective than placebo (response rate 64% v 44%).[49] In another Chinese trial the selective serotonin reuptake inhibitor sertraline was not superior to placebo (28% experienced complete symptom resolution in both treatment arms).[50] Finally, in a placebo controlled trial of the tricyclic antidepressant amitriptyline or the selective serotonin reuptake inhibitor escitalopram, only amitriptyline showed a significant benefit over placebo.[51] Withdrawal owing to adverse events was more common with antidepressants in all three trials. These findings suggest that, if an antidepressant is used, a tricyclic is preferable.

A Cochrane review of the efficacy of psychological interventions in functional dyspepsia identified four trials.[52] Formal meta-analysis was not possible because of incomplete data reporting. The authors concluded that insufficient evidence existed for any benefit. Little has been published since this systematic review. A small randomised controlled trial of patients in whom conventional treatments had failed compared cognitive behavioural therapy (CBT) as an adjunct to intensive medical treatment (including testing for and targeting motor and sensory abnormalities) with intensive medical treatment alone or standard medical treatment.[53] A response was significantly more likely with intensive medical therapy combined with CBT compared with standard treatment (54% v 17%), but response rates were similar with intensive medical treatment alone (46%), suggesting that CBT may have no additive benefit. Despite the lack of evidence for any benefit, it seems reasonable to consider psychological treatments in patients with troublesome symptoms who have coexistent anxiety or depression.

Alternative therapies
In a randomised controlled trial that compared acupuncture with a sham procedure in functional dyspepsia, response rates were significantly higher with true acupuncture (71% v 35%).[54] A smaller sham controlled trial,[55] which included neurological imaging studies, found that acupuncture led to deactivation of the anterior cingulate cortex, insula, thalamus, and hypothalamus, which are all involved in processing painful visceral stimuli, perhaps explaining its therapeutic mechanism.

The herbal preparation iberogast, also known as STW5, which is a combination of plant extracts, has been tested in several trials of functional dyspepsia. Iberogast significantly improved symptom scores compared with placebo in one trial,[56] and in another 43% of patients randomised to iberogast reported resolution of symptoms at eight weeks compared with only 3% with placebo.[57] A single placebo controlled trial also found that peppermint oil, combined with caraway oil, was beneficial in functional dyspepsia.[58] At the time of writing, no randomised controlled trials have investigated probiotics in dyspepsia.

Contributors: Both authors conceived and designed the article, drafted the manuscript, and approved the final version. ACF is guarantor.

Competing interests: We have read and understood the BMJ Group policy on declaration of interests and declare the following interests: ACF has received speaker's fees from Shire Pharmaceuticals; PM has

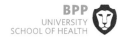

TIPS FOR NON-SPECIALISTS

- Treat peptic ulcer disease with eradication therapy if *Helicobacter pylori* is present or proton pump inhibitors if non-steroidal anti-inflammatory drugs are implicated

- Eradication therapy may be beneficial in *H pylori* positive functional dyspepsia, although the effect is modest

- Proton pump inhibitors, H2 antihistamines, and prokinetics may be beneficial in *H pylori* negative functional dyspepsia or in patients who do not benefit from eradication therapy

- Proton pump inhibitors are beneficial in patients with functional dyspepsia who mainly have reflux symptoms or epigastric pain, but not in those with dysmotility-like symptoms

- Increasing evidence suggests that tricyclic antidepressants, but not selective serotonin reuptake inhibitors, are beneficial in functional dyspepsia

- There is no evidence that psychological treatments are of benefit in functional dyspepsia

- Alternative therapies should be reserved for patients with functional dyspepsia whose symptoms are not relieved by conventional treatments

ADDITIONAL EDUCATIONAL RESOURCES BOX

Resources for healthcare professionals

- Leontiadis GI, Moayyedi P, Ford AC. Helicobacter pylori infection. *Clin Evid (Online)* 2009;pii:0406. An up-to-date summary of the evidence for the eradication of *Helicobacter pylori* in various situations

- National Institute for Clinical Excellence. Dyspepsia. Managing dyspepsia in adults in primary care. www.nice.org.uk/nicemedia/live/10950/29460/29460.pdf . NICE clinical guideline

Resources for patients

- Patient.co.uk (www.patient.co.uk/health/dyspepsia-indigestion)—Patient information on dyspepsia (indigestion)

- NHS Choices (www.nhs.uk/Conditions/Indigestion/Pages/Introduction.aspx)—Information from the NHS on indigestion

QUESTIONS FOR FUTURE RESEARCH

- Are psychological treatments of benefit in functional dyspepsia?

- Does dietary manipulation have a role to play in the management of functional dyspepsia?

- Is non-coeliac gluten sensitivity implicated in symptom generation in a proportion of patients with presumed functional dyspepsia?

received speakers fees from Shire Pharmaceuticals, Forest Canada, and AstraZeneca; his chair is funded in part by an unrestricted donation from AstraZeneca to McMaster University.

Provenance and peer review: Commissioned; externally peer reviewed.

1 Ford AC, Forman D, Bailey AG, Axon ATR, Moayyedi P. Effect of dyspepsia on survival: a longitudinal 10-year follow-up study. *Am J Gastroenterol*2012;107:912-21.

2 Ford AC, Forman D, Bailey AG, Axon ATR, Moayyedi P. Initial poor quality of life and new onset of dyspepsia: Results from a longitudinal 10-year follow-up study. *Gut*2007;56:321-7.

3 Mahadeva S, Yadav H, Rampal S, Everett SM, Goh K-L. Ethnic variation, epidemiological factors and quality of life impairment associated with dyspepsia in urban Malaysia. *Aliment Pharmacol Ther*2010;31:1141-51.

4 Brook RA, Kleinman NL, Choung RS, Melkonian AK, Smeeding JE, Talley NJ. Functional dyspepsia impacts absenteeism and direct and indirect costs. *Clin Gastroenterol Hepatol*2010;8:498-503.

5 Moayyedi P, Mason J. Clinical and economic consequences of dyspepsia in the community. *Gut*2002;50(suppl 4):10-2.

6 Marwaha A, Ford AC, Lim A, Moayyedi P. Worldwide prevalence of dyspepsia: Systematic review and meta-analysis. *Gastroenterology*2009;136(suppl 1):A182.

7 Moayyedi P, Forman D, Braunholtz D, Feltbower R, Crocombe W, Liptrott M, et al. The proportion of upper gastrointestinal symptoms in the community associated with Helicobacter pylori, lifestyle factors, and nonsteroidal anti-inflammatory drugs. *Am J Gastroenterol*2000;95:1448-55.

8 Aro P, Talley NJ, Ronkainen J, Storskrubb T, Vieth M, Johansson SE, et al. Anxiety is associated with uninvestigated and functional dyspepsia (Rome III criteria) in a Swedish population-based study. *Gastroenterology*2009;137:94-100.

9 Mujakovic S, ter Linde JJ, de Wit NJ, van Marrewijk CJ, Fransen GA, Onland-Moret NC, et al. Serotonin receptor 3A polymorphism c.-42C > T is associated with severe dyspepsia. *BMC Med Genet*2011;12:140.

10 Ford AC, Marwaha A, Lim A, Moayyedi P. Systematic review and meta-analysis of the prevalence of irritable bowel syndrome in individuals with dyspepsia. *Clin Gastroenterol Hepatol*2010;8:401-9.

11 Choung RS, Locke III GR, Schleck CD, Zinsmeister AR, Talley NJ. Overlap of dyspepsia and gastroesophageal reflux in the general population: one disease or distinct entities? *Neurogastroenterol Motil*2012;24:229-34.

12 Ford AC, Marwaha A, Lim A, Moayyedi P. What is the prevalence of clinically significant endoscopic findings in subjects with dyspepsia? Systematic review and meta-analysis. *Clin Gastroenterol Hepatol*2010;8:830-7.

13 Tack J, Talley NJ, Camilleri M, Holtmann G, Hu P, Malagelada JR, et al. Functional gastroduodenal disorders. *Gastroenterology*2006;130:1466-79.

14 Moayyedi P, Talley NJ. Gastro-oesophageal reflux disease. *Lancet*2006;367:2086-100.

15 Moayyedi P. Dyspepsia. *Curr Opin Gastroenterol*2012;28:602-7.

16 Zhou G, Qin W, Zeng F, Liu P, Yang X, von Deneem KM, et al. White-matter microstructural changes in functional dyspepsia: a diffusion tensor imaging study. *Am J Gastroenterol*2013;108:260-9.

17 Zeng F, Qin W, Liang F, Liu J, Tang Y, Liu X, et al. Abnormal resting brain activity in patients with functional dyspepsia is related to symptom severity. *Gastroenterology* 2011;141:499-506.

18 Liebregts T, Adam B, Bredack C, Gururatsakul M, Pilkington KR, Brierley SM, et al. Small bowel homing T cells are associated with symptoms and delayed gastric emptying in functional dyspepsia. *Am J Gastroenterol*2011;106:1089-98.

19 Talley NJ, Walker MM, Aro P, Ronkainen J, Storskrubb T, Hindley LA, et al. Non-ulcer dyspepsia and duodenal eosinophilia: an adult endoscopic population-based case-control study. *Clin Gastroenterol Hepatol*2007;5:1175-83.

20 Ford AC, Thabane M, Collins SM, Moayyedi P, Garg AX, Clark WF, et al. Prevalence of uninvestigated dyspepsia 8 years after a large waterborne outbreak of bacterial dysentery: a cohort study. *Gastroenterology*2010;138:1727-36.

21 Moayyedi P, Talley NJ, Fennerty MB, Vakil N. Can the clinical history distinguish between organic and functional dyspepsia? *JAMA*2006;295:1566-76.

22 Vakil N, Moayyedi P, Fennerty MB, Talley NJ. Limited value of alarm features in the diagnosis of upper gastrointestinal malignancy: systematic review and meta-analysis. *Gastroenterology*2006;131:390-401.

23 National Institute for Health and Clinical Excellence. Referral guidelines for suspected cancer. 2005. www.nice.org.uk/nicemedia/live/10968/29814/29814.pdf.

24 American Gastroenterological Association. American Gastroenterological Association technical review on the evaluation of dyspepsia. *Gastroenterology* 2005;129:1756-80.

25 Talley NJ, Locke GR III, Lahr BD, Zinsmeister AR, Tougas G, Ligozio G,, et al. Functional dyspepsia, delayed gastric emptying, and impaired quality of life. *Gut*2006;55:933-9.

26 Ford AC, Qume M, Moayyedi P, Arents NLA, Lassen AT, Logan RFA, et al. Helicobacter pylori "test and treat" or endoscopy for managing dyspepsia? An individual patient data meta-analysis. *Gastroenterology*2005;128:1838-44.

27 Ford AC, Moayyedi P, Jarbol DE, Logan RFA, Delaney BC. Meta-analysis: Helicobacter pylori "test and treat" compared with empirical acid suppression for managing dyspepsia. *Aliment Pharmacol Ther*2008;28:534-44.

28 National Institute for Clinical Excellence. Dyspepsia. Managing dyspepsia in adults in primary care. 2004. www.nice.org.uk/nicemedia/pdf/CG017fullguideline.pdf.

29 Van Marrewijk CJ, Mujakovic S, Fransen GAJ, Numans ME, de Wit NJ, Muris JWM, et al. Effect and cost-effectiveness of step-up versus step-down treatment with antacids, H2-receptor antagonists, and proton pump inhibitors in patients with new onset dyspepsia (DIAMOND study): a primary-care-based randomised controlled trial. *Lancet*2009;373:215-25.

30 Raghunath AS, Hungin AP, Mason J, Jackson W. Helicobacter pylori eradication in long-term proton pump inhibitor users in primary care: A randomized controlled trial. *Aliment Pharmacol Ther*2007;25:585-92.

31 Ford AC, Forman D, Bailey AG, Axon ATR, Moayyedi P. A community screening program for Helicobacter pylori saves money: ten-year follow-up of a randomised controlled trial. *Gastroenterology*2005;129:1910-7.

32 Harvey RF, Lane JA, Nair P, Egger M, Harvey I, Donovan J, et al. Clinical trial: prolonged beneficial effect of Helicobacter pylori eradication on dyspepsia consultations—the Bristol helicobacter project. *Aliment Pharmacol Ther*2010;32:394-400.

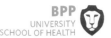

33 Ford AC, Delaney BC, Forman D, Moayyedi P. Eradication therapy in Helicobacter pylori positive peptic ulcer disease: systematic review and economic analysis. *Am J Gastroenterol*2004;99:1833-55.

34 Malfertheiner P, Megraud F, O'Morain CA, Atherton J, Axon AT, Bazzoli F, et al; European Helicobacter Study Group. Management of Helicobacter pylori infection: the Maastricht IV Florence consensus report. *Gut*2012;61:646-64.

35 Yeomans ND, Tulassay Z, Juhasz L, Racz I, van Rensburg CJ, Swannell AJ, et al. A comparison of omeprazole with ranitidine for ulcers associated with nonsteroidal antiinflammatory drugs. Acid Suppression Trial: Ranitidine versus Omeprazole for NSAID-associated Ulcer Treatment (ASTRONAUT) study group. *N Engl J Med*1998;338:719-26.

36 Agrawal NM, Campbell DR, Safdi MA, Lukasik NL, Huang B, Haber MM. Superiority of lansoprazole vs ranitidine in healing nonsteroidal anti-inflammatory drug-associated gastric ulcers: results of a double-blind, randomized, multicenter study. NSAID-Associated Gastric Ulcer Study Group. *Ann Intern Med*2000;160:1455-61.

37 Pilichiewicz AN, Horowitz M, Holtmann G, Talley NJ, Feinle-Bisset C. Relationship between symptoms and dietary patterns in patients with functional dyspepsia. *Clin Gastroenterol Hepatol* 2009;7:317-22.

38 Ford AC, Chey WD, Talley NJ, Malhotra A, Spiegel BMR, Moayyedi P. Yield of diagnostic tests for celiac disease in subjects with symptoms suggestive of irritable bowel syndrome: Systematic review and meta-analysis. *Arch Intern Med*2009;169:651-8.

39 Ford AC, Ching E, Moayyedi P. Meta-analysis: yield of diagnostic tests for coeliac disease in dyspepsia. *Aliment Pharmacol Ther*2009;30:28-36.

40 Feinle-Bisset C, Azpiroz F. Dietary and lifestyle factors in functional dyspepsia. *Nat Rev Gastroenterol Hepatol*2013;10:150-7.

41 Moayyedi P, Soo S, Deeks J, Delaney B, Innes M, Forman D. Pharmacological interventions for non-ulcer dyspepsia. *Cochrane Database Syst Rev*2006;4:CD001960.

42 Moayyedi P, Delaney BC, Vakil N, Forman D, Talley NJ. The efficacy of proton pump inhibitors in non-ulcer dyspepsia: a systematic review and economic analysis. *Gastroenterology*2004;127:1329-37.

43 Moayyedi P, Leontiadis GI. The risks of PPI therapy. *Nat Rev Gastroenterol Hepatol*2012;9:132-9.

44 Ngamruengphong S, Leontiadis GI, Radhi S, Dentino A, Nugent K. Proton pump inhibitors and risk of fracture: a systematic review and meta-analysis of observational studies. *Am J Gastroenterol* 2011;106:1209-18.

45 Moayyedi P, Soo S, Deeks J, Delaney B, Harris A, Innes M, et al. Eradication of Helicobacter pylori for non-ulcer dyspepsia. *Cochrane Database Syst Rev*2006;2:CD002096.

46 Abraham NS, Moayyedi P, Daniels B, Veldhuyzen Van Zanten SJO. The methodological quality of trials affects estimates of treatment efficacy in functional (non-ulcer) dyspepsia. *Aliment Pharmacol Ther*2004;19:631-41.

47 Koloski NA, Jones M, Kalantar J, Weltman M, Zaguirre J, Talley NJ. The brain-gut pathway in functional gastrointestinal disorders is bidirectional: a 12-year prospective population-based study. *Gut*2012;61:1284-90.

48 Ford AC, Talley NJ, Schoenfeld PS, Quigley EMM, Moayyedi P. Efficacy of antidepressants and psychological therapies in irritable bowel syndrome: systematic review and meta-analysis. *Gut* 2009;58:367-378.

49 Wu JC, Cheong PK, Chan Y, Lai LH, Ching J, Chan A, et al. A randomized, double-blind, placebo-controlled trial of low dose imipramine for treatment of refractory functional dyspepsia. *Gastroenterology*2011;140(suppl 1):S50.

50 Tan VP, Cheung TK, Wong WM, Pang R, Wong BC. Treatment of functional dyspepsia with sertraline: a double-blind randomized placebo-controlled pilot study. *World J Gastroenterol*2012;18:6127-33.

51 Locke GR, Bouras EP, Howden CW, Brenner DM, Lacy BE, Dibaise JK, et al. The functional dyspepsia treatment trial (FDTT) key results. *Gastroenterology*2013;144(suppl 1):S140.

52 Soo S, Moayyedi P, Deeks JJ, Delaney B, Lewis M, Forman D. Psychological interventions for non-ulcer dyspepsia. *Cochrane Database Syst Rev*2005;2:CD002301.

53 Haag S, Senf W, Tagay S, Langkafel M, Braun-Lang U, Pietsch A, et al. Is there a benefit from intensified medical and psychological interventions in patients with functional dyspepsia not responding to conventional therapy? *Aliment Pharmacol Ther*2007;25:973-86.

54 Ma TT, Yu SY, Li Y, Liang FR, Tian XP, Zheng H, et al. Randomised clinical trial: an assessment of acupuncture on specific meridian or specific acupoint vs sham acupuncture for treating functional dyspepsia. *Aliment Pharmacol Ther*2012;35:552-61.

55 Zeng F, Qin W, Ma T, Sun J, Tang Y, Yuan K, et al. Influence of acupuncture treatment on cerebral activity in functional dyspepsia patients and its relationship with efficacy. *Am J Gastroenterol*2012;107:1236-47.

56 Von Arnim U, Peitz U, Vinson B, Gundermann KJ, Malfertheiner P. STW 5, a phytopharmacon for patients with functional dyspepsia: results of a multicenter, placebo-controlled double-blind study. *Am J Gastroenterol*2007;102:1268-75.

57 Madisch A, Holtmann G, Mayr G, Vinson B, Hotz J. Treatment of functional dyspepsia with a herbal preparation. A double-blind, randomized, placebo-controlled, multicenter trial. *Digestion*2004;69:45-52.

58 May B, Kohler S, Schneider B. Efficacy and tolerability of a fixed combination of peppermint oil and caraway oil in patients suffering from functional dyspepsia. *Aliment Pharmacol Ther*2000;14:1671-7.

Related links

bmj.com
- Get CME credits with this article

bmj.com/archive
Previous articles in this series
- Tourette's syndrome (2013;347:f4964)
- Developing role of HPV in cervical cancer prevention (2013;347:f4781)
- Frontotemporal dementia (2013;347:f4827)
- Strongyloides stercoralis infection (2013;347:f4610)
- An introduction to patient decision aids (2013;347:f4147)

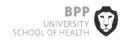

The diagnosis and management of hiatus hernia

Sabine Roman, associate professor[1], Peter J Kahrilas, professor[2]

[1]Digestive Physiology, Hospices Civils de Lyon, Lyon I University, and Labtau, INSERM 1032, Lyon, France

[2]Department of Medicine, Division of Gastroenterology, Northwestern University, Chicago, IL 60611-2951, USA

Correspondence to: P J Kahrilas
p-kahrilas@northwestern.edu

Cite this as: BMJ 2014;349:g6154

DOI: 10.1136/bmj.g6154

http://www.bmj.com/content/349/bmj.g6154

Hiatus hernia is a condition involving herniation of the contents of the abdominal cavity, most commonly the stomach, through the diaphragm into the mediastinum. In the United States, hiatus hernia was listed as a primary or secondary cause of hospital admissions in 142 of 10000 inpatients between 2003 and 2006.[1] However, the exact prevalence of hiatus hernia is difficult to determine because of the inherent subjectivity in diagnostic criteria. Consequently, estimates vary widely—for example, from 10% to 80% of the adult population in North America.[2] It is, however, accepted that the prevalence of hiatus hernia parallels that of obesity and that it increases with age. The typical symptom of hiatus hernia is gastroesophageal reflux (heartburn, regurgitation). Less common symptoms are dysphagia, epigastric or chest pain, and chronic iron deficiency anaemia. This clinical review summarises the current evidence for the diagnosis and management of hiatus hernia.

What is hiatus hernia and how is it classified?

The esophagus enters the abdomen through the diaphragmatic hiatus, anchored at the level of the esophagogastric junction by the phrenoesophageal membrane, which also fills the potential space within the hiatus. The hiatus is vulnerable to visceral herniation because it is directly subject to pressure stress between the abdomen and the chest. The diaphragmatic margin of the hiatus is formed by the right diaphragmatic crus. The right crus and lower esophageal sphincter together form the esophagogastric junction, which acts as a barrier against the reflux of gastric content into the esophagus.

Hiatus hernias are subdivided into sliding hernias (85-95%) and paraesophageal hernias (5-15% overall). In cases of sliding hiatus hernia, the diaphragmatic hiatus dilates allowing the cardia of the stomach to herniate upward (fig 1). Paraesophageal hernias are less common (5-15% of all hiatus hernias, fig 1). The defining characteristic of a paraesophageal hernia is asymmetry, such that the herniated viscera, be that stomach, colon, spleen, pancreas, or small intestine, herniates adjacent to the native course of the esophagus. Most paraesophageal hernias also have a sliding component, making them "mixed."

SOURCES AND SELECTION CRITERIA

We based this review on articles identified through a search of PubMed using the term "hiatal hernia" on 12 August 2014. Largely because of the extensive literature on reflux disease and the overlap between reflux disease and hiatus hernia, the search returned over 4500 citations, even when limited to publications in the English language. We favoured what we judged to be topics of interest in primary care.

What are the risk factors?

Age and obesity are the major risk factors for the development of hiatus hernia.[3][4][5] People who are overweight or obese compared with people of normal body mass index experience a progressive increase in intra-abdominal pressure, which promotes herniation.[6] In a recent meta-analysis, the odds ratio for hiatus hernia in people with a body mass index greater than 25 was 1.93 (95% confidence interval 1.10 to 3.39), with risk increasing in parallel with body mass index.[7] In a case-control study of patients who underwent upper gastrointestinal endoscopy, the controls had a body mass index of less than 20; the relative risk of hiatus hernia in participants of a healthy weight (body mass index 20-25) was 1.9 (95% confidence interval 1.1 to 3.2), in those who were overweight (25-30) was 2.5 (1.5 to 4.3), and in those who were obese (30-35) was 4.2 (2.4 to 7.6). Recently, researchers found that even a tightened belt around the abdomen of healthy participants induced herniation of the esophagogastric junction within the diaphragmatic hiatus and increased exposure of the distal esophagus to acid.[8] The same phenomenon was observed in those with central obesity. Laxity of the phrenoesophageal membrane, which increases with age, also plays an important role in this susceptibility to hernia.[7]

Paraesophageal hernias are associated with previous gastroesophageal surgery (antireflux procedures, esophagomyotomy, partial gastrectomy). Thoracoabdominal trauma (for example, motor vehicle incidents or falls from a height[9]) might also lead to paraesophageal hernias, with some patients presenting with symptoms months to years after the injury. Skeletal deformities and congenital conditions such as scoliosis, kyphosis, and pectus excavatum, predispose people to hernias. Scoliosis and kyphosis can distort the anatomy of the diaphragm; scoliosis is present in almost a third of patients with giant paraesophageal hernia.[10] Congenital defects are the most common cause of paraesophageal hernia in children, sometimes associated with other malformations, such as intestinal malrotation.[11]

What are the symptoms?

Hiatus hernia can exacerbate gastroesophageal reflux by several mechanisms. Separation between the lower esophageal sphincter and crus can lead to an impaired antireflux barrier,[12] particularly in circumstances of acute intra-abdominal pressure, as occurs with bending or coughing. Acidic gastric juice layered on top of recently ingested food and extending into the hernia, the "acid

SUMMARY POINTS

- Hiatus hernia refers to herniation of the contents of the abdominal cavity, most commonly the stomach, through the esophageal hiatus of the diaphragm into the mediastinum
- The prevalence of hiatus hernia increases with age and body mass index
- In the absence of symptoms, there is no indication to diagnose or treat hiatus hernia
- Gastroesophageal reflux disease is the main clinical manifestation of hiatus hernia
- Endoscopy, radiology with barium swallow, or high resolution manometry can detect most cases of hiatus hernia
- Surgical treatment of hiatus hernia, usually coupled with an antireflux procedure, can be complicated, making a critical risk-benefit assessment mandatory

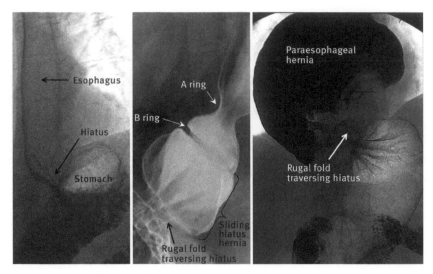

Fig 1 Barium swallow examination. (Left) Normal esophagogastric junction. (Middle) Sliding hiatus hernia with luminal distension distorting the native anatomy. A muscular ring at the proximal margin of the lower esophageal sphincter called the A ring may be visible during swallowing, as well as a second ring, the B ring, that corresponds to the squamocolumnar junction. A hiatus hernia is a .2 cm separation between the B ring and the hiatus (distance indicated by black bracket). The B ring is variably present; in its absence the demonstration of rugal folds traversing the diaphragm is used as the defining criterion for hiatus hernia. In paraesophageal hernia (right) the leading edge is the gastric fundus, and the squamnocolumnar junction maintains its native position unless it is a mixed type, in which case there are both sliding and paraesophageal elements. Note the rugal folds traversing the hiatus and that the herniated stomach is asymmetrical and is twisted

pocket," may then reflux into the esophagus.[13] Once reflux has occurred, hiatus hernia impairs the mechanism of esophageal acid clearance. Hence, increasing size of the hernia is associated with greater exposure to esophageal acid both by increasing the occurrence of reflux and by impairing the process of esophageal acid clearance.[14]

No symptom is specific for hiatus hernia. However, the presence of hernia might be suspected with symptoms of gastroesophageal reflux, including heartburn, regurgitation, or dysphagia. In cases of paraesophageal hernia, dysphagia may be caused by the herniated stomach compressing the distal esophagus, resulting in an extrinsic mechanical obstruction. Sliding hiatus hernia may also promote dysphagia secondary to stasis in the herniated stomach, or functional obstruction at the level of the crural diaphragm, or both.[15]

Though the major importance of sliding hernias is their association with gastroesophageal reflux disease (GERD), the main clinical importance of paraesophageal hernias lies in their potential for obstruction, ischemia, or volvulus.[2] Paraesophageal hernias either cause no symptoms or are associated with non-specific, intermittent symptoms such as chest pain, epigastric pain, postprandial fullness, nausea, and retching; symptoms potentially related to ischemia or obstruction.

Sliding hiatus hernias may also lead to bleeding and chronic iron deficiency anemia as a consequence of Cameron erosions.[16 17] These linear gastric erosions can occur on the rugae where they cross the hiatal constriction, especially with large hernias.

When should patients with suspected hiatus hernia be referred?

In the absence of symptoms potentially related to hiatus hernia there is no indication to pursue a diagnosis of hiatus hernia. Even with typical symptoms of GERD (heartburn, regurgitation), but no alarm signs (dysphagia, weight loss, bleeding, anemia), empiric treatment with proton pump inhibitors without diagnostic testing is standard practice.[18] Specialist referral is necessary if symptomatic

treatment is ineffective or there are alarm signs that might be experienced by patients with hiatus hernia but could be related to ulcers, tumours, or strictures. Hence affected patients should be evaluated using upper endoscopy. Indications for non-urgent upper endoscopy include age greater than 50 years with longstanding symptoms of reflux and atypical symptoms of GERD (chest pain, epigastric pain, postprandial fullness, nausea, or retching).

How is hiatus hernia diagnosed?

Typically, hiatus hernia is intermittent, especially when small. Intermittency coupled with an element of subjectivity in distinguishing a small hernia from normal with all investigational techniques results in a circumstance in which no investigational technique has a definable sensitivity or specificity for the detection of hiatus hernia. The main indication for these investigations is to rule out potential complications of hiatus hernia and to detect other possible diagnoses such as ulcers, strictures, or tumours.

Endoscopy

The clinical indications for endoscopy of the upper gastrointestinal tract include symptoms typical of GERD but that are refractory to treatment, alarm signs (dysphagia, bleeding, weight loss, anemia), or symptoms in patients older than 50 years.[18] In the absence of symptoms, there is no clinical indication to systematically search for hiatus hernia. There is no absolute contraindication for upper gastrointestinal endoscopy. Major complications such as perforation or aspiration are rare, occurring in less than 1 per 1000 cases.

Sliding hiatus hernia is diagnosed when the apparent separation between the squamocolumnar junction (the transition from esophageal to gastric epithelium) and the constriction formed as the stomach traverses the hiatus is greater than 2 cm. Asking patients to inspire while the proximal stomach is observed might help to localize the hiatus. Dilation of the hiatus can also be seen from a retroflexed view. However, the endoscopic diagnosis of hiatus hernia has limitations: the esophagogastric junction is mobile (for example, with swallowing, breathing, and straining), which may lead to intermittent hernia; metaplasia (Barrett's esophagus) or inflammation can make it difficult to localize the native squamocolumnar junction; and excess air insufflation of the stomach might exaggerate the size of the hernia.

Upper gastrointestinal endoscopy is essential in the evaluation of potential complications from hiatus hernia that may explain symptoms (bleeding, dysphagia, pain). The size of the hiatus hernia is the main determinant of the presence and severity of esophagitis.[19] Cameron erosions should be considered in cases of chronic anemia or bleeding, or both. Even without visualization of these, the finding of a large hiatus hernia in association with a normal colonoscopy result, otherwise normal upper gastrointestinal endoscopy result, and normal capsule endoscopy (small bowel endoscopy using the ingestion of a capsule) result might be considered an adequate explanation for iron deficiency anemia, with intermittent Cameron erosions being a diagnosis of exclusion.

Radiologic imaging

Hiatus hernia can be diagnosed by radiology of the upper gastrointestinal tract (fig 1), albeit with poor sensitivity for mucosal complications. Radiology is usually indicated in the presurgical evaluation. Risks are related to radiation exposure and allergy to barium or iodine. Pregnancy is a contraindication. Computed tomography is not a standard procedure in patients with hiatus hernia. It might be useful in the assessment of gastric volvulus in cases of paraesophageal hernia and the detection of other herniated organs. Hiatus hernia might also be found by chance during computed tomography for another indication.

High resolution manometry and reflux monitoring

Functional esophageal testing using manometry (assessment of esophageal contractile function using an esophageal catheter) and reflux monitoring (assessment of reflux of gastric content into the esophagus using an esophageal catheter) is indicated when surgery is being considered to control symptoms of gastroesophageal reflux related to a hiatus hernia. Risks of functional testing are minimal. High resolution manometry with topographic pressure plotting depicts the pressure profile across the esophagogastric junction (fig 2), helping to locate the crural diaphragm and the lower esophageal sphincter[20] in real time, potentially making it a more accurate depiction of the relation between these structures; a separation greater than 2 cm between these defines hiatus hernia. However, separation between lower esophageal sphincter and the crural diaphragm might also be intermittent. Hence, as with endoscopy and radiology, the accuracy of high resolution manometry in the diagnosis of hiatus hernia is not perfect. Manometry also verifies the integrity of esophageal peristalsis, which is considered essential before undergoing fundoplication surgery. Reflux monitoring is not useful in diagnosing hiatus hernia, but it is indicated to verify the presence of pathological GERD in the absence of high grade reflux esophagitis.

What are the treatment options?

Not all hiatus hernias cause symptoms and in the absence of symptoms, treatment is rarely indicated. Paraesophageal hernias might be considered for treatment because of potential catastrophic complications.[21] Otherwise, drug treatment of hiatus hernia aims to limit the consequences

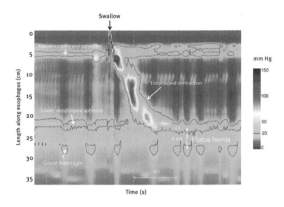

Fig 2 High resolution manometry showing pressure variations recorded along the esophagus (represented as pressure topography plots). Three high pressure zones are identified: upper esophageal sphincter, lower esophageal sphincter, and crural diaphragm. Swallow is followed by a propagated contraction along the esophagus. Lower esophageal sphincter and crural diaphragm are separated by more than 2 cm, defining hiatus hernia

of GERD. The surgical approach consists of restoring the stomach into the abdominal cavity and compensating for anatomic abnormalities to approximate normal physiology of the esophagogastric junction.

Medical approach

Alleviation of the symptoms of GERD is the cornerstone for treatment of hiatus hernia. This is usually achieved indirectly with drugs that inhibit gastric acid secretion, thereby preventing symptoms or complications related to the reflux of gastric acid into the esophagus. Proton pump inhibitors (PPIs) are the most potent inhibitors of gastric acid secretion and the most effective drugs to treat reflux esophagitis and typical symptoms of GERD.[22 23 24] Histamine 2 receptor antagonists and antacids are alternatives to PPIs, though they are substantially less effective.[22 23 24] As reflux is usually a chronic problem and the treatment approach of inhibiting acid secretion is compensatory rather than curative, long term PPI treatment of GERD is more the rule than the exception. The usual recommendation is to use the minimal PPI dose that is sufficient to control symptoms. Some patients even prefer on-demand treatment for intermittent symptoms, a practice common in the United States, where PPIs are now available without prescription. Adverse effects of PPIs include headache (<5%), diarrhea (<5%), and an increased susceptibility to gastrointestinal pathogens, including infectious gastroenteritis, and colitis caused by *Clostridium difficile*.[25] Severe adverse events include rare cases of acute interstitial nephritis and reversible severe hypomagnesemia. Long term treatment may predispose to osteopenia and small intestinal bacterial overgrowth, although supportive evidence for this is weak.

Histamine 2 receptor antagonists, antacids, and alginate-antacid combinations can reduce postprandial exposure of the esophagus to acid[26] and thus decrease the symptoms of GERD.[22] These treatments might be utilized in an on-demand fashion by patients with moderate symptoms or as add-on treatment if symptoms occur despite PPI treatment.

Minimal evidence supports the efficacy of prokinetic drugs as monotherapy or as add-on treatment in patients with GERD. Guidelines do not recommend the use of metoclopramide or domperidone in uncomplicated GERD and even advise against metoclopramide because of potential

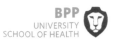

neurologic side effects, including tardive dyskinesia.[23] QT prolongation possibly leading to lethal cardiac arhythmias is another potentially dangerous side effect limiting the usefulness of dopaminergic or serotonergic prokinetics (domperidone, cisapride) in the treatment of GERD.[24]

Though modifications to lifestyle are routinely advocated, evidence supporting their effectiveness is generally weak.[22] None the less, they should be selectively advised according to patients' circumstances. Lifestyle modifications entail weight loss, avoidance of specific "trigger" foods, smaller meals, not eating late in the evening, and postural adjustments such as remaining upright after eating and elevating the head of the bed for sleep. Raising the head of the bed by 6-8 inches (15-20 cm) and avoidance of food three hours before bedtime are especially pertinent for patients who are prone to symptoms at night.

Surgical approach

Surgery is the only way to restore herniated organs into the abdominal cavity and to compensate for the functional abnormalities associated with hiatus hernia. The standard procedure is currently laparoscopic fundoplication. The essential components of this technique are mobilization of the distal esophagus, reduction of the associated hiatus hernia, and either partial (Toupet 270°) or complete (Nissen 360°) fundoplication around the esophagus (fig 3).[27] Recent guidelines emphasize that surgical repair of a sliding hernia is not necessary in the absence of GERD.[28] When symptoms of GERD and sliding hiatus hernia are present, surgical treatment might be considered for patients with persistent regurgitation despite medical treatment, symptoms such as chronic cough that prove refractory to PPI treatment, intolerance to PPIs, or (rarely) refractory esophagitis. The main side effects of fundoplication are dysphagia and bloating, which vary in severity from mild to severe. The risk of major complications or death is about 1-2%. Importantly, efficacy data from community practice report that up to 30% of patients resume treatment with PPIs within five years

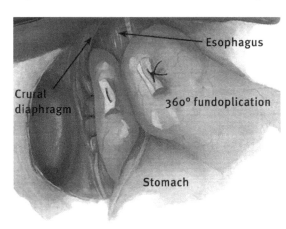

Fig 3 Nissen fundoplication. The essential features of fundoplication are to mobilize the lower esophagus, reduce the hiatus hernia, and wrap the gastric fundus around the esophagus. During the procedure the proximal stomach is wrapped 360° around the gastroesophageal junction. Adapted from Peters and DeMeester[32]

QUESTIONS FOR FUTURE RESEARCH

- Should surgery be routinely advised for paraesophageal hernia in patients without symptoms?
- When should bariatric surgery be used instead of a fundoplication to treat gastroesophageal reflux disease?

TIPS FOR NON-SPECIALISTS

- Hiatus hernia is prevalent in the general population
- Hiatus hernia can be asymptomatic
- Hiatus hernia should be investigated in patients with gastroesophageal reflux disease incompletely controlled by medical treatment, bleeding, weight loss, dysphagia, or chronic iron deficiency anaemia
- Paraesophageal hernia should be considered in patients with non-specific and troublesome dyspeptic symptoms
- Medical treatment for gastroesophageal reflux symptoms is the preferred management strategy, irrespective of hiatus hernia

---

ADDITIONAL EDUCATIONAL RESOURCES

Information for healthcare professionals

- Roman S, Kahrilas PJ. Hiatal hernia. In: Principles of deglutition: a multidisciplinary text for swallowing and its disorders. Springer, 2013:753-68—Provides details of physiopathology and diagnosis of hiatus hernia

Information for patients

- The following resources explain the causes and symptoms of hiatus hernia and provide an overview of tests and treatment
- National Institutes of Health. Hiatal hernia (www.ncbi.nlm.nih.gov/pubmedhealth/PMH0002122/)
- Mayo Clinic. Hiatus hernia (www.mayoclinic.org/diseases-conditions/hiatal-hernia/basics/definition/con-20030640)
- UpToDate: patient information. Hiatus hernia (www.uptodate.com/contents/hiatal-hernia-the-basics?source=search_result&search=hiatus±hernia&selectedTitle=2~75)

of antireflux surgery,[29] and accumulating evidence suggests that the risk of recurrence is much greater in the presence of abdominal obesity.[30] Redo fundoplication is also common, accounting for up to 50% of operations performed at some referral centres.[31]

Laparoscopic repair of paraesophageal hernia is a complex operation because in many cases the associated anatomic distortion is severe.[33] Surgery includes complete resection of the hernia sac from the mediastinum, mobilization of the esophagus, closure of the hiatus (sometimes using mesh), and fundoplication. Given this complexity, the risk of surgery must be balanced against the underlying risk of complications from paraesophageal hernia,[28] currently a topic of considerable controversy. Few data are available on the risk of progression from asymptomatic to symptomatic paraesophageal hernia: it might be around 14% per year.[28] However, the risk of developing acute symptoms that require emergency surgery is less than 2%. Finally, the mortality rate associated with repair of paraesophageal hiatus hernia might be up to 5% when surgery is performed in an emergency situation. The recurrence rate for paraesophageal hernia after repair is up to 50% at five years.

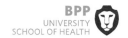
Competing interests: We have read and understood the BMJ policy on declaration of interests and declare the following interests: SR carries out consultancy work for Given Imaging, sits on its advisory board, and has received a grant from the company for a study entitled "Normal values for 3D ano-rectal high resolution manometry."

Provenance and peer review: Commissioned; externally peer reviewed.

1 Thukkani N, Sonnenberg A. The influence of environmental risk factors in hospitalization for gastro-oesophageal reflux disease-related diagnoses in the United States. *Aliment Pharmacol Ther*2010;31:852-61.

2 Skinner DB, ed. Hernia (hiatal, traumatic, and congenital). 4th ed. Saunders, 1985.

3 Sakaguchi M, Oka H, Hashimoto T, Asakuma Y, Takao M, Gon G, et al. Obesity as a risk factor for GERD in Japan. *J Gastroenterol*2008;43:57-62.

4 Wilson LJ, Ma W, Hirschowitz BI. Association of obesity with hiatal hernia and esophagitis. *Am J Gastroenterol*1999;94:2840-4.

5 Stene-Larsen G, Weberg R, Froyshov Larsen I, Bjortuft O, Hoel B, Berstad A. Relationship of overweight to hiatus hernia and reflux oesophagitis. *Scand J Gastroenterol*1988;23:427-32.

6 Pandolfino JE, El-Serag HB, Zhang Q, Shah N, Ghosh SK, Kahrilas PJ. Obesity: a challenge to esophagogastric junction integrity. *Gastroenterology*2006;130:639-49.

7 Menon S, Trudgill N. Risk factors in the aetiology of hiatus hernia: a meta-analysis. *Eur J Gastroenterol Hepatol*2011;23:133-8.

8 Lee YY, Wirz AA, Whiting JG, Robertson EV, Smith D, Weir A, et al. Waist belt and central obesity cause partial hiatus hernia and short-segment acid reflux in asymptomatic volunteers. *Gut*2014;63:1053-60.

9 Eren S, Ciris F. Diaphragmatic hernia: diagnostic approaches with review of the literature. *Eur J Radiol*2005;54:448-59.

10 Schuchert MJ, Adusumilli PS, Cook CC, Colovos C, Kilic A, Nason KS, et al. The impact of scoliosis among patients with giant paraesophageal hernia. *J Gastrointest Surg*2011;15:23-8.

11 Karpelowsky JS, Wieselthaler N, Rode H. Primary paraesophageal hernia in children. *J Pediatr Surg*2006;41:1588-93.

12 Kahrilas PJ, Lin S, Chen J, Manka M. The effect of hiatus hernia on gastro-oesophageal junction pressure. *Gut*1999;44:476-82.

13 Beaumont H, Bennink RJ, de Jong J, Boeckxstaens GE. The position of the acid pocket as a major risk factor for acidic reflux in healthy subjects and patients with GORD. *Gut*2010;59:441-51.

14 Jones MP, Sloan SS, Jovanovic B, Kahrilas PJ. Impaired egress rather than increased access: an important independent predictor of erosive oesophagitis. *Neurogastroenterol Motil*2002;14:625-31.

15 Pandolfino JE, Kwiatek MA, Ho K, Scherer JR, Kahrilas PJ. Unique features of esophagogastric junction pressure topography in hiatus hernia patients with dysphagia. *Surgery*2010;147:57-64.

16 Annibale B, Capurso G, Chistolini A, D'Ambra G, DiGiulio E, Monarca B, et al. Gastrointestinal causes of refractory iron deficiency anemia in patients without gastrointestinal symptoms. *Am J Med*2001;111:439-45.

17 Maganty K, Smith RL. Cameron lesions: unusual cause of gastrointestinal bleeding and anemia. *Digestion*2008;77:214-7.

18 Shaheen NJ, Weinberg DS, Denberg TD, Chou R, Qaseem A, Shekelle P. Upper endoscopy for gastroesophageal reflux disease: best practice advice from the clinical guidelines committee of the American College of Physicians. *Ann Intern Med*2012;157:808-16.

19 Jones MP, Sloan SS, Rabine JC, Ebert CC, Huang CF, Kahrilas PJ. Hiatal hernia size is the dominant determinant of esophagitis presence and severity in gastroesophageal reflux disease. *Am J Gastroenterol*2001;96:1711-7.

20 Pandolfino JE, Kim H, Ghosh SK, Clarke JO, Zhang Q, Kahrilas PJ. High-resolution manometry of the EGJ: an analysis of crural diaphragm function in GERD. *Am J Gastroenterol*2007;102:1056-63.

21 Poulose BK, Gosen C, Marks JM, Khaitan L, Rosen MJ, Onders RP, et al. Inpatient mortality analysis of paraesophageal hernia repair in octogenarians. *J Gastrointest Surg*2008;12:1888-92.

22 Kahrilas PJ, Shaheen NJ, Vaezi MF, Hiltz SW, Black E, Modlin IM, et al. American Gastroenterological Association medical position statement on the management of gastroesophageal reflux disease. *Gastroenterology*2008;135:1383-91, 91 e1-5.

23 Katz PO, Gerson LB, Vela MF. Guidelines for the diagnosis and management of gastroesophageal reflux disease. *Am J Gastroenterol*2013;108:308-28; quiz 29.

24 Fuchs KH, Babic B, Breithaupt W, Dallemagne B, Fingerhut A, Furnee E, et al. EAES recommendations for the management of gastroesophageal reflux disease. *Surg Endosc*2014;28:1753-73.

25 Yang YX, Metz DC. Safety of proton pump inhibitor exposure. *Gastroenterology*2010;139:1115-27.

26 Rohof WO, Bennink RJ, Smout AJ, Thomas E, Boeckxstaens GE. An alginate-antacid formulation localizes to the acid pocket to reduce acid reflux in patients with gastroesophageal reflux disease. *Clin Gastroenterol Hepatol*2013;11:1585-91; quiz e90.

27 Rydberg L, Ruth M, Lundell L. Mechanism of action of antireflux procedures. *Br J Surg*1999;86:405-10.

28 Kohn GP, Price RR, DeMeester SR, Zehetner J, Muensterer OJ, Awad Z, et al. Guidelines for the management of hiatal hernia. *Surg Endosc*2013;27:4409-28.

29 Vakil N, Shaw M, Kirby R. Clinical effectiveness of laparoscopic fundoplication in a US community. *Am J Med*2003;114:1-5.

30 Morgenthal CB, Lin E, Shane MD, Hunter JG, Smith CD. Who will fail laparoscopic Nissen fundoplication? Preoperative prediction of long-term outcomes. *Surg Endosc*2007;21:1978-84.

31 Hunter JG, Smith CD, Branum GD, Waring JP, Trus TL, Cornwell M, et al. Laparoscopic fundoplication failures: patterns of failure and response to fundoplication revision. *Ann Surg*1999;230:595-604; discussion 04-6.

32 Peters JH, DeMeester TR, eds. Minimally invasive surgery of the foregut. Quality Medical Publishing, 1994.

33 Morrow EH, Oelschlager BK. Laparoscopic paraesophageal hernia repair. *Surg Laparosc Endosc Percutan Tech*2013;23:446-8.

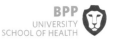

Diagnosis and management of Barrett's oesophagus

Janusz Jankowski, James Black fellow[1] James Black professor[2] consultant gastroenterologist[3],
Hugh Barr, professor[4] oesophagogastric resection surgeon[5],
Ken Wang, professor of gastroenterology[6],
Brendan Delaney, Guy's and St Thomas' charity chair of primary care research[7]

[1]Gastrointestinal Oncology Group, University of Oxford, Oxford

[2]Centre for Digestive Disease, Blizard Institute, Queen Mary University of London, London

[3]Digestive Disease Centre, University Hospitals of Leicester, Leicester

[4]Cranfield Health, Cranfield University, Cranfield, Bedfordshire

[5]Department of Surgery, Gloucestershire Royal Hospital, Gloucestershire

[6]Advanced Endoscopy Group and Esophageal Neoplasia, Mayo Clinic, Rochester, Minnesota, USA

[7]Department of Primary Care and Public Health Sciences, King's College London, London

Correspondence to: J Jankowski
j.a.jankowski@qmul.ac.uk

Cite this as: BMJ 2010;341:c4551

DOI: 10.1136/bmj.c4551

http://www.bmj.com/content/341/bmj.c4551

Barrett's oesophagus affects 2% of the adult population in the West, which makes it one of the most common premalignant lesions after colorectal polyps. Conversion to oesophageal adenocarcinoma is the most important complication of the condition, with a lifetime risk of 5% in men and 3% in women.[1 2 3 4] Several large trials investigating surveillance (Barrett's Oesophagus Surveillance Study (BOSS)), chemoprevention (the Aspirin Esomeprazole Chemoprevention Trial (AspECT)), genetic stratification (EArly Genetics and Lifecourse Epidemiology (EAGLE) consortium), and endotherapy for high risk individuals are under way to determine the best way to prevent progression to adenocarcinoma.

There are now several endoscopic alternatives to the long established technique of radical surgical oesophagectomy for treating high grade dysplasia and early mucosal cancer, which avoid the mortality and morbidity of surgery. Recently consensus on optimal management of the condition was reached after a National Institute of Health and Clinical Excellence (NICE) review. It is recommended that clinicians, after discussion within the multidisciplinary team, consider offering endoscopic ablative therapy as an alternative to oesophagectomy for patients with high grade dysplasia and intramucosal cancer.[1 2 5]

A diagnosis of Barrett's oesophagus has important ramifications for the patient because of the uncertainty of prognosis, possible anxiety about cancer in the future, the need for repeated endoscopy in a surveillance programme, and the costs of drugs and repeated investigations.[2 4] We review evidence from epidemiological studies, observational studies, and randomised trials, and draw on expert opinion to discuss the importance of early recognition and optimal treatment of Barrett's oesophagus.

What is Barrett's oesophagus and who gets it?

Barrett's oesophagus is a change in the lining of the oesophagus from normal stratified (multilayered) squamous mucosa to single layered, inflamed, premalignant, mucin secreting mucosa with variable degrees of goblet cell differentiation, termed intestinal metaplasia.[3]

Barrett's oesophagus develops in 5% of people with gastro-oesophageal reflux disease, which affects as many as 30% of adults in the Western world.[6 7] Evidence from one case series suggests that at least 60% of patients with Barrett's oesophagus develop the disease as a result of chronic reflux, although other forms of mucosal inflammation in the lower oesophagus (such as from damage by chemotherapy, non-steroidal anti-inflammatory drugs, and viral infections) could be linked to the condition.[3 7 8]

Community studies have estimated the prevalence of Barrett's oesophagus to be just under 2% among adults in the West, which corresponds with approximately one million cases in the United Kingdom and four million in the United States. It is especially prevalent in middle aged to older men of Anglo-Saxon origin.[3 8]

The annual incidence of Barrett's oesophagus in the adult population is probably around 0.1% (1 new case a year for every 1000 people)—approximately 60000 new cases in the UK and 240000 in the US a year—but evidence from case series suggests that the global rate of diagnosis of Barrett's oesophagus is increasing by 2% a year.[7 8 9] This high rate may be in part because of increased endoscopic recognition, but it probably reflects a true increased incidence.[7 9]

What is the natural history of the condition?

Complete resolution of Barrett's oesophagus rarely occurs except in very small segments, despite early reports suggesting otherwise. However, it is not uncommon to see modest shrinkage of the segment length in patients treated with acid suppression. The majority of cases stay constant, neither progressing to oesophageal adenocarcinoma nor regressing.

Case series have indicated that the risk of patients with Barrett's oesophagus developing oesophageal adenocarcinoma is small in absolute terms (~5% lifetime risk in men and ~3% in women).[1 2 3 10 11] A recent decision analysis has suggested that in secondary referral centres this risk could be higher at 14% lifetime risk—a 30-100-fold higher risk of adenocarcinoma of the oesophagus compared with the general population's risk of 0.1%.[1 2 3 11] The rates of oesophageal adenocarcinoma related to Barrett's oesophagus in west Scotland are the highest in the world (16 per 100000 population) compared with lower rates in eastern Europe, Africa, and Asia.[11 12] Once a patient is in a surveillance programme, the risk of developing oesophageal adenocarcinoma varies from 0.4% a year in the US to 1% a year in the UK.[11]

SUMMARY POINTS

- Barrett's oesophagus usually occurs as a consequence of chronic gastro-oesophageal reflux disease

- The incidence of Barrett's oesophagus is increasing: the condition is present in 2% of the adult population in the West

- The incidence of oesophageal adenocarcinoma related to Barrett's oesophagus is also increasing. In the United Kingdom, especially Scotland, oesophageal adenocarcinoma rates are higher than anywhere else in the world

- Patients detected with early cancer related to Barrett's oesophagus might have surgically or endoscopically curable disease. Endoscopic therapy is recommended as an alternative to oesophagectomy for patients with dysplasia

- The value of protocol based endoscopic surveillance to detect early cancer is yet to be established and is the subject of a major randomised clinical trial

- Other cancer prevention strategies being tested are chemoprevention of Barrett's oesophagus by aspirin in the 2513 patient AspECT trial and genome-wide identification of inherited risk factors in the 4500 patient EAGLE consortium study

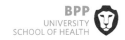

which decrease their function.[13] [14] However, none of these biological alterations can yet replace conventional histology for diagnosis and staging, because their exact relation with clinical progression has not been robustly tested in large randomised clinical trials.[15]

What influences the risk of developing adenocarcinoma?

The major factors associated with progression to cancer are: male gender; white ethnicity; length of Barrett's segment in centimetres, as seen during endoscopy (higher risk for length greater than 8 cm); diet poor in vegetables and fruit and high in fats; cigarette smoking; and obesity.[3]

Case-control studies have shown that symptoms of gastro-oesophageal reflux disease are associated with a significant increase in the risk of developing cancer (odds ratio 40±15), but also that as many as 40% of those with adenocarcinoma do not report a history of reflux symptoms.[8] [9] [12]

How is Barrett's oesophagus diagnosed?

Current evidence based guidelines on the management of dyspepsia from the National Institute for Health and Clinical Excellence advise that patients with long term symptoms of reflux (more than 5-10 years) should be referred for screening endoscopy to check for Barrett's oesophagus or its complications.[16] [17] On endoscopy, if the distal oesophagus looks pink or crimson in colour and is clearly distinguishable from the appearance of a hiatal hernia (fig 2) using accepted criteria such as the Prague endoscopic criteria,[17] then mucosal biopsies should be performed and the samples examined histopathologically. Biopsy samples are graded as "diagnostic of Barrett's oesophagus," "corroborative of Barrett's oesophagus," "consistent with Barrett's oesophagus," or "Barrett's oesophagus not present." The first

How does Barrett's oesophagus progress to adenocarcinoma of the oesophagus?

Figure 1 illustrates the stages of progression of Barrett's oesophagus, from oesophagitis through metaplasia and dysplasia to adenocarcinoma.[13] [14] [15] The sequence is thought to involve damage to stem cells deep in the oesophageal mucosa, an increase in number of abnormal but non-malignant cells, development of precancerous (dysplastic) cells, and, finally, progression to invasive cancer.

The steps of progression to cancer all involve genetic (damage to the DNA in cells) and epigenetic (reversible alterations to cell function) changes. For example, the development of metaplasia is associated with alterations in genes controlling stem cells, and progression to dysplasia is reflected by loss of heterozygosity or methylation of the adenomatous polyposis coli (APC) gene. Further progression entails loss of expression or mutations in P16 and P53,

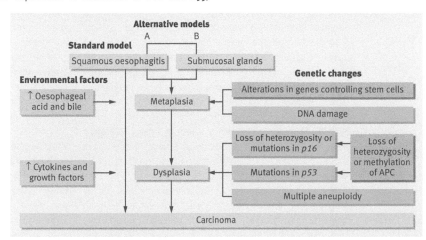

Fig 1 The standard and alternative models of progression of Barrett's oesophagus to adenocarcinoma of the oesophagus. The standard pathway to cancer is through the oesophagitis-metaplasia-dysplasia-adenocarcinoma sequence. Recently, however, it has been recognised that submucosal glands can also develop into metaplastic cells (alternative pathway A). In addition, squamous oesophagitis can conceivably develop directly into adenocarcinoma via "microscopic metaplasia" without apparently transitioning through endoscopically evident metaplasia (alternative pathway B). The column on the left shows the environmental factors that help facilitate progression of the Barrett's oesophagus. The column on the right shows the genetic (blue) and epigenetic (red) changes in the evolution of cancer. APC, adenomatous polyposis coli gene

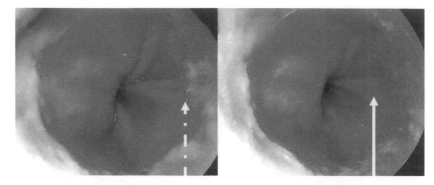

Fig 2 Endoscopic image of Barrett's oesophagus. The two pictures are from the same patient but were taken five seconds apart. The panel on the right shows correct air insufflation during endoscopy, whereas the panel on the left shows the oesophagus suboptimally distended. As a consequence, the picture on the left may be misdiagnosed by inexperienced endoscopists as a hiatal hernia, because the folds in the oesophageal lining extend to the gastro-oesophageal junction (broken arrow). The panel on the right indicates circumferential Barrett's oesophagus, which can easily be seen above the folds of the hiatal hernia (solid arrow). Pictures taken with full informed written consent

three classifications should qualify the patient for entry into an endoscopic surveillance programme.[18]

The exact protocol for surveillance programmes varies, but they conventionally consist of biennial endoscopies (that is, every two years) with random circumferential biopsies, ideally four quadrants every 2 cm for flat mucosa and additional targeted biopsies for any areas that appear abnormal on endoscopy. The vast majority of patients will be assessed according to this protocol unless dysplasia is found, when more frequent intervals of endoscopy a few months apart coupled with more intensive endoscopic pinch biopsies should be used. Alternatively, those who are no longer fit for any intervention may be discharged. However, age alone should not be the sole criterion for removing patients from surveillance, because even octogenarians can cope easily with endoscopy.[9 18 19 20 21 22]

Does surveillance prevent the development of adenocarcinoma?

Data from several medium sized case series suggest that patients with Barrett's oesophagus enrolled in surveillance programmes have cancer detected at an earlier (and hence more curable) stage than patients not in a surveillance programme who present with symptoms of oesophageal cancer.[19 20] Other evidence suggests that most patients with cancer related to Barrett's oesophagus do not benefit from surveillance endoscopy.[23 24] BOSS is a randomised trial aimed at identifying both the objective value of endoscopic surveillance and the best protocol. Data from the 2500 patient trial will be used to explore the benefits, in terms of preventing oesophageal cancer, of a regular two year upper gastrointestinal endoscopic surveillance programme versus endoscopy at time of need.[20] Without evidence from randomised trials such as the BOSS trial to guide surveillance, current empirical random biopsy protocols may be suboptimal. In addition, several audits have shown that many specialists do not adhere to international surveillance guidelines.[23 24]

The cost effectiveness of surveillance is still highly uncertain in the absence of real cost estimates from randomised controlled trials such as BOSS. Costs have been estimated to be about £40 000 (50 000; $60 000) per cancer diagnosed for less than one quality adjusted life year (QALY) gained.[25 26] The cost effectiveness is arguably better in the US. Although the country has a lower incidence of oesophageal adenocarcinoma than in the UK, endoscopic surveillance is undertaken less often (three yearly in the US v two yearly in the UK). In addition, in the US endoscopic

surveillance is undertaken only in patients with proven intestinal metaplasia on biopsy, because such patients are threefold more likely to develop cancer than those without proven intestinal metaplasia.[1 23 24 26]

Surveillance related prevention of oesophageal adenocarcinoma, even if optimised, might not dramatically increase the longevity of patients because Barrett's oesophagus has also been associated with an increased risk of other potentially fatal conditions. For example, Barrett's oesophagus might be associated with obesity and gastropulmonary aspiration, which increase the risk of ischaemic heart disease and bronchopneumonia, respectively.[10] The principal concern for health systems is how to manage patients at greatest risk of oesophageal cancer and distinguish them from those who are more likely to die of other causes.

What treatments can prevent progression of Barrett's oesophagus to adenocarcinoma?

Case series have suggested that as many as 10% of patients with Barrett's oesophagus develop high grade dysplasia in their lifetime.[3] Cohort studies have shown that such patients have an increased risk of progression to adenocarcinoma compared with those who have non-dysplastic Barrett's oesophagus (30-55% in 8 years).[18]

Data from several case control series indicate that management of multifocal areas of high grade dysplasia can be technically difficult and may require multiple interventions.[19 20] Expert consensus indicates that because of their increased risk of cancer, such patients warrant intervention with either several sessions of endoscopic ablation therapy or, in exceptional cases, oesophagectomy.[4 5 18] Arguably these patients represent a bigger burden to healthcare providers than those with cancer [4].

Proton pump inhibitors

A recent large randomised controlled trial found that early effective therapy for gastro-oesophageal reflux disease with proton pump inhibitors both manages symptoms effectively and heals oesophageal ulceration.[27] These findings have given rise to a strategy whereby acid suppressant drugs such as proton pump inhibitors are used not only to heal and maintain healing of oesophagitis but also for "chemoprevention" in patients with Barrett's oesophagus. Proton pump inhibitor therapy for Barrett's oesophagus has been shown to be well tolerated and safe in both case-control studies and randomised controlled trials.[28] They do not seem to promote elongation of Barrett's

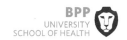

oesophagus, which was an initial fear following reports of hypergastrinaemia caused by proton pump inhibitors.[29]

However, case reports have speculated about a possible link between use of proton pump inhibitors and intestinal infections—especially *Clostridium difficile*—deficiencies of nutrients like folate and vitamin B12, and osteoporosis. Proton pump inhibitors also reduce the effectiveness of clopidogrel, and co-administration of the two drugs should be avoided if possible.

Some practitioners have attempted to reduce costs and potential for side effects of proton pump inhibitors by treating patients who have gastro-oesophageal reflux disease with on demand medication.[18] However, this approach might be the worst of all options because intermittent treatment could in fact increase the risk of Barrett's oesophagus and adenocarcinoma. Partial treatment might prevent the oesophagitis from healing completely and might also conceivably regulate the inflammation sufficiently for the metaplastic Barrett's cells at the ulcer base, which can tolerate a low pH, to colonise the residual ulcerated oesophageal mucosa.[30] [31] Selective mechanisms that allow Barrett's cells to grow preferentially in low inflammatory conditions when compared with native oesophageal squamous cells have already been demonstrated.[31]

Detecting significant differences between interventions for relatively rare outcomes in Barrett's oesophagus such as adenocarcinoma would need a controlled study with a very large number of subjects. Future developments in linking routine clinical data with research in the community could potentially facilitate this type of large scale study. A large randomised trial in secondary care, AspECT, —is currently evaluating the long term value of low dose (20 mg) esomeprazole (a proton pump inhibitor) compared with high dose (80 mg) esomeprazole, either with or without aspirin.[32] Aspirin is arguably the best drug to prevent cancer of the gastrointestinal tract, such as cancers of the colon, stomach, and oesophagus. So far 2513 patients have been recruited into the AspECT trial, and an interim analysis in one large centre has found a low rate of major side effects, suggesting that any interaction between esomeprazole and aspirin is acceptable.[32]

Nissen fundoplication

Moderately sized randomised controlled trials have shown that surgical repair of the oesophageal sphincter by buttressing the stomach onto the oesophagus (fundoplication) offers good symptom control in patients with severe reflux disease and Barrett's oesophagus. In addition, this approach might be cheaper than proton pump inhibitors when drug use over many years is anticipated.[27] Other randomised trials have confirmed that surgery controls reflux more completely than does medical therapy.

Furthermore, fundoplication may prevent all constituents of the refluxate from entering the oesophagus, in particular the contents of the duodenum such as bile. Evidence from case series has suggested that these agents may not be suppressed by proton pump inhibitor therapy.[3]

Newer endoscopic therapies

Endoscopic mucosal resection for the eradication of early cancers (by definition confined to the mucosal lining) is highly effective—five year survival is 98% in patients with early adenocarcinoma confined to the mucosa and high grade dysplasia.[1] [19] [21] [24] [25] The type of epithelium that re-grows is in part determined by the depth of injury that occurs as a consequence of treatment. In order to ensure squamous cell regeneration as opposed to recurrence of Barrett's oesophagus, some of the superficial squamous lined ducts of the oesophageal mucous glands must survive.[30]

Photodynamic therapy comprises systemic administration of photosensitising agents that are retained selectively in malignant tissue. When exposed to appropriate wavelength laser light, a cytotoxic reaction occurs that causes cellular destruction. The strongest evidence for the effectiveness of photodynamic therapy comes from the five year follow-up of a randomised, multicentre, multinational, pathology blinded trial that evaluated the usefulness of the technique to eradicate dysplasia. Photodynamic therapy was significantly more effective at eradicating high grade dysplasia than omeprazole only (odds ratio 2±0.7) and reduced the likelihood of developing cancer by half, with a significantly longer time to progression in the photodynamic therapy group compared with the omeprazole group.[33] It may be necessary to repeat ablation at intervals, and patients treated this way should remain in lifelong surveillance.[4]

A further randomised trial compared thermal ablation and argon plasma coagulation with surveillance in 40 patients who had undergone surgical reflux control.[34] Significant reversal of Barrett's oesophagus occurred in patients treated with argon plasma coagulation ablation (63% v 15% in patients under surveillance (odds ratio 4.1±1.2)). Most recently, a randomised trial of radiofrequency ablation showed that this strategy is very effective in ablating both non-dysplastic and dysplastic Barrett's oesophagus, with complete eradication in 90.5% and 81.0% of cases, respectively.[21] The immediate side effects of ablation are minor retrosternal discomfort in 30% of patients, but full functional activity is possible in almost all patients. Stricture, bleeding, and perforation occur in 10%, 1%, and less than 1% of patients, respectively.

Recently published National Institute of Health and Clinical Excellence guidelines from the UK recommend that clinicians consider offering endoscopic ablative therapy as an alternative to oesophagectomy for people with high grade dysplasia and intramucosal cancer, according to individual patient preferences and their suitability for the procedure.[4] [5] National Institute of Health and Clinical Excellence guidelines consider endoscopic therapy—especially endoscopic resection and radiofrequency ablation—to be particularly suitable for patients who are considered unsuitable for surgery and those who do not wish to undergo oesophagectomy.[5] [21]

What does the future hold?

Consensus has not yet been reached on the value of either tissue or blood biomarkers to stratify patients with Barrett's oesophagus in terms of risk of developing cancer.[14] [15] However, researchers hope that data from genome-wide association studies may assist with the understanding of the inherited basis of Barrett's oesophagus and its progression. Such knowledge might allow patient centred stratification of already known risk factors such as ethnicity, gender, and mucosal phenotype and facilitate individual tailoring of management. In fact, diagnosis and stratification may very well move to another level when the first genome-wide assessment study of Barrett's oesophagus is published in 2011. Several genetic consortiums are being set up to replicate these genetic data once published and validate them for clinical use. Perhaps the largest in Europe is the Esophageal Adenocarcinoma Genetic LinkagE (EAGLE) consortium, which incorporates both the Chemoprevention Of Premalignant Intestinal Neoplasia

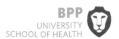

TIPS FOR NON-SPECIALISTS

Who should be referred for routine endoscopy?

- Patients with reflux for more than five years and who are aged over 50 years[16 22]

What are the alarm symptoms for immediate referral for endoscopy?

- Dysphagia[16 22]
- Weight loss[16 22]
- Vomiting blood[16 22]
- Anaemia[16 22]

What other comorbid diseases should be screened for?

- Ischaemic heart disease[4 35]
- Hypercholesterolaemia[4 35]

What is the best treatment approach for patients diagnosed with Barrett's oesophagus?

- 90% can be managed by acid suppression therapy[1 6 27]
- 5% may benefit from Nissen fundoplication[1 6 27]
- 5% may develop oesophageal adenocarcinoma after at least 15 years[1 3 27]

What dose of proton pump inhibitors should be used?

- Use the lowest effective dose that suppresses symptoms so that heartburn occurs less than once a week[16 22]

When should patients be reviewed?

- **Primary care physician**—Dose of proton pump inhibitors should be reviewed annually, and healthy living messages—such as maintaining a low fat diet, exercising, and maintaining a BMI of less than 30—should be reinforced regularly
- **Secondary care physician**—Patients should be reviewed endoscopically every two years in the UK and every three years elsewhere (because of higher incidence of cancer in the UK)[22]

ADDITIONAL EDUCATIONAL RESOURCES

For healthcare professionals

- CORE (www.corecharity.org.uk)—Charity specifically geared towards funding research into gastrointestinal diseases
- National Institute for Health and Clinical Excellence (www.nice.org.uk)—National body providing evidence based guidance on specific diseases and conditions
- Barrett's Dysplasia and Cancer Taskforce (www.worldgastroenterology.org/international-consensus-of-management-of-dysplastic-barretts-and-cancer.html)—Taskforce producing evidence based guidelines for best clinical and cost effective management of high grade dysplasia and early mucosal cancer in Barrett's oesophagus

For patients

- Oesophageal Patients Association (www.opa.org.uk)—Largest patients' support group dedicated to oesophageal cancer
- Patient UK (www.patient.co.uk)—Comprehensive source of health and disease information for patients
- Fight Oesophageal Reflux Together (refluxhelp.org)—Largest UK patient support group, with online resources
- American College of Gastroenterology (www.gi.org/patients/patientinfo/barretts.asp)—Patient information on Barrett's oesophagus from one of the largest clinical organisations dealing with digestive care
- MacMillan Cancer Support and Cancer Backup (www.macmillan.org.uk/Cancerinformation/Cancertypes/Gulletoesophagus/Pre-cancerousconditions/Barrettsoesophagus.aspx)—Patient information from one of the largest cancer patient information websites
- British Society of Gastroenterology (www.bsg.org.uk/patients/patients/general/oesophageal-cancer.html)—Patient information from one of the largest gastroenterology organisations in Europe

(ChOPIN) trial and the Inherited Predisposition of Oesophageal Diseases (IPOD) study.

Conclusion

From diagnosis through to management of all stages of Barrett's oesophagus, early prompt action is important. Expert consensus and evidence based guidelines recommend that for patients with Barrett's oesophagus confirmed on histology, two yearly endoscopic surveillance is warranted along with either medical or surgical treatment to prevent gastric reflux. In patients with confirmed dysplasia, ablation therapy should be considered with endoscopic resection either alone or coupled with ablation therapy. For patients with non-dysplastic disease, the risk-benefit equation for ablation therapy has not yet determined and stratification of the likelihood of progression should be undertaken using conventional histological and endoscopic criteria. A large specialist and patient international consensus on the management of high grade dysplasia (BArretts's Dysplasia and CAncer Taskforce (BAD CAT)) is due in 2011, and the National Institute of Health and Clinical Excellence has published management guidelines this year. In the meantime patients with Barrett's oesophagus are strongly recommended to join patient support organisations with expertise in this disease, such as Fight Oesophageal Reflux Together (FORT), so they can be helped to have an informed opinion of their options at each stage in the pathway.[35]

We thank Cathy Bennett of the Cochrane Collaboration Upper Gastrointestinal and Pancreatic Diseases Group and the BArrett's Dysplasia Cancer Taskforce (BAD CAT) for her help. We also thank Rebecca Harrison, Leicester, UK, for discussions during writing and proof reading.

Contributors: JJ came up with the concept for this article and undertook the research, writing, and coordination. HB contributed to researching and writing the article, whereas KW and BD both contributed to the writing. JJ and HB contributed equally to the manuscript. JJ acts as the guarantor and accepts full responsibility for the work, had full access to the data, and controlled the decision to publish.

Funding: The authors received funding for this review from the following organisations: AstraZeneca; Cancer Research UK; the National Institute for Health Research Health Technology Assessment programme; National Institutes of Health; BAD CAT; Queen Mary University of London; and the Wellcome Trust.

Competing interests: All authors have completed the Unified Competing Interest form at www.icmje.org/coi_disclosure.pdf (available on request from the corresponding author) and declare: (1) Financial support from AstraZeneca; Cancer Research UK; the National Institute for Health Research Health Technology Assessment programme; National Institutes of Health; BAD CAT; Queen Mary University of London; and the Wellcome Trust for the submitted work. (2) JJ has acted as a consultant to AstraZeneca, has received educational grants, and is chief investigator for the AspECT and ChOPIN trials; HB has been a consultant for AstraZeneca and Axcan Pharma, and is chief investigator for the BOSS trial; and KW is a consultant to various companies. (3) No spouses, partners, or children with relationships with commercial entities that might have an interest in the submitted work. (4) No non-financial interests that may be relevant to the submitted work.

Provenance and peer review: Commissioned; externally peer reviewed.

1   Shaheen NJ, Richter JE. Barrett'soesophagus. *Lancet*2009 7;373:850-61.
2   Spechler SJ, Fitzgerald RC, Prasad GA, Wang KK. History, molecular mechanisms, and endoscopic treatment of Barrett's esophagus. *Gastroenterology*2010;138:854-69.
3   Jankowski J, Harrison RF, Perry I, Balkwill F, Tselepis C. Seminar: Barrett's metaplasia. *Lancet*2000;356:2079-85.
4   Barrett's Dysplasia and Cancer Taskforce 'BAD CAT' consensus group. *International consensus of the management of dysplastic Barrett's and cancer.* World Gastroenterology Organisation. http://www.worldgastroenterology.org/international-consensus-of-management-of-dysplastic-barretts-and-cancer.html.

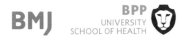

5   National Institute for Health and Clinical Excellence. *Ablative therapy for the treatment of Barrett's oesophagus* (clinical guideline CG106). NICE, 2010.

6   Moayyedi P, Talley NJ. Gastro-oesophageal reflux disease. *Lancet*2006;367:2086-100.

7   Ronkainen J, Pertti A, Storskrubb T, Johansson SE, Lind T, Bolling-Sternevald E, et al. Prevalence of Barrett's esophagus in the general population: an endoscopic study. *Gastroenterology*2005;129:1825-31.

8   Vakil N, van Zanten SV, Kahrilas P, Dent J, Jones R for the Global Consensus Group. The Montreal definition and classification of gastroesophageal reflux disease: a global evidence-based consensus. *Am J Gastroenterol*2006;101:1900-20.

9   Gerson LB, Banerjee S. Screening for Barrett's esophagus in asymptomatic women. *Gastrointest Endosc*2009;70:867-73.

10   Moayyedi P, Burch N, Akhtar-Danesh N, Enaganti SK, Harrison R, Talley NJ, et al. Mortality rates in patients with Barrett's oesophagus. *Aliment Pharmacol Ther*2008;27:316-20.

11   Jankowski JA, Provenzale D, Moayyedi P. Esophageal adenocarcinoma arising from Barrett's metaplasia has regional variations in the West. *Gastroenterology*2002;122:588-90.

12   Peng S, Cui Y, Xiao YL, Xiong LS, Hu PJ, Li CJ, et al. Prevalence of erosive esophagitis and Barrett's esophagus in the adult Chinese population. *Endoscopy*2009;41:1011-7.

13   Jankowski J, Wright NA, Meltzer S, Triadafilopoulos G, Geboes K, Casson A, et al. Molecular evolution of the metaplasia dysplasia adenocarcinoma sequence in the esophagus (MCS). *Am J Pathol*1999;154:965-74.

14   Robertson EV, Jankowski JA. Genetics of gastroesophageal cancer: paradigms, paradoxes and prognostic utility. *Am J Gastroenterol*2008;103:443-9.

15   Jankowski J, Odze R. Biomarkers in gastroenterology; between hype and hope comes histopathology. *Am J Gastroenterol*2009;104:1093-6.

16   National Institute for Health and Clinical Excellence. *Dyspepsia: managing dyspepsia in adults in primary care* (clinical guideline CG17). NICE, 2005.

17   Sharma P, Dent J, Armstrong D, Bergman J, Gossner L, Hoshihara Y, et al. The development and validation of an endoscopic grading system for Barrett's esophagus—the Prague C and M criteria. *Gastroenterology*2006;131:1392-9.

18   Sharma P, McQuaid K, Dent J, Fennerty MB, Sampliner R, Spechler S, et al. A critical review of the diagnosis and management of Barrett's esophagus. *Gastroenterology*2004;127:310-30.

19   Wong T, Tian J, Nagar AB. Barrett's surveillance identifies patients with early esophageal adenocarcinoma. *Am J Med*2010;123:462-7.

20   Rubenstein JH, Sonnenberg A, Davis J, McMahon L, Inadomi JM. Effect of a prior endoscopy on outcomes of esophageal adenocarcinoma among United States veterans. *Gastrointest Endosc*2008;68:849-55.

21   Shaheen NJ, Sharma P, Overholt BF, Wolfsen HC, Sampliner RE, Wang KK, et al. Radiofrequency ablation in Barrett's esophagus with dysplasia. *N Engl J Med*2009;360:2277-88.

22   British Society of Gastroenterology. *Guidelines for the diagnosis and management of Barrett's columnar-lined oesophagus.* BSG, 2005.

23   Das D, Ishaq S, Harrison R, Kosuri K, Harper E, deCaestecker J, et al. Management of Barrett's oesophagus in the UK: over treated, and under biopsied but improved by a national randomised trial. *Am J Gastroenterol*2008;103:1079-89.

24   Wang KK, Sampliner RE. Updated guidelines 2008 for the diagnosis, surveillance and therapy of Barrett's esophagus. *Am J Gastroenterol*2008;103:788-97.

25   Inadomi JM, Somsouk M, Madanick RD, Thomas JP, Shaheen NJ. A cost-utility analysis of ablative therapy for Barrett's esophagus. *Gastroenterology*2009;136:2101-14.

26   Cook MB, Wild CP, Everett SM, Hardie LJ, Bani-Hani KE, Martin IG, et al. Risk of mortality and cancer incidence in Barrett's esophagus. *Cancer Epidemiol Biomarkers Prev*2007;16:2090-6.

27   Epstein D, Bojke L, Sculpher MJ for the REFLUX trial group. Laparoscopic fundoplication compared with medical management for gastro-oesophageal reflux disease: cost effectiveness study. *BMJ*2009;339:b2576.

28   Obszynska J, Atherfold P, Nanji M, Glancy D, Santander S, Graham T, et al. Long-term proton pump induced hypergastrinaemia does induce lineage-specific restitution but not clonal expansion in benign Barrett's oesophagus *in vivo*. *Gut*2010;59:156-63.

29   Leedham S, Jankowski J. The evidence base of proton pump inhibitor chemopreventative agents in Barrett's esophagus: the good, the bad and the flawed. *Am J Gastroenterol*2007;102:21-3.

30   Leedham SJ, Preston SL, McDonald SAC, Elia G, Bhandari P, Poller D, et al. Individual crypt genetic heterogeneity and the origin of metaplastic glandular epithelium in human Barrett's oesophagus. *Gut*2008;57:1041-8.

31   Tselepis C, Perry I, Dawson C, Hardy R, Darnton J, McConkey C, et al. Tumour necrosis factor alpha in Barrett's metaplasia: a novel mechanism of action. *Oncogene*2002;39:6071-81.

32   Das D, Chilton A, Jankowski J. Oesophageal cancer prevention and the AspECT trial. In: Senn HJ, Kapp U, Otto F eds. *Cancer Prevention II.* Springer, 2009. pp 161-72.

33   Overholt BF, Wang KK, Burdick JS, Lightdale CJ, Kimmey M, Nava HR, et al for the International Photodynamic Group for High-Grade Dysplasia in Barrett's Esophagus. Five-year efficacy and safety of photodynamic therapy with Photofrin in Barrett's high-grade dysplasia. *Gastrointest Endosc*2007;66:460-8.

34   Hage M, Siersema PD, van Dekken H, Steyerberg EW, Haringsma J, van de Vrie W, et al. 5-aminolevulinic acid photodynamic therapy versus argon plasma coagulation for ablation of Barrett's oesophagus: a randomised trial. *Gut*2004;53:785-90.

35   Fight Oesophageal Reflux Together (FORT). http://refluxhelp.org/.

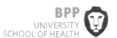

Oesophageal cancer

Jesper Lagergren, professor and consultant of surgery[1][2],
Pernilla Lagergren, associate professor and senior lecturer in healthcare science[1]

[1]Upper Gastrointestinal Research, Department of Molecular Medicine and Surgery, Karolinska Institutet, Stockholm SE-171 76, Sweden

[2]Division of Cancer Studies, King's College London, UK

Correspondence to:
jesper.lagergren@ki.se

Cite this as: BMJ 2010;341:c6280

DOI: 10.1136/bmj.c6280

http://www.bmj.com/content/341/bmj.c6280

The incidence of oesophageal cancer is increasing. While the incidence of squamous cell carcinoma of the oesophagus has recently been stable or declined in Western societies, the incidence of oesophageal adenocarcinoma has risen more rapidly than that of any other cancer in many countries since the 1970s, particularly among white men.[1] The UK has the highest reported incidence worldwide, for reasons yet unknown.[2] Overall, the prognosis for patients diagnosed with oesophageal cancer is poor, but those whose tumours are detected at an early stage have a good chance of survival. We outline strategies for prevention and describe presenting features of oesophageal cancer to assist generalists in diagnosing and referring patients early. Treatment is often highly invasive and alters patients' quality of life. We review the evidence from large randomised clinical trials, meta-analyses, and large cohort and case-control studies (preferably those of population based design, since they carry a lower risk of selection bias).

Who gets oesophageal cancer?

The two main histological types of oesophageal cancer, adenocarcinoma and squamous cell carcinoma (fig 1), have different causes and patterns of incidence.[1] Although the incidence of adenocarcinoma has surpassed that of squamous cell carcinoma in many Western countries, squamous cell carcinoma still represents 90% of all oesophageal cancer cases in most Eastern countries. Register based cohort studies have found that the incidence of oesophageal cancer increases with age and the average age of onset is about 65 to 70 years. Generally, men are more affected than women: the striking 7:1 male predominance of oesophageal adenocarcinoma remains unexplained.[1]

The origins of oesophageal cancer are multifactorial, including interactions among environmental risk exposures and nucleotide polymorphisms of inflammatory and tumour growth promoting pathways. The two main risk factors for oesophageal adenocarcinoma are gastro-oesophageal reflux and obesity.[3] Some gene-environment interaction patterns differ between patients with and without reflux.[4] Polymorphisms of genes coding for the obesity linked insulin-like growth factor may also be markers of risk.[5]

SOURCES AND SELECTION CRITERIA

We searched PubMed to identify peer reviewed original articles, meta-analyses, and reviews. Search terms were oesophageal cancer, cancer of the oesophagus, oesophageal adenocarcinoma, oesophageal squamous cell carcinoma, neoplasm and oesophagus, and oesophageal neoplasm. Only papers written in English were considered. We mainly included studies published during the recent few years where we deemed the scientific validity to be adequate.

The two main risk factors for squamous cell carcinoma of the oesophagus are tobacco smoking and high alcohol consumption, particularly in combination. The 3:1 male predominance is explained by differences in such exposures between the sexes. Infection with the bacterium *Helicobacter pylori*, which commonly occurs in the gastric mucosa, seems to reduce the risk of oesophageal adenocarcinoma by about half.[6] A possible mechanism is that the gastric atrophy that might follow such infection reduces the acidity and volume of the gastric juice, thereby lowering the risk of gastro-oesophageal reflux.[7]

Use of aspirin or non-steroidal anti-inflammatory drugs (NSAIDs) might decrease the risk of oesophageal cancer. A recent meta-analysis, mainly including case-control studies, showed a 35% decrease in the risk of oesophageal cancer among users of NSAIDs compared with non-users.[8] Factors affecting the choice of using NSAIDs, however, constitute a threat to the validity of observational studies, as highlighted in some investigations.[8][9]

How does a patient with oesophageal cancer present?

The cardinal symptoms of oesophageal cancer are progressive dysphagia and weight loss. The dysphagia is typically linked with vomiting of undigested food. Earlier symptoms may include discomfort or occasionally pain when swallowing. If such symptoms persist they should prompt an upper endoscopy. However, elasticity of the oesophagus means that onset of symptoms may not occur until the tumour is at an advanced stage. Late symptoms include hoarseness, caused by tumour overgrowth of the left laryngeal nerve, severe cough linked with tumour fistula between the oesophagus and the respiratory tract, and signs of metastatic disease—for example, ascites or palpable lymph node metastases.

How is the diagnosis made?

Figure 2 shows a flowchart for diagnosis.

Referral

Patients presenting with symptoms indicative of oesophageal cancer should undergo urgent endoscopy, preferably within one week. Patients with typical symptoms together with macroscopic signs of tumour on endoscopy require immediate referral (without need for histological confirmation) to a unit with relevant experience, usually an upper gastrointestinal surgery unit.

SUMMARY POINTS

- The incidence of oesophageal adenocarcinoma has increased during the past few decades, particularly among white men in the UK
- Oesophageal adenocarcinoma is associated with gastro-oesophageal reflux and obesity, whereas squamous cell carcinoma is associated with use of tobacco and alcohol
- Diagnosis is confirmed by endoscopy with biopsies, precise tumour stage is defined by more sophisticated radiological examinations
- A multidisciplinary approach is recommended in decision making and treatment
- Curatively intended treatment usually includes chemotherapy or radiochemotherapy followed by extensive surgery
- The overall prognosis for oesophageal cancer patients remains poor and several palliative options are available where cure is not possible

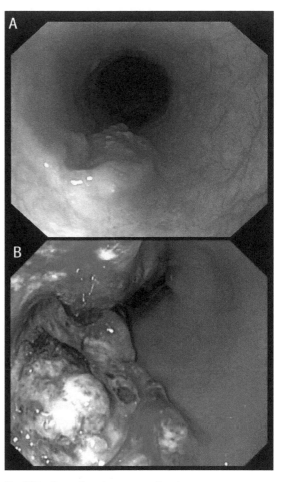

Primary tumour

The diagnosis is made by visualising a mass on endoscopy and by histological confirmation using biopsy samples collected from the mass and adjacent tissue. Figure 1 shows typical oesophageal cancer lesions as seen on endoscopy.

The importance of staging

Accurate staging allows for individually tailored treatment and the tumour needs to be staged before a treatment decision can be made. Recent advances in imaging techniques have contributed to more accurate staging. Cohort studies have shown that fluorodeoxyglucose combined positron emission tomography combined with computed tomography can be used to visualise early distant spread of tumours.[10] This tool has also shown promising results in the evaluation of the effects of preoperative oncological treatment.[11] Endoscopic ultrasonography can accurately measure the extent of local and regional tumour growth, which helps with staging.[12] More recently, endoscopic mucosal resection has become a useful staging technique for early intramucosal tumours. These tools have led to improved staging and less referral of patients with advanced or incurable disease for aggressive treatment.

Can oesophageal cancer be prevented?

Primary prevention

Avoidance of obesity, tobacco smoking, and alcohol intake decrease the risk of oesophageal cancer. Gastro-oesophageal reflux could also be reduced by controlling obesity and tobacco smoking, which are the two main established risk factors for reflux.

Secondary prevention

The hypothesis that antireflux medication and antireflux surgery reduce the incidence of oesophageal adenocarcinoma in people with reflux has been addressed mainly in uncontrolled studies. Robust data (from randomised trials, for example) supporting a preventive effect of antireflux medication against cancer are limited.[13 14] A large population based cohort study found no reduction in the risk of oesophageal adenocarcinoma with time after antireflux surgery.[15] The potential preventive effect of NSAIDs needs to be evaluated in randomised trials.

Is there a role for endoscopic screening?

Endoscopic screening for early oesophageal cancer requires selection of an easily identifiable high risk group. One such group might be white men with severe reflux and obesity. However, the feasibility of screening has to be based on the individual's absolute risk, which takes the incidence of the cancer into account. The high prevalence of reflux and the low incidence of oesophageal adenocarcinoma make endoscopic screening programmes of people with reflux symptoms, with or without known risk factors, unfeasible.[3] Moreover, there are no data showing a reduction in deaths from oesophageal adenocarcinoma resulting from endoscopic screening.[16] A better defined and much smaller, truly high risk group needs to be identified before any endoscopic screening can be considered. Measures other than endoscopy could be used for such screening in the future—for example, ingestible oesophageal sampling devices such as the Cytosponge.[17] The role of endoscopic surveillance of Barrett's oesophagus, a metaplasia associated with oesophageal adenocarcinoma, has been addressed in a recent review.[18]

Fig 1 (A) Small oesophageal squamous cell carcinoma seen on endoscopy. (B) Large necrotic and bleeding oesophageal adenocarcinoma seen on endoscopy. Used with permission from Dr Edgar Jaramillo

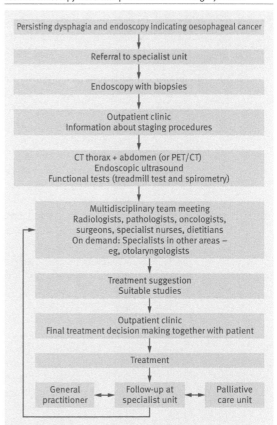

Persisting dysphagia and endoscopy indicating oesophageal cancer

↓

Referral to specialist unit

↓

Endoscopy with biopsies

↓

Outpatient clinic
Information about staging procedures

↓

CT thorax + abdomen (or PET/CT)
Endoscopic ultrasound
Functional tests (treadmill test and spirometry)

↓

Multidisciplinary team meeting
Radiologists, pathologists, oncologists, surgeons, specialist nurses, dietitians
On demand: Specialists in other areas – eg, otolaryngologists

↓

Treatment suggestion
Suitable studies

↓

Outpatient clinic
Final treatment decision making together with patient

↓

Treatment

General practitioner ↔ Follow-up at specialist unit ↔ Palliative care unit

Fig 2 Diagnosis with multidisciplinary team for cancer of the oesophagus suitable for curatively intended surgery

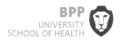

What is the approach to making a decision about treatment?

Patients with invasive oesophageal cancer need to be thoroughly evaluated regarding fitness and tumour stage. Tumours with local overgrowth into adjacent tissues or organs (T4) or with distant metastases (M1) are usually not eligible for curatively intended treatment. Physical activity, biological age, and comorbidities are considered when patient fitness is evaluated, and treadmill tests and spirometry are used whenever needed to objectively assess fitness. The final treatment recommendation should be based on a multidisciplinary meeting, as shown in figure 2, in which experienced doctors representing surgery, oncology, radiology, and pathology should participate. A multidisciplinary review of the radiology examinations, pathology reports, and the objective and subjective fitness of the patient could improve the accuracy of the treatment decisions and facilitate inclusion into clinical trials.[19] [20] The final decision must thereafter be taken together with the patient. The doctor responsible for the patient must thoroughly explain the reasons for the recommendation of the meeting. If there are doubts about this recommendation, a second opinion from a multidisciplinary team in another hospital is valuable.

What is the best approach to organisation of care?

The optimal treatment of patients with oesophageal cancer requires the resources and skills of a well coordinated multidisciplinary team (fig 2). Increased centralisation of treatment for patients with cancer of the oesophagus puts additional strain on resources at large centres, and these patients have high needs for supportive care.[21] Such circumstances emphasise the need for good coordination and continuity of the complex care pathway. A randomised clinical trial has emphasised the important role of specialised contact nurses in maintaining and coordinating the care pathway.[22] These nurses ideally keep in close contact with each patient and take part in all appointments with them.

Treatment with intent to cure—what are the options?

Treatment with a curative intent is undertaken only in patients who are considered fit enough to undergo extensive surgery and who have a tumour without any signs of overgrowth or distant metastases. The most common tumour stages among resected oesophageal cancer patients are advanced primary cancer without invasion into surrounding tissue or organs (T2-T3) with local or regional lymph node metastases (N1).[23]

Surgical resection remains the main option for curative treatment. Whether to offer chemotherapy or chemoradiotherapy before surgery is controversial because underpowered trials have produced contradictory results. Although the majority of individual studies do not show any benefit from such a strategy, data from more recent and larger randomised clinical trials indicate that preoperative chemotherapy or chemoradiotherapy improve survival compared with surgery alone.[24] [25] Moreover, data from case series indicate a curative potential for chemoradiotherapy alone without surgery, particularly in older non-surgical candidate patients, but randomised trials are needed to support a nonsurgical strategy.[26] Nevertheless, chemoradiotherapy alone is used in many patients who are not fit enough for surgery or in those who choose not to undergo surgery. Currently, a typical treatment strategy in fit patients with the most commonly occurring tumour stages (II-III) is chemotherapy followed by surgery.[25]

Surgical resection

Which is the preferred surgical approach?
Oesophageal cancer surgery is an extensive procedure with substantial risk of postoperative complications and long term morbidity.[27] A recent review concluded that fit patients are possibly best treated by a transthoracic oesophagectomy with removal of local and regional lymph nodes and vessels along with the oesophageal specimen (extended en bloc, two field lymphadenectomy). However, for patients who are less fit or those with junctional tumours or tumours of the gastric cardia, a transhiatal approach with a partly blunt dissection in the chest (through an abdominal and neck incision, without opening the thoracic wall) with a neck anastomosis may be a better option.[28]

Where to have surgery?
Since the in-hospital mortality after oesophagectomy is lower when centres and surgeons are experienced in this procedure, centralisation to high volume units has taken place in recent years.[21] Much of the lower risk of mortality at centres dealing with high volumes of such cases seems to be explained by better handling of complications.[29] The risk of complications seems, however, to be more related to the skills of the individual surgeon than to volume alone.[30]

How to improve quality of life outcomes?
Large, population based cohort studies have shown that patients who undergo surgical resection of an oesophageal tumour have poor health related quality of life in the short and long term.[27] These findings highlight a need to improve the procedure—for example, by better tailoring of surgery, and through the development of less invasive techniques such as minimally invasive, robotic, and vagal nerve preserving oesophagectomy.[31] [32] [33] Such developments must, however, be based on results from large multicentre randomised clinical trials that are well designed rather than on case series. Generally, patients undergoing surgical resection should be enrolled in a randomised trial when possible.

Endoscopic treatments

Various endoscopic approaches are emerging as potential alternatives to surgical treatment in the highly selected group of patients with high grade dysplastic mucosa and early intramucosal oesophageal cancer.[34] [35] Such local procedures might be justified in view of the low likelihood of lymph node metastases in early tumours, but more research is needed before general clinical recommendations can be given. Endoscopic mucosal resection, photodynamic therapy, argon plasma coagulation, and radiofrequency ablation can all induce regression of dysplasia.[14] A large randomised trial found that radiofrequency ablation resulted in eradication rates of 94% in patients with dysplasia, compared with a sham treatment,[35] and it might become the endoscopic treatment of choice, combined with endoscopic mucosal resection for visible, focal lesions. Until longer term trials become available, however, radiofrequency ablation should only be used in expert centres with careful follow-up.[14] For the vast majority of patients with an invasive tumour, endoscopic therapy is, at least currently, not a treatment option.

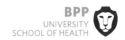

Who will get palliative care and what will it involve?

Large population based cohort studies estimate that up to 75% of patients with oesophageal cancer are never treated with a curative intent, mainly because of advanced tumour stage or poor physical condition.[23] For incurable disease, patients need the support of expert palliative care professionals who are familiar with the pros and cons of the available palliative treatments. Several approaches can improve health related quality of life in patients who are ineligible for surgery (box), and the best approach involves treatment that is tailored to offer the best possible outcome for the patient. Patients with advanced oesophageal cancer have a short median survival and thus are no longer offered surgical resection for palliation only. A major challenge is to relieve dysphagia as effectively as possible. A recent Cochrane systematic review of interventions aimed at relieving dysphagia concluded that self expanding metallic stents and intraluminal brachytherapy (local radiotherapy) seem to offer the best palliation.[36] Chemotherapy and external beam radiotherapy can also palliate dysphagia. We stress that a well functioning care pathway is just as important for patients in whom the aim of therapy is palliation, as it is for those where curatively intended treatment is possible. Support from a palliative care team, including, for example, pain therapy, feeding, or general support, is valuable for these patients.

Is the prognosis for patients with oesophageal cancer improving?

Population based cohort studies have shown that the overall prognosis for patients with cancer of the oesophagus has improved slightly during the past 20 years.[37] However, despite efforts to improve surveillance, diagnostic procedures, and treatment, the overall five year survival in oesophageal adenocarcinoma remains lower than 15%.[37] Population based studies from Europe have shown the five year survival after curatively intended surgery for oesophageal adenocarcinoma to be 30-35%, a figure that has improved substantially during the past few years, whereas the population based five year survival for stage specific tumours has been reported to be 67%, 33%, and 8% in stages 0-I, II, and III, respectively.[23] Unfortunately, patients with tumour recurrence after surgery cannot usually be cured because of the lack of effective second line treatment.

Which might be the future directions?

Primary prevention by avoidance of preventable risk exposures might help to reduce the incidence of oesophageal cancer in the future. It should also be possible to identify true high risk patients for oesophageal cancer who might benefit from tailored surveillance strategies, possibly by combining risk factor information with future genetic markers that might predict a risk of progression.

Improvements in the treatment of oesophageal cancer, in regard to survival and to health related quality of life, are best achieved through large randomised clinical trials to investigate new chemotherapeutic agents and new, less invasive, surgical approaches.

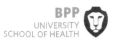

Contributors: JL and PL contributed to the concept and writing of this article.

Funding: JL and PL are funded by the Swedish Research Council and the Swedish Cancer Society.

Competing interests: Both authors have completed the Unified Competing Interest form and declare no support for the submitted work; no relationships that might have an interest in the submitted work; and no non-financial interests that may be relevant to the submitted work.

Provenance and peer review: Not commissioned; externally peer reviewed.

1   Cook MB, Chow WH, Devesa SS. Oesophageal cancer incidence in the United States by race, sex, and histologic type, 1977-2005. Br J Cancer2009;101:855-9.

2   Bollschweiler E, Wolfgarten E, Gutschow C, Holscher AH. Demographic variations in the rising incidence of esophageal adenocarcinoma in white males. Cancer2001;92:549-55.

3   Lagergren J, Ye W, Bergstrom R, Nyren O. Utility of endoscopic screening for upper gastrointestinal adenocarcinoma. JAMA2000;284:961-2.

4   Zhai R, Chen F, Liu G, Su L, Kulke MH, Asomaning K, et al. Interactions among genetic variants in apoptosis pathway genes, reflux symptoms, body mass index, and smoking indicate two distinct etiologic patterns of esophageal adenocarcinoma. J Clin Oncol2010;28:2445-51.

5   McElholm AR, McKnight AJ, Patterson CC, Johnston BT, Hardie LJ, Murray LJ. A population-based study of IGF axis polymorphisms and the esophageal inflammation, metaplasia, adenocarcinoma sequence. Gastroenterology2010;139:204-12.e3.

6   Rokkas T, Pistiolas D, Sechopoulos P, Robotis I, Margantinis G. Relationship between Helicobacter pylori infection and esophageal neoplasia: a meta-analysis. Clin Gastroenterol Hepatol2007;5:1413-7, 1417.e1-2.

7   Anderson LA, Murphy SJ, Johnston BT, Watson RG, Ferguson HR, Bamford KB, et al. Relationship between Helicobacter pylori infection and gastric atrophy and the stages of the oesophageal inflammation, metaplasia, adenocarcinoma sequence: results from the FINBAR case-control study. Gut2008;57:734-9.

8   Abnet CC, Freedman ND, Kamangar F, Leitzmann MF, Hollenbeck AR, Schatzkin A. Non-steroidal anti-inflammatory drugs and risk of gastric and oesophageal adenocarcinomas: results from a cohort study and a meta-analysis. Br J Cancer2009;100:551-7.

9   Heath EI, Canto MI, Piantadosi S, Montgomery E, Weinstein WM, Herman JG, et al. Secondary chemoprevention of Barrett's esophagus with celecoxib: results of a randomized trial. J Natl Cancer Inst2007;99:545-57.

10 Meyers BF, Downey RJ, Decker PA, Keenan RJ, Siegel BA, Cerfolio RJ, et al. The utility of positron emission tomography in staging of potentially operable carcinoma of the thoracic esophagus: results of the American College of Surgeons Oncology Group Z0060 trial. J Thorac Cardiovasc Surg2007;133:738-45.

11 Lordick F, Ott K, Krause BJ, Weber WA, Becker K, Stein HJ, et al. PET to assess early metabolic response and to guide treatment of adenocarcinoma of the oesophagogastric junction: the MUNICON phase II trial. Lancet Oncol2007;8:797-805.

12 Kelly S, Harris KM, Berry E, Hutton J, Roderick P, Cullingworth J, et al. A systematic review of the staging performance of endoscopic ultrasound in gastro-oesophageal carcinoma. Gut2001;49:534-9.

13 Nguyen DM, El-Serag HB, Henderson L, Stein D, Bhattacharyya A, Sampliner RE. Medication usage and the risk of neoplasia in patients with Barrett's esophagus. Clin Gastroenterol Hepatol2009;7:1299-304.

14 Rees JR, Lao-Sirieix P, Wong A, Fitzgerald RC. Treatment for Barrett's oesophagus. Cochrane Database Syst Rev2010;1:CD004060.

15 Lagergren J, Ye W, Lagergren P, Lu Y. The risk of esophageal adenocarcinoma after antireflux surgery. Gastroenterology2010;138:1297-301.

16 Rubenstein JH, Sonnenberg A, Davis J, McMahon L, Inadomi JM. Effect of a prior endoscopy on outcomes of esophageal adenocarcinoma among United States veterans. Gastrointest Endosc2008;68:849-55.

17 Kadri SR, Lao-Sirieix P, O'Donovan M, Debiram I, Das M, Blazeby JM, et al. Acceptability and accuracy of a non-endoscopic screening test for Barrett's oesophagus in primary care: cohort study. BMJ2010;341:c4372.

18 Jankowski J, Barr H, Wang K, Delaney B. Diagnosis and management of Barrett's oesophagus. BMJ2010;341:c4551.

19 Stephens MR, Lewis WG, Brewster AE, Lord I, Blackshaw GR, Hodzovic I, et al. Multidisciplinary team management is associated with improved outcomes after surgery for esophageal cancer. Dis Esophagus2006;19:164-71.

20 McNair AG, Choh CT, Metcalfe C, Littlejohns D, Barham CP, Hollowood A, et al. Maximising recruitment into randomised controlled trials: the role of multidisciplinary cancer teams. Eur J Cancer2008;44:2623-6.

21 Stitzenberg KB, Sigurdson ER, Egleston BL, Starkey RB, Meropol NJ. Centralization of cancer surgery: implications for patient access to optimal care. J Clin Oncol2009;27:4671-8.

22 Verschuur EM, Steyerberg EW, Tilanus HW, Polinder S, Essink-Bot ML, Tran KT, et al. Nurse-led follow-up of patients after oesophageal or gastric cardia cancer surgery: a randomised trial. Br J Cancer2009;100:70-6.

23 Rouvelas I, Zeng W, Lindblad M, Viklund P, Ye W, Lagergren J. Survival after surgery for oesophageal cancer: a population-based study. Lancet Oncol2005;6:864-70.

24 Medical Research Council Oesophageal Cancer Working Group. Surgical resection with or without preoperative chemotherapy in oesophageal cancer: a randomised controlled trial. Lancet2002;359:1727-33.

25 Gebski V, Burmeister B, Smithers BM, Foo K, Zalcberg J, Simes J. Survival benefits from neoadjuvant chemoradiotherapy or chemotherapy in oesophageal carcinoma: a meta-analysis. Lancet Oncol2007;8:226-34.

26 Morgan MA, Lewis WG, Casbard A, Roberts SA, Adams R, Clark GW, et al. Stage-for-stage comparison of definitive chemoradiotherapy, surgery alone and neoadjuvant chemotherapy for oesophageal carcinoma. Br J Surg2009;96:1300-7.

27 Djarv T, Lagergren J, Blazeby JM, Lagergren P. Long-term health-related quality of life following surgery for oesophageal cancer. Br J Surg2008;95:1121-6.

28 Lagarde SM, Vrouenraets BC, Stassen LP, van Lanschot JJ. Evidence-based surgical treatment of esophageal cancer: overview of high-quality studies. Ann Thorac Surg2010;89:1319-26.

29 Ghaferi AA, Birkmeyer JD, Dimick JB. Variation in hospital mortality associated with inpatient surgery. N Engl J Med2009;361:1368-75.

30 Rutegard M, Lagergren J, Rouvelas I, Lagergren P. Surgeon volume is a poor proxy for skill in esophageal cancer surgery. Ann Surg2009;249:256-61.

31 Gemmill EH, McCulloch P. Systematic review of minimally invasive resection for gastro-oesophageal cancer. Br J Surg2007;94:1461-7.

32 Galvani CA, Gorodner MV, Moser F, Jacobsen G, Chretien C, Espat NJ, et al. Robotically assisted laparoscopic transhiatal esophagectomy. Surg Endosc2008;22:188-95.

33 Pring C, Dexter S. A laparoscopic vagus-preserving Merendino procedure for early esophageal adenocarcinoma. Surg Endosc2010;24:1195-9.

34 Prasad GA, Wu TT, Wigle DA, Buttar NS, Wongkeesong LM, Dunagan KT, et al. Endoscopic and surgical treatment of mucosal (T1a) esophageal adenocarcinoma in Barrett's esophagus. Gastroenterology2009;137:815-23.

35 Shaheen NJ, Sharma P, Overholt BF, Wolfsen HC, Sampliner RE, Wang KK, et al. Radiofrequency ablation in Barrett's esophagus with dysplasia. N Engl J Med2009;360:2277-88.

36 Sreedharan A, Harris K, Crellin A, Forman D, Everett SM. Interventions for dysphagia in oesophageal cancer. Cochrane Database Syst Rev2009;4:CD005048.

37 Sundelof M, Ye W, Dickman PW, Lagergren J. Improved survival in both histologic types of oesophageal cancer in Sweden. Int J Cancer2002;99:751-4.

Related links

bmj.com/archive
- Managing frostbite (2010;341:c5864)
- Management of venous ulcer disease (2010;341:c6045)
- Translating genomics into improved healthcare (2010;341:c5945)
- Extracorporeal life support (2010;341:c5317)
- Managing diabetic retinopathy (2010;341:c5400)

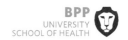

The diagnosis and management of gastric cancer

Sri G Thrumurthy, honorary research fellow[1], M Asif Chaudry, oesophagogastric surgeon[2], Daniel Hochhauser, Kathleen Ferrier professor of medical oncology[3], Muntzer Mughal, honorary clinical professor and head [1]

[1]Department of Upper Gastrointestinal Surgery, University College London Hospital, London NW1 2BU, UK

[2]Department of Upper Gastrointestinal Surgery, St Thomas' Hospital, London, UK

[3]UCL Cancer Institute, University College London, London, UK

Correspondence to: M Mughal
muntzer.mughal@uclh.nhs.uk

Cite this as: BMJ 2013;347:f6367

DOI: 10.1136/bmj.f6367

http://www.bmj.com/content/347/bmj.f6367

Age standardised mortality rates for gastric cancer are 14.3 per 100 000 in men and 6.9 per 100 000 in women worldwide.[1] Incidence shows clear regional and sex variations—rates are highest in eastern Asia, eastern Europe, and South America and lowest in northern and southern Africa.[1] Early diagnosis is crucial because of the possibility of early metastasis to the liver, pancreas, omentum, oesophagus, bile ducts, and regional and distant lymph nodes.[2] Using evidence from large randomised controlled trials, meta-analyses, cohort studies, and case-control studies this review aims to outline preventive strategies, highlight the presenting features of gastric cancer, and guide generalists in early diagnosis, referral, and treatment.

What is gastric cancer?

Gastric cancer refers to tumours of the stomach that arise from the gastric mucosa (adenocarcinoma), connective tissue of the gastric wall (gastrointestinal stromal tumours), neuroendocrine tissue (carcinoid tumours), or lymphoid tissue (lymphomas). This review will focus on gastric adenocarcinoma (>90% of all gastric cancers), which may be polypoid, ulcerating, or diffuse infiltrative (linitis plastica) in macroscopic form.

Who gets gastric cancer?

Epidemiological data from the American Cancer Society suggest that gastric cancer is the fourth most common cancer in men (after lung, prostate, and colorectal cancer) and the fifth most common cancer In women (after breast, cervical, colorectal, and lung cancer) globally.[3] Gastric cancer accounts for 8% of the total number of cases of cancer and 10% of annual deaths from cancer worldwide.

SOURCES AND SELECTION CRITERIA

We searched PubMed to identify peer reviewed original articles, meta-analyses, and reviews. Search terms were gastric cancer, cancer of the stomach, gastric adenocarcinoma, gastro-oesophageal cancer, gastric neoplasm, and neoplasm of the stomach. We considered only those papers that were written in English, published within the past 10 years, and which described studies that had adequate scientific validity.

It has a significantly higher fatality to case ratio (70%) than prostate (30%) and breast (33%) cancer.[4]

Men are twice as likely as women to develop gastric cancer,[3] with an expected worldwide incidence of 640 000 cases in men and 350 000 cases in women in 2011[3] (fig 1) and peak age of incidence of 60-84 years.[5][6] The global incidence of gastric cancer has decreased significantly over time—the age standardised incidence in the United Kingdom decreased from 44 per 100 000 in 1975-77 to 18 per 100 000 in 2006-08).[7] This is partly because of reductions in chronic Helicobacter pylori infection and smoking in the developed world and partly the result of increased use of refrigeration, availability of fresh fruit and vegetables, and decreased reliance on salted or preserved foods.[3][8]

What are the risk factors for gastric cancer?

Helicobacter pylori

H pylori infection is widely regarded as the most important modifiable risk factor for gastric cancer. More than 2 billion people are infected worldwlde, although fewer than 0.5% will develop gastric adenocarcinoma.[4] A meta-analysis of 34 cohort and case-control studies found that H pylori carried a relative risk of gastric cancer of 3.02 (95% confidence interval 1.92 to 4.74) in high risk settings (China, Japan, and Korea) and 2.56 (1.99 to 3.29) in low risk settings (western Europe, Australia, and United States).[10]

Cigarette smoking

A meta-analysis of 42 cohort, case-cohort, and nested case-control studies across Asia, Europe, and the US found a relative risk of 1.53 (1.42 to 1.65) of developing gastric cancer in people who smoked.[11] Results from a retrospective cohort study of 699 patients, of whom 59% were current or ex-smokers, showed that tobacco use was associated with a 43% increase in disease recurrence and death from gastric cancer (hazard ratio 1.43, 1.08 to1.91; P=0.01).[12] Smoking was also an independent and significant risk factor for other measures of recurrence and survival, including five year disease-free survival (1.46; P=0.007) and overall survival (1.48; P=0.003).[12]

SUMMARY POINTS

- The incidence of gastric cancer is highest in eastern Asia, eastern Europe, and South America, and it affects twice as many men as women
- Risk factors for gastric cancer include *Helicobacter pylori* infection, cigarette smoking, high alcohol intake, excess dietary salt, lack of refrigeration, inadequate fruit and vegetable consumption, and pernicious anaemia
- Patients present with weight loss and abdominal pain, although those with proximal or gastro-oesophageal junction tumours may present with dysphagia
- Upper gastrointestinal endoscopy with biopsy is used to confirm the diagnosis; precise tumour stage is defined by more sophisticated radiological investigations
- Multidisciplinary approach to treatment: early gastric cancer is treated with surgery alone, whereas advanced disease is usually managed with chemotherapy before and after surgery, or postoperative chemoradiation
- Metastatic disease is managed with chemotherapy or chemoradiation as well as supportive care measures

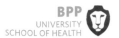

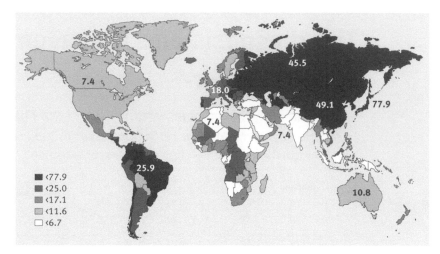

Fig 1 Worldwide annual incidence (per 100 000) of gastric cancer in men. Numbers on the map indicate regional average values. Adapted, with permission, from an article by the International Agency for Research on Cancer[9]

In a Norwegian prospective cohort study with 69 962 participants, the absolute lifetime risk of gastric cancer was 0.776% in heavy smokers (.20 cigarettes/day), 1.511% in long term smokers (.30 years), and 0.658% in those who had never smoked.[13]

Alcohol
A meta-analysis of 44 case-control and 15 cohort studies of 34 557 cases of gastric cancer found a slightly increased risk (relative risk 1.07, 1.01 to 1.13) in people with light to moderate alcohol consumption and a greater increase (1.20, 1.01 to 1.44) for heavy alcohol drinkers (.4 drinks/day).[14] A prospective European cohort study estimated that a high alcohol intake (>60 g/day) carried a relative risk of gastric cancer of 1.65 (1.06 to 2.58) and an absolute lifetime risk of 0.256%.[15]

Dietary salt and food preservation
A meta-analysis of cohort studies from the World Cancer Research Fund found that each gram of salt consumed each day increased the relative risk of gastric cancer by a factor of 1.08 (1.00 to 1.17).[16] A Japanese prospective cohort study with 2467 participants found an independent association between salt intake and incidence of gastric cancer. Compared with people who consumed less than 10 g of salt per day, those who consumed more than 16 g per day had a relative risk of 2.98 (1.53 to 5.82) of developing gastric cancer.[17] This correlation was stronger in the presence of *H pylori* infection and atrophic gastritis, suggesting that mucosal damage induced by salt intake increases the risk of persistent *H pylori* infection.[4]

The lack of refrigeration and use of salt based food preservatives have been associated with an increased risk of gastric cancer in socioeconomically deprived regions.[18] A cross sectional Korean study of multiple national statistics databases found a threefold decrease in age standardised mortality from gastric cancer between 1983 and 2007 (46.1/1 000 000 v 16.9/100 000), which was significantly and independently correlated with an increase in the number of refrigerators per household.[19]

Dietary fruit and vegetables
A Swedish cohort study of 82 002 participants and a total of 139 cases of gastric cancer found that an intake of two to five servings of fruit and vegetables a day decreased the risk of gastric cancer when compared with less than one serving a day (hazard ratio 0.56, 0.34 to 0.93). This suggested a 44% reduction in the incidence of gastric cancer with increased fruit and vegetable intake.[20] A meta-analysis of cohort studies from the World Cancer Research Fund suggested a relative risk of 0.81 (0.58 to 1.14) per 100 g per day of non-starchy vegetables and fruit consumed.[16]

Pernicious anaemia
A recent meta-analysis of 27 cohort and case-control studies found an overall relative risk for gastric cancer in pernicious anaemia of 6.8 (2.6 to 18.1).[21] Although heterogeneity between the studies was not significant at the 5% level, the quality of the studies was variable, so further high quality studies are needed to confirm this higher risk before instigating surveillance for these patients.

Genetic syndromes
Hereditary diffuse gastric cancer is a syndrome caused by a germline mutation in the *CDH1* gene, which encodes E-cadherin, a calcium dependent cell adhesion protein involved in cell-cell interaction and cell polarity. The condition is characterised by early onset (age <40 years) of diffuse gastric adenocarcinoma, an autosomal dominant inheritance pattern, and increased risk of lobular breast cancer and signet ring cell colon cancer.[22] Prospective analysis of a genetic database showed that this mutation carries a cumulative risk of gastric cancer of 67% in men and 83% in women.[23]

Lynch syndrome, an autosomal dominant syndrome involving defective DNA mismatch repair and an increased risk of colorectal and other visceral cancers, is also associated with a higher incidence of gastric cancer.[24] A Dutch prospective cohort study of 2014 people found an increased lifetime risk of gastric cancer in both men (8%) and women (5.3%),[25] prompting consideration of surveillance gastroscopy for patients with this syndrome who carry an *MLH1* or *MSH2* mutation.

How do patients with gastric cancer present?
Because patients with gastric cancer often present with vague and non-specific symptoms, the diagnosis is challenging. Data from the US National Cancer Institute suggest that patients are typically male smokers aged 60-84 years,[5] who exhibit the cardinal symptoms of upper abdominal pain and weight loss.[26] Less common symptoms

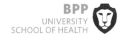

Common conditions that can mimic the symptoms of gastric cancer

Differential diagnosis	Features suggestive of cancer	Differentiating investigations
Benign oesophageal stricture	No history of gastro-oesophageal reflux disease	Endoscopy and biopsy
Peptic ulcer disease	Overt gastrointestinal bleeding, weight loss, early satiety, palpable masses or lymphadenopathy, jaundice, progressive dysphagia, recurrent vomiting	Endoscopy and biopsy; patients with peptic ulcers should undergo repeat endoscopy after treatment to assess healing
	Family history of cancer	
	Age of symptom onset >55 years	
Achalasia*	Duration of symptoms <6 months	Oesophageal manometry, endoscopy, and biopsy*
	Age at presentation >60 years	
	Substantial weight loss relative to symptom duration	

Gastro-oesophageal cancer that initially presents with the clinical and investigative findings of achalasia is known as pseudoachalasia.

BOX 1 ALARM FEATURES SUGGESTIVE OF GASTRIC CANCER[26]

- New onset dyspepsia (in patients aged >55 years)
- Family history of upper gastrointestinal cancer
- Unintended weight loss
- Upper or lower gastrointestinal bleeding
- Progressive dysphagia
- Odynophagia
- Unexplained iron deficiency anaemia
- Persistent vomiting
- Palpable mass or lymphadenopathy
- Jaundice

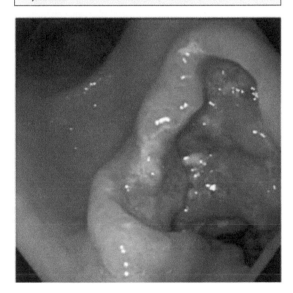

Fig 2 Endoscopic image of an advanced ulcerated gastric tumour

are nausea, dysphagia (in proximal and gastro-oesophageal junction tumours), and evidence of melaena. Typical textbook descriptions such as Virchow's node (prominent left supraclavicular node) and Sister Mary Joseph's nodule (periumbilical nodule) are rarely seen in primary care.

A meta-analysis of 15 studies with 57 363 patients found that "alarm" features (box 1) had a pooled sensitivity of 67% (54% to 83%), pooled specificity of 66% (55% to 79%), and a pooled positive likelihood ratio of 2.74 (1.47 to 5.24).[27] The National Cancer Institute study suggested that although these symptoms have limited predictive value, their identification will probably remain part of dyspepsia management strategies in the United Kingdom[28] and US[26] until better approaches emerge.

The table lists the common differential diagnoses of gastric cancer.

Who should be referred for further investigations?

UK consensus guidelines in 2011 recommended that patients aged 55 years or more with new onset dyspepsia and all those with alarm symptoms should undergo urgent (within two weeks) upper gastrointestinal endoscopy.[28] If macroscopic signs of tumour (ulceration, masses, or mucosal changes) are found on endoscopy, immediate referral to a specialist upper gastrointestinal surgery unit is warranted.

How is gastric cancer diagnosed?

Endoscopy and biopsy of primary tumour

British consensus guidelines recommend that the diagnosis is made by visualising a mass on endoscopy and by histological confirmation using at least six biopsy samples from the mass and adjacent tissue (fig 2).[28] If the biopsy result of a suspicious lesion is negative, a repeat biopsy is needed. Pathological examination may include immunohistochemistry for HER2/neu, which is overexpressed in a subset of gastric cancers,[29] because targeted treatment may be an option for these tumours.[30]

Staging of confirmed gastric cancer

Recent advances in imaging have enabled more accurate staging, and fewer patients with advanced or incurable disease are now referred for aggressive treatment. A meta-analysis of 54 studies of 5601 patients suggested that endoscopic ultrasonography had a sensitivity and specificity of 86% and 91% for T stage tumours and 69% and 84% for N stage tumours, respectively (box 2).[31] However, owing to the limited capacity of this technique for staging mucosal disease, current UK guidelines advocate its use only for gastro-oesophageal junction tumours and selected gastric cancers.[28]

A meta-analysis of 33 patients showed that computed tomography of the abdomen detected liver metastases with a sensitivity of 74% (59% to 85%) and specificity of 99% (97% to 100%) and peritoneal metastases with a sensitivity of 33% (16% to 56%) and specificity of 99% (98% to 100%). Computed tomography of the chest is indicated only in patients with proximal or gastro-oesophageal junction tumours. Positron emission tomography combined with computed tomography has become increasingly available in tertiary centres. A recent prospective cohort study of 113 patients found that this technique detected metastatic disease with a sensitivity of 35% (19% to 55%) and specificity of 99% (93% to 100%).[32]

When imaging investigations are negative, staging laparoscopy should be used to detect peritoneal and metastatic disease under 5 mm in diameter, which may be missed even with high quality radiological imaging. Laparoscopy also enables peritoneal cytology and biopsies to be obtained from suspicious lesions and should be considered before definitive treatment. A retrospective review of 511 patients found that staging laparoscopy effectively changed treatment decisions in 28.0% of patients with gastric cancer after computed tomography and endoscopic ultrasonography.[33]

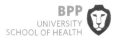

BOX 2 AMERICAN JOINT COMMITTEE ON CANCER (AJCC) CANCER STAGING, 2010

Primary tumour (T)

- TX: primary tumour cannot be assessed
- T0: no evidence of primary tumour
- Tis: carcinoma in situ, intra-epithelial tumour
- T1: tumour invades lamina propria, muscularis mucosae, or submucosa
- T2: tumour invades muscularis propria
- T3: tumour penetrates subserosal connective tissue
- T4: tumour invades serosa (visceral peritoneum) or adjacent structures

Regional lymph nodes (N)

- NX: regional lymph node(s) cannot be assessed
- N0: no regional lymph node metastases
- N1: metastasis in 1-2 regional lymph nodes
- N2 = metastasis in 3-6 regional lymph nodes
- N3: metastasis in ≥7 regional lymph nodes

Distant metastasis (M)

- M0: no distant metastasis
- M1: distant metastasis

Stage grouping

- Stage 0: Tis N0 M0
- Stage IA: T1 N0 M0
- Stage IB: T2 N0 M0; T1 N1 M0
- Stage IIA: T3 N0 M0; T2 N1 M0; T1 N2 M0
- Stage IIB: T4a N0 M0; T3 N1 M0; T2 N2 M0; T1 N3 M0
- Stage IIIA: T4a N1 M0; T3 N2 M0; T2 N3 M0
- Stage IIIB: T4b N0 M0; T4b N1 M0; T4a N2 M0; T3 N3 M0
- Stage IIIC: T4b N2 M0; T4b N3 M0; T4a N3 M0
- Stage IV: any T any N M1

What is the approach to making a decision about treatment?

Thorough oncological staging and preoperative evaluation of fitness are vital for patients with invasive gastric cancer. Tumours that show local invasion (T4) or distant metastases (M1) are typically not amenable to curative treatment. The patient's fitness is determined by physical activity status, biological age, and comorbidities. It can be measured objectively by lung function and cardiopulmonary exercise testing. Final treatment recommendations are made at a multidisciplinary team meeting involving experienced surgeons, radiologists, pathologists, and oncologists. The final decision should be made together with the patient after the clinician carefully explains the recommended treatment.

Treatment with intent to cure—what are the options?

Surgical resection

Current UK and US guidelines recommend that all medically fit patients with regionally confined disease undergo primary surgical resection for up to stage IA tumours and surgery after neoadjuvant therapy for stage II-III tumours.[28] [34] The extent of surgical resection usually depends on tumour location. Although total gastrectomy is routinely performed for proximal tumours, multicentre randomised controlled trials have shown similar survival rates after subtotal gastrectomy for distal tumours.[35] [36]

The extent of lymph node dissection is a key consideration during surgery. Recent randomised controlled trials have advocated D2 lymph node dissection (perigastric nodes and nodes along the coeliac trunk) over D1 dissection (perigastric nodes only) because D2 dissection results in lower rates of locoregional recurrence and cancer related death, despite increased rates of early morbidity and mortality.[37] [38] Most high volume centres currently perform modified (spleen preserving) D2 dissections.

Randomised trials of minimally invasive gastrectomy versus open surgery suggest that long term outcomes are similar, although laparoscopic procedures offer better pain control and are associated with reduced blood loss and postoperative complication rates.[39] [40]

A prospective study of 827 patients found that robotic gastrectomy produced better short term and comparable oncological outcomes compared with laparoscopic gastrectomy.[41]

Early gastric cancer (T1a) can be treated with endoscopic mucosal resection if it is confined to the mucosa, less than 2 cm in diameter, of low or moderate differentiation, and exhibits no ulceration or lymphovascular involvement.[28] [42]

Neoadjuvant and adjuvant treatment

Systemic treatment is given before definitive surgery (neoadjuvant) or after resection (adjuvant) to treat micrometastases and improve outcome. The pivotal Medical Research Council Adjuvant Gastric Infusional Chemotherapy (MAGIC) trial randomised 503 patients with cancer of the gastro-oesophageal junction or gastric body to surgery alone or three preoperative cycles of chemotherapy (epirubicin, cisplatin, 5-fluorouracil), followed when possible by three cycles after surgery.[43] Chemotherapy resulted in a significantly greater five year survival than surgery alone (36% v 23%; P=0.009), indicating significant benefit for patients with stage 2 disease or higher, although the necessity for six cycles was unresolved. This has become the standard of care for resectable gastric cancer in the UK. A later multi-centre randomised trial in patients with advanced disease, which found that oxaliplatin can replace cisplatin and that oral fluoropyrimidine capecitabine can replace the inconvenient 5-fluorouracil infusion, has resulted in wider neoadjuvant use of these agents.[44]

Adjuvant chemoradiation also showed benefit in a randomised trial of 556 patients with resected adenocarcinoma of the stomach or gastro-oesophageal junction, who were randomly assigned to surgery plus postoperative chemoradiation (fluorouracil/calcium folinate for five days then 4500 cGy radiation at 180 cGy/day, five days a week for five weeks) or surgery alone.[45] One month after completing radiotherapy, two five day cycles of fluorouracil plus calcium folinate were given. The median survival of the adjuvant chemoradiation group was 36 months compared with 27 months in the surgery alone group (P=0.005). The trial was criticised for poor survival in the surgery alone arm, with only 10% of patients in the surgery arm receiving a D2 resection and D0 resection in more than 50% of patients. In addition, toxicity was high, and this regimen—although used in the US—has not been widely adopted in the UK.

A meta-analysis of adjuvant chemotherapy trials suggests that such treatment is beneficial, although the size of the effect is small and the optimal agents are unclear. Adjuvant chemotherapy was associated with a significant benefit on overall survival (hazard ratio 0.82, 0.76 to 0.90; P <0.001) and disease-free survival (0.82, 0.75 to 0.90; P<0.001), with five year overall survival increasing from 49.6% to 55.3% with chemotherapy.[46]

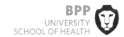
Patients who undergo chemotherapy for gastric cancer may develop fatigue, nausea, vomiting, alopecia, neuropathy, and other side effects specific to the agents used.[43] [44] Neutropenic sepsis is potentially life threatening and may present with fever alone. Its recognition and management are crucial in the primary care setting.[47]

Where to have surgery for gastric cancer?

In recent years, cancer services have become centralised to high volume units, and studies have shown improved in-hospital outcomes when centres and surgeons are experienced at major cancer surgery.[48] Prospective nationwide data from the American College of Surgeons' national surgical quality improvement programme attributed the lower mortality rates at high volume centres to better management of postoperative complications.[49] Large prospective studies suggest that, although postoperative mortality and mid-term survival are better in high volume centres,[50] long term survival and recurrence may be independent of hospital volume.[51]

What does palliative care involve and what are the considerations?

Up to half of all patients with gastric cancer present with incurable disease and require palliative treatment.[28] Best supportive care aims to prevent or alleviate symptoms such as bleeding, obstruction, pain, nausea, and vomiting and to improve quality of life for patients and caregivers. This should be a key focus of the multidisciplinary team, taking into account performance status and patient preference, with early direct involvement of the palliative care team and clinical nurse specialists.

Treatment of advanced disease

Chemotherapy and chemoradiotherapy

Randomised trials have shown that chemotherapy improves quality of life over best supportive care alone in patients with metastatic gastric cancer.[52] [53] In the UK, the epirubicin, cisplatin, and 5-fluorouracil regimen or variants including oxaliplatin and capecitabine are most widely used. In the REAL-2 study, which compared similar regimens, median survival was 9.3-11.2 months.[44]

A randomised Korean trial of patients after initial chemotherapy showed a small survival benefit from second line treatment with taxane or irinotecan based chemotherapy—5.3 months for 33 patients in the chemotherapy arm and 3.8 months in 69 patients in the best supportive care arm (hazard ratio 0.657, 0.485 to 0.891; one sided P=0.007).[52] Patient preference, performance status, and potential side effects must be factored into decisions to administer such treatment.

A fifth of patients with gastric cancer have tumours with amplification of *HER2* (erbB2).[54] The randomised ToGA (Trastuzumab with Chemotherapy in HER2-Positive Advanced Gastric Cancer) study of 594 patients showed that targeted treatment with herceptin (trastuzumab) plus chemotherapy (cisplatin with capecitabine or 5-fluorouracil) was superior to chemotherapy alone, with a median survival of 13.8 versus 11.1 months, respectively (P=0.0048).[54] For patients whose tumours showed high *HER2* expression, median overall survival was 16.0 months (15 to 19) in those assigned to trastuzumab plus chemotherapy versus 11.8 months (10 to 13) in those assigned to chemotherapy alone. The ToGA trial established this treatment as standard for *HER2* positive patients with advanced cancer.

Palliative surgery

Palliative gastrectomy may benefit patients with obstruction of the gastric outlet secondary to antral tumours, or for incomplete dysphagia caused by tumours of the cardia. The decision to manage patients palliatively should not limit the extent of surgery; a large retrospective study has shown that more radical procedures may improve survival and quality of life in eligible patients.[55] A gastrojejunostomy, which can often be performed laparoscopically, and endoscopic stenting can be performed in those who are not eligible for first line surgical procedures.

How should patients be followed up after treatment?

Routine blood tests are needed to monitor bone marrow function during chemotherapy, and nutritional monitoring is recommended after surgery (for example, vitamin B12 monitoring after proximal or total gastrectomy). Despite the lack of randomised evidence evaluating follow-up strategies,[28] most UK based tertiary centres review patients every four months for three years, and annually thereafter; with radiographic imaging and endoscopy performed as clinically indicated. Patients with recurrent disease may benefit from surgery if complete resection is possible, although most patients undergo salvage chemotherapy, provided they have adequate performance status.[56]

Can gastric cancer be prevented?

Primary prevention

A meta-analysis of seven randomised trials conducted in high risk regions for gastric cancer (six in Asia) showed that eradication of *H pylori* reduced the risk of gastric cancer from 1.7% to 1.1% (relative risk 0.65, 0.43 to 0.98).[57] An intention to treat analysis of a recent Chinese randomised trial of 3365 participants found that a two week course of omeprazole and amoxicillin reduced the incidence of gastric cancer by 39% within 15 years of randomisation, with similar but not significant reductions in mortality from gastric cancer.[58] The cost effectiveness of *H pylori* vaccination as long term prophylaxis against gastric cancer in the US has been extrapolated by simulation studies,[59] but evidence for the benefit of *H pylori* eradication in low risk regions is lacking.

A meta-analysis of case-control studies (14 442 cases and 73 918 controls) found that people who had ever smoked had a 43% greater risk of developing gastric cancer (odds ratio 1.43, 1.24 to 1.66) than never smokers, whereas current smokers had a 57% greater risk (1.57, 1.24 to 2.01).[60] This suggests that efforts to prevent cigarette smoking, and help people quit, would reduce the incidence of gastric cancer.

Secondary prevention

A multi-centre open label randomised controlled trial of 544 patients found that eradication of *H pylori* (with lansoprazole, amoxicillin, and clarithromycin) after endoscopic resection for early gastric cancer decreased the risk of developing metachronous gastric carcinoma (hazard ratio 0.339, 0.157 to 0.729; P=0.003) at three years' follow-up.[61] It recommended prophylactic eradication of *H pylori* after endoscopic resection of early gastric cancer to prevent the development of metachronous gastric carcinoma.

Is there a role for screening?

Screening for early gastric cancer requires the presence of an easily identifiable group with a high absolute risk. One such group might be middle aged male smokers with a history of

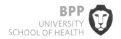

Helicobacter pylori infection or other pre-malignancy, such as Barrett's oesophagus. However, absolute risk also takes into account the incidence of cancer. The large numbers of potentially high risk people and the low incidence of gastric cancer make screening programmes unfeasible in all regions but those with a high incidence of gastric cancer (such as Japan and Chile).[62] In such regions, serological screening techniques involving pepsinogens, gastrin-17 and anti-*H pylori* (or anti-Cag-A, or both) antibodies are being evaluated, in addition to photofluorography and endoscopy.[63][64] Nanomaterial based breath testing has also recently been evaluated as a screening tool—a pilot study to a large multicentre trial found that this test has a sensitivity of 89% and specificity of 90% in distinguishing gastric cancer from benign gastric disease.[65]

Is the prognosis for patients with gastric cancer improving?

A single centre Korean study of 12 026 patients with gastric cancer found that the five year overall survival rate increased from 64.0% to 73.2% (P<0.001) from 1986 to 2006.[66] A large European study of 10 cancer registries across seven countries showed similar improvements but also detected marked variation in survival rates (28.0-44.3%) between certain countries, which could not be explained by operative mortality alone.[67]

Greater access to care; better diagnostic techniques for early detection; more rational surgical strategies; lower complication rates; advances in anaesthesia, perioperative care, and nutritional care; and wider use of systemic chemotherapy have been deemed responsible for such improvements in prognosis. These factors may also partly explain the discrepancies in postoperative survival rates across the world, although quantitative data are lacking for this.[66][67]

What treatment strategies lie on the horizon?

Novel targeted biological agents are being investigated in the treatment of gastric cancer. The role of anti-angiogenic agents such as bevacizumab (a monoclonal antibody targeting vascular endothelial growth factor) combined with chemotherapy is the subject of a randomised trial.[68] No targeted small molecules or antibodies have yet shown benefit in the management of gastric cancer, but greater understanding of the underlying molecular basis of the disease will undoubtedly suggest strategies for treatment in the future.

Contributors: SGT conceived the review, extracted evidence, and drafted the manuscript. MAC, DH, and MM coauthored the article (including article direction, interpreting the literature, and editing the manuscript). MM is guarantor.

Funding: Supported by the National Institute for Health Research University College London Hospitals Biomedical Research Centre. DH was supported by CRUK grant C2259/A16569.

Competing interests: We have read and understood the BMJ Group policy on declaration of interests and declare the following interests: None.

Provenance and peer review: Not commissioned; externally peer reviewed.

1 Ferlay J, Shin HR, Bray F, Forman D, Mathers C, Parkin DM. Estimates of worldwide burden of cancer in 2008: GLOBOCAN 2008. *Int J Cancer*2010;127:2893-917.
2 Coupland VH, Allum W, Blazeby JM, Mendall MA, Hardwick RH, Linklater KM, et al. Incidence and survival of oesophageal and gastric cancer in England between 1998 and 2007, a population-based study. *BMC Cancer*2012;12:11.
3 Jemal A, Bray F, Center MM, Ferlay J, Ward E, Forman D. Global cancer statistics. *CA Cancer J Clin*2011;61:69-90.
4 Guggenheim DE, Shah MA. Gastric cancer epidemiology and risk factors. *J Surg Oncol*2013;107:230-6.
5 Anderson WF, Camargo MC, Fraumeni JF Jr, Correa P, Rosenberg PS, Rabkin CS. Age-specific trends in incidence of noncardia gastric cancer in US adults. *JAMA*2010;303:1723-8.
6 Crew KD, Neugut AI. Epidemiology of gastric cancer. *World J Gastroenterol*2006;12:354-62.
7 Office for National Statistics. Cancer statistics registrations: registrations of cancer diagnosed in 2008, England. Series MB1 no 39. 2010. www.ons.gov.uk/ons/rel/vsob1/cancer-statistics-registrations--england--series-mb1-/no--39--2008/index.html .
8 Bertuccio P, Chatenoud L, Levi F, Praud D, Ferlay J, Negri E, et al. Recent patterns in gastric cancer: a global overview. *Int J Cancer*2009;125:666-73.
9 International Agency for Research on Cancer. Pathology and genetics of tumours of the digestive system. 2000. www.iarc.fr/en/publications/pdfs-online/pat-gen/bb2/bb2-cover.pdf
10 Cavaleiro-Pinto M, Peleteiro B, Lunet N, Barros H. Helicobacter pylori infection and gastric cardia cancer: systematic review and meta-analysis. *Cancer Causes Control*2011;22:375-87.
11 Ladeiras-Lopes R, Pereira AK, Nogueira A, Pinheiro-Torres T, Pinto I, Santos-Pereira R, et al. Smoking and gastric cancer: systematic review and meta-analysis of cohort studies. *Cancer Causes Control*2008;19:689-701.
12 Smyth EC, Capanu M, Janjigian YY, Kelsen DK, Coit D, Strong VE, et al. Tobacco use is associated with increased recurrence and death from gastric cancer. *Ann Surg Oncol*2012;19:2088-94.
13 Sjodahl K, Lu Y, Nilsen TI, Ye W, Hveem K, Vatten L, et al. Smoking and alcohol drinking in relation to risk of gastric cancer: a population-based, prospective cohort study. *Int J Cancer*2007;120:128-32.
14 Tramacere I, Negri E, Pelucchi C, Bagnardi V, Rota M, Scotti L, et al. A meta-analysis on alcohol drinking and gastric cancer risk. *Ann Oncol*2012;23:28-36.
15 Duell EJ, Travier N, Lujan-Barroso L, Clavel-Chapelon F, Boutron-Ruault MC, Morois S, et al. Alcohol consumption and gastric cancer risk in the European Prospective Investigation into Cancer and Nutrition (EPIC) cohort. *Am J Clin Nutr*2011;94:1266-75.
16 World Cancer Research Fund. Food, nutrition, physical activity, and the prevention of cancer: a global perspective. 2007. www.dietandcancerreport.org/cancer_resource_center/downloads/Second_Expert_Report_full.pdf
17 Shikata K, Kiyohara Y, Kubo M, Yonemoto K, Ninomiya T, Shirota T, et al. A prospective study of dietary salt intake and gastric cancer incidence in a defined Japanese population: the Hisayama study. *Int J Cancer*2006;119:196-201.

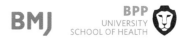

18 Kim J, Park S, Nam BH. Gastric cancer and salt preference: a population-based cohort study in Korea. *Am J Clin Nutr*2010;91:1289-93.

19 Park B, Shin A, Park SK, Ko KP, Ma SH, Lee EH, et al. Ecological study for refrigerator use, salt, vegetable, and fruit intakes, and gastric cancer. *Cancer Causes Control*2011;22:1497-502.

20 Larsson SC, Bergkvist L, Wolk A. Fruit and vegetable consumption and incidence of gastric cancer: a prospective study. *Cancer Epidemiol Biomarkers Prev*2006;15:1998-2001.

21 Vannella L, Lahner E, Osborn J, Annibale B. Systematic review: gastric cancer incidence in pernicious anaemia. *Aliment Pharmacol Ther*2013;37:375-82.

22 Fitzgerald RC, Hardwick R, Huntsman D, Carneiro F, Guilford P, Blair V, et al. Hereditary diffuse gastric cancer: updated consensus guidelines for clinical management and directions for future research. *J Med Genet*2010;47:436-44.

23 Pharoah PD, Guilford P, Caldas C. Incidence of gastric cancer and breast cancer in CDH1 (E-cadherin) mutation carriers from hereditary diffuse gastric cancer families. *Gastroenterology*2001;121:1348-53.

24 Lynch HT, Grady W, Suriano G, Huntsman D. Gastric cancer: new genetic developments. *J Surg Oncol*2005;90:114-33; discussion 33.

25 Capelle LG, Van Grieken NC, Lingsma HF, Steyerberg EW, Klokman WJ, Bruno MJ, et al. Risk and epidemiological time trends of gastric cancer in Lynch syndrome carriers in the Netherlands. *Gastroenterology*2010;138:487-92.

26 Talley NJ, Vakil NB, Moayyedi P. American gastroenterological association technical review on the evaluation of dyspepsia. *Gastroenterology*2005;129:1756-80.

27 Vakil N, Moayyedi P, Fennerty MB, Talley NJ. Limited value of alarm features in the diagnosis of upper gastrointestinal malignancy: systematic review and meta-analysis. *Gastroenterology*2006;131:390-401; quiz 659-60.

28 Allum WH, Blazeby JM, Griffin SM, Cunningham D, Jankowski JA, Wong R. Guidelines for the management of oesophageal and gastric cancer. *Gut*2011;60:1449-72.

29 Gravalos C, Jimeno A. HER2 in gastric cancer: a new prognostic factor and a novel therapeutic target. *Ann Oncol*2008;19:1523-9.

30 National Institute for Health and Care Excellence. Trastuzumab for the treatment of HER2-positive metastatic gastric cancer. TA208. 2010. http://guidance.nice.org.uk/TA208.

31 Mocellin S, Marchet A, Nitti D. EUS for the staging of gastric cancer: a meta-analysis. *Gastrointest Endosc*2011;73:1122-34.

32 Smyth E, Schoder H, Strong VE, Capanu M, Kelsen DP, Coit DG, et al. A prospective evaluation of the utility of 2-deoxy-2-[(18) F]fluoro-D-glucose positron emission tomography and computed tomography in staging locally advanced gastric cancer. *Cancer*2012;118:5481-8.

33 de Graaf GW, Ayantunde AA, Parsons SL, Duffy JP, Welch NT. The role of staging laparoscopy in oesophagogastric cancers. *Eur J Surg Oncol*2007;33:988-92.

34 National Comprehensive Cancer Network. Gastric cancer. Version 2. 2013. www.nccn.org/professionals/physician_gls/pdf/gastric.pdf.

35 Bozzetti F, Marubini E, Bonfanti G, Miceli R, Piano C, Gennari L. Subtotal versus total gastrectomy for gastric cancer: five-year survival rates in a multicenter randomized Italian trial. Italian Gastrointestinal Tumor Study Group. *Ann Surg*1999;230:170-8.

36 Gouzi JL, Huguier M, Fagniez PL, Launois B, Flamant Y, Lacaine F, et al. Total versus subtotal gastrectomy for adenocarcinoma of the gastric antrum. A French prospective controlled study. *Ann Surg*1989;209:162-6.

37 Songun I, Putter H, Kranenbarg EM, Sasako M, van de Velde CJ. Surgical treatment of gastric cancer: 15-year follow-up results of the randomised nationwide Dutch D1D2 trial. *Lancet Oncol*2010;11:439-49.

38 Sasako M, Sano T, Yamamoto S, Kurokawa Y, Nashimoto A, Kurita A, et al. D2 lymphadenectomy alone or with para-aortic nodal dissection for gastric cancer. *N Engl J Med*2008;359:453-62.

39 Kim HH, Hyung WJ, Cho GS, Kim MC, Han SU, Kim W, et al. Morbidity and mortality of laparoscopic gastrectomy versus open gastrectomy for gastric cancer: an interim report—a phase III multicenter, prospective, randomized Trial (KLASS Trial). *Ann Surg*2010;251:417-20.

40 Ohtani H, Tamamori Y, Noguchi K, Azuma T, Fujimoto S, Oba H, et al. A meta-analysis of randomized controlled trials that compared laparoscopy-assisted and open distal gastrectomy for early gastric cancer. *J Gastrointest Surg*2010;14:958-64.

41 Woo Y, Hyung WJ, Pak KH, Inaba K, Obama K, Choi SH, et al. Robotic gastrectomy as an oncologically sound alternative to laparoscopic resections for the treatment of early-stage gastric cancers. *Arch Surg*2011;146:1086-92.

42 Bennett C, Wang Y, Pan T. Endoscopic mucosal resection for early gastric cancer. *Cochrane Database Syst Rev*2009;4:CD004276.

43 Cunningham D, Allum WH, Stenning SP, Thompson JN, Van de Velde CJ, Nicolson M, et al. Perioperative chemotherapy versus surgery alone for resectable gastroesophageal cancer. *N Engl J Med*2006;355:11-20.

44 Cunningham D, Starling N, Rao S, Iveson T, Nicolson M, Coxon F, et al. Capecitabine and oxaliplatin for advanced esophagogastric cancer. *N Engl J Med*2008;358:36-46.

45 Macdonald JS, Smalley SR, Benedetti J, Hundahl SA, Estes NC, Stemmermann GN, et al. Chemoradiotherapy after surgery compared with surgery alone for adenocarcinoma of the stomach or gastroesophageal junction. *N Engl J Med*2001;345:725-30.

46 Paoletti X, Oba K, Burzykowski T, Michiels S, Ohashi Y, Pignon JP, et al. Benefit of adjuvant chemotherapy for resectable gastric cancer: a meta-analysis. *JAMA*2010;303:1729-37.

47 National Institute for Health and Care Excellence. Neutropenic sepsis: prevention and management of neutropenic sepsis in cancer patients. CG151. 2012. http://publications.nice.org.uk/neutropenic-sepsis-prevention-and-management-of-neutropenic-sepsis-in-cancer-patients-cg151.

48 Coupland VH, Lagergren J, Luchtenborg M, Jack RH, Allum W, Holmberg L, et al. Hospital volume, proportion resected and mortality from oesophageal and gastric cancer: a population-based study in England, 2004-2008. *Gut*2013;62:961-6.

49 Ghaferi AA, Birkmeyer JD, Dimick JB. Variation in hospital mortality associated with inpatient surgery. *N Engl J Med*2009;361:1368-75.

50 Dikken JL, Dassen AE, Lemmens VE, Putter H, Krijnen P, van der Geest L, et al. Effect of hospital volume on postoperative mortality and survival after oesophageal and gastric cancer surgery in the Netherlands between 1989 and 2009. *Eur J Cancer*2012;48:1004-13.

51 Enzinger PC, Benedetti JK, Meyerhardt JA, McCoy S, Hundahl SA, Macdonald JS, et al. Impact of hospital volume on recurrence and survival after surgery for gastric cancer. *Ann Surg*2007;245:426-34.

52 Wagner AD, Unverzagt S, Grothe W, Kleber G, Grothey A, Haerting J, et al. Chemotherapy for advanced gastric cancer. *Cochrane Database Syst Rev*2010;3:CD004064.

53 Kang JH, Lee SI, Lim do H, Park KW, Oh SY, Kwon HC, et al. Salvage chemotherapy for pretreated gastric cancer: a randomized phase III trial comparing chemotherapy plus best supportive care with best supportive care alone. *J Clin Oncol*2012;30:1513-8.

54 Bang YJ, Van Cutsem E, Feyereislova A, Chung HC, Shen L, Sawaki A, et al. Trastuzumab in combination with chemotherapy versus chemotherapy alone for treatment of HER2-positive advanced gastric or gastro-oesophageal junction cancer (ToGA): a phase 3, open-label, randomised controlled trial. *Lancet*2010;376:687-97.

55 Zhang JZ, Lu HS, Huang CM, Wu XY, Wang C, Guan GX, et al. Outcome of palliative total gastrectomy for stage IV proximal gastric cancer. *Am J Surg*2011;202:91-6.

56 Song KY, Park SM, Kim SN, Park CH. The role of surgery in the treatment of recurrent gastric cancer. *Am J Surg*2008;196:19-22.

57 Fuccio L, Zagari RM, Laterza LH, Cennamo V, Ceroni L, et al. Meta-analysis: can Helicobacter pylori eradication treatment reduce the risk for gastric cancer? *Ann Intern Med*2009;151:121-8.

58 Ma JL, Zhang L, Brown LM, Li JY, Shen L, Pan KF, et al. Fifteen-year effects of Helicobacter pylori, garlic, and vitamin treatments on gastric cancer incidence and mortality. *J Natl Cancer Inst*2012;104:488-92.

59 Rupnow MF, Chang AH, Shachter RD, Owens DK, Parsonnet J. Cost-effectiveness of a potential prophylactic Helicobacter pylori vaccine in the United States. *J Infect Dis*2009;200:1311-7.

60 La Torre G, Chiaradia G, Gianfagna F, De Lauretis A, Boccia S, Mannocci A, et al. Smoking status and gastric cancer risk: an updated meta-analysis of case-control studies published in the past ten years. *Tumori*2009;95:13-22.

61 Fukase K, Kato M, Kikuchi S, Inoue K, Uemura N, Okamoto S, et al. Effect of eradication of Helicobacter pylori on incidence of metachronous gastric carcinoma after endoscopic resection of early gastric cancer: an open-label, randomised controlled trial. *Lancet*2008;372:392-7.

62 Lagergren J, Ye W, Bergstrom R, Nyren O. Utility of endoscopic screening for upper gastrointestinal adenocarcinoma. *JAMA*2000;284:961-2.

63 Rugge M. Secondary prevention of gastric cancer. *Gut*2007;56:1646-7.

64 Kato M, Asaka M. Recent development of gastric cancer prevention. *Jpn J Clin Oncol*2012;42:987-94.

65 Xu ZQ, Broza YY, Ionsecu R, Tisch U, Ding L, Liu H, et al. A nanomaterial-based breath test for distinguishing gastric cancer from benign gastric conditions. *Br J Cancer*2013;108:941-50.

66 Ahn HS, Lee HJ, Yoo MW, Jeong SH, Park DJ, Kim HH, et al. Changes in clinicopathological features and survival after surgery for gastric cancer over a 20-year period. *Br J Surg*2011;98:255-60.

67 Lepage C, Sant M, Verdecchia A, Forman D, Esteve J, Faivre J. Operative mortality after gastric cancer resection and long-term survival differences across Europe. *Br J Surg*2010;97:235-9.

68 Van Cutsem E, de Haas S, Kang YK, Ohtsu A, Tebbutt NC, Ming Xu J, et al. Bevacizumab in combination with chemotherapy as first-line therapy in advanced gastric cancer: a biomarker evaluation from the AVAGAST randomized phase III trial. *J Clin Oncol*2012;30:2119-27.

Related links

bmj.com
- Get Cleveland Clinic CME credits for this article

bmj.com/archive
Previous articles in this series
- The diagnosis and management of gastric cancer (BMJ 2013;347:f6367)
- An introduction to advance care planning in practice (BMJ 2013;347:f6064)
- Post-mastectomy breast reconstruction (BMJ 2013;347:f5903)
- Identifying brain tumours in children •and young adults (BMJ 2013;347:f5844)
- Gout (BMJ 2013;347:f5648)

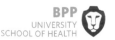

Percutaneous endoscopic gastrostomy (PEG) feeding

Matthew Kurien, specialty registrar 4 in gastroenterology[1],
Mark E McAlindon, consultant gastroenterologist[2],
David Westaby, consultant gastroenterologist[3],
David S Sanders, consultant gastroenterologist[2]

[1]Department of Gastroenterology, Chesterfield Royal Hospital, Chesterfield S44 5BL

[2]Department of Gastroenterology, Royal Hallamshire Hospital, Sheffield S10 2JF

[3]Department of Gastroenterology, Imperial College Healthcare NHS Trust, London, UK

Correspondence to: M Kurien
matthew.kurien@chesterfieldroyal.nhs.uk

Cite this as: BMJ 2010;340:c2414

DOI: 10.1136/bmj.c2414

http://www.bmj.com/content/340/bmj.c2414

Percutaneous endoscopic gastrostomy (PEG) feeding, introduced into clinical practice in 1980,[1] is now established as an effective way of providing enteral feeding to patients who have functionally normal gastrointestinal tracts but who cannot meet their nutritional needs because of inadequate oral intake.[2] It is the preferred method of feeding when nutritional intake is likely to be inadequate for more than four to six weeks, and when enteral feeding is likely to prevent further weight loss, correct nutritional deficiencies, and stop the decline in quality of life in patients caused by insufficient nutritional intake.[3] [4] The beneficial effects of gastrostomy feeding on morbidity and mortality have been described only in certain subgroups of patients.[5] [6] Randomised studies in patients after stroke who received gastrostomy feeding have shown improved nutritional outcomes, higher likelihood of survival, and earlier discharge.[6] [7] However, gastrostomy tubes are increasingly being requested and inserted for indications where long term outcomes are uncertain.[8] In this review we discuss the indications for, controversies surrounding, and complications of gastrostomy feeding and provide practical advice on the management of percutaneous endoscopic gastrostomies.

What is a percutaneous endoscopic gastrostomy?

This is a procedure for placing a feeding tube directly into the stomach via a small incision through the abdominal wall. After aseptic preparation of the abdominal wall and prophylactic antibiotics, an endoscope is passed via the oesophagus into the stomach.[w1 w2] A powerful light source within the endoscope and insufflation of air allows the position of the endoscope to be identified through the abdominal wall. Use of the finger invagination technique may also help identify the optimal site. After local anaesthetic infiltration, a needle is inserted through the abdominal wall (fig 1A) into the stomach, along with a guide wire and grasped using a snare via the endoscope (fig 1B). The guide wire, the snare, and the endoscope are

SOURCES AND SELECTION CRITERIA

We searched the Cochrane database of systematic reviews and did a PubMed search (from January 1980 until January 2010) using the keywords "percutaneous endoscopic gastrostomy" and "enteral feeding". We selected well conducted systematic reviews, meta-analyses, and large randomised controlled trials. When no study of these types was available, we considered small randomised control trials, cohort studies, observational studies, and guidelines.

then retracted. The guide wire is attached to the end of a gastrostomy tube (fig 1C), pulled back down through the oesophagus and stomach, and brought out through the hole in the abdominal wall (fig 1D). The end of the PEG tube is retained within the stomach cavity, by a wide internal bumper (fig 1E). An external bumper is then fixed to the tube to prevent the internal bumper from moving distally in the alimentary canal. The procedure is usually performed under sedation and takes about 15-20 minutes. Gastrostomy feeding tubes may also be placed using radiological or surgical methods, depending on technical considerations or local availability.[w3 w4]

What are the benefits of gastrostomy feeding?

Malnutrition determines disease outcomes because it affects every system in the body, leading to both physical and psychological disability.[w5] Percutaneous endoscopic gastrostomy feeding aims to improve nutritional status. Gastrostomy feeding reduces mortality, length of hospital stay, and complications in carefully selected patients who are likely to be or later become nutritionally depleted for longer than four to six weeks.[9] [10] Clinical studies have shown clear benefits of PEG feeding after stroke[6] [7] (in terms of improving nutritional status and reducing mortality) and in patients with oropharyngeal cancer (in terms of improving nutritional status).[11] [12] When compared with other methods of enteral nutrition, such as nasogastric feeding, gastrostomy feeding caused less discomfort and had lower rates of complications such as bleeding, blockage, and dislodgment of the tube.[13] [14] Although gastrostomy feeding does not prevent reflux or aspiration, rates may be lower than in patients fed by a nasogastric tube.[w6]

Who should have a percutaneous endoscopic gastrostomy?

Cohort studies have shown that 20-50% of hospital patients are malnourished.[15] [16] Box 1 provides a broad list of indications for which patients are currently being referred for percutaneous endoscopic gastrostomy. Although clinical studies have shown benefits for PEG feeding in stroke[6] [7] and oropharyngeal cancer,[11] [12] the appropriateness of gastrostomy insertion in other patient subgroups is controversial. The National Confidential Enquiry into Patient

---

SUMMARY POINTS

- Percutaneous endoscopic gastrostomy feeding presents complex moral and ethical problems
- Gastrostomy feeding has mortality and nutritional benefits in carefully selected patients
- There is no evidence of improved mortality in patients with dementia who are gastrostomy fed
- Patient selection can be improved by the use of guidelines, protocols, and a multidisciplinary team approach
- Patients referred for gastrostomy should be considered on the basis of their individual needs
- After gastrostomy insertion, signs of a serious complication—pain on feeding and bleeding around or within the gastrostomy tube—should prompt urgent referral to a specialist

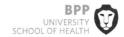
> **BOX 1 CONDITIONS FOR WHICH PATIENTS ARE COMMONLY REFERRED FOR INSERTION OF A PERCUTANEOUS ENDOSCOPIC GASTROSTOMY TUBE**
>
> **Neurological indications**
> - Cerebrovascular disease
> - Motor neurone disease
> - Multiple sclerosis
> - Parkinson's disease
> - Cerebral palsy
> - Dementia
>
> **Reduced level of consciousness or cognition**
> - Head injury
> - Intensive care patients
>
> **Obstruction**
> - Oropharyngeal cancer
> - Oesophageal cancer
>
> **Miscellaneous**
> - Burns
> - Fistulae
> - Cystic fibrosis
> - Short bowel syndromes (such as Crohn's disease)

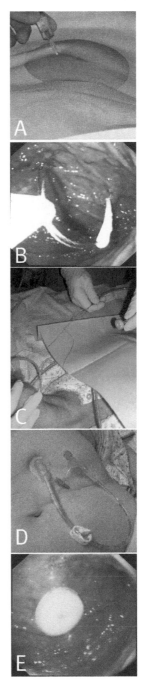

Insertion of percutaneous endoscopic gastrostomy

Outcome and Death (NCEPOD) undertook the largest study in the United Kingdom to date, which reviewed mortality after PEG insertion between April 2002 and March 2003. This study found a 6% mortality in a cohort of 16 648 patients. Of those who died, 43% died within one week of PEG insertion, and in 19% of patients PEG insertion was thought to have been futile.[8] We believe that the decision making process for gastrostomy feeding should not be based solely on the referral indication, but that each patient must be considered according to their individual needs.

What is the role of PEG feeding in dementia?
We currently have insufficient evidence to support PEG feeding in dementia and other neurodegenerative diseases.[w7-w9] Patients with advanced dementia commonly develop feeding problems that lead to weight loss and nutritional deficiencies. Whether or not to use percutaneous gastrostomies to feed patients with dementia is an emotive and controversial question. This controversy is compounded by the fact that in the late stages of the illness people lack capacity to express their wishes. The British artificial nutrition survey (BANS) found that in 2007, 109 new patients and 582 established patients with dementia were being artificially fed in the community, most by gastrostomy feeding.[17] However, a recent Cochrane review showed no evidence of increased survival; reduced pressure ulcers; or improved quality of life, nutritional status, function, behaviour, or psychiatric symptoms of dementia in patients with advanced dementia who were fed using gastrostomy tubes.[18]

No large prospective studies have examined outcomes of PEG feeding in patients with dementia. A retrospective study of 361 patients found that patients with dementia who had a PEG inserted had higher mortality than other patient subgroups (54% 30 day mortality and 90% at one year).[19] These findings have been reproduced by other investigators, who found that eating problems occurred in 85.8% of patients with dementia before death, which suggests that difficulties with feeding are an end stage problem.[20]

Optimising referral for PEG insertion
One method used internationally to optimise referral practice is to employ institutional guidelines that use a standardised referral protocol. Use of a multidisciplinary team in assessing patients and dissemination of evidence allows carers and health professionals to make informed decisions. This approach has been shown (in observational studies) to improve the selection of patients referred for gastrostomy.[21 22 23]

When considering whether insertion of a gastrostomy tube is appropriate, the question that must be asked is whether gastrostomy feeding would maintain or improve a patient's quality of life. This question must be answered in the context of the underlying diagnosis and prognosis, considering moral and ethical issues, as well as respecting the patient's wishes. Guidelines exist to aid clinicians in making decisions on PEG feeding, but the decision to insert a PEG tube should always be made on an individual basis.[4 w10]

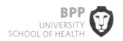

BOX 2 COMPLICATIONS OF INSERTION OF A PERCUTANEOUS ENDOSCOPIC GASTROSTOMY (PEG) TUBE

Immediate (<72 hours)

Endoscopy related
- Haemorrhage or perforation
- Aspiration
- Oversedation

Procedure related
- Ileus
- Pneumoperitoneum*
- Wound infection
- Wound bleeding
- Injury to the liver, bowel, or spleen

Delayed
- Gastric outlet obstruction
- Buried bumper syndrome
- Dislodged PEG tube
- Peritonitis
- Peristomal leakage or infection
- Skin or gastric ulceration
- Blocked PEG tube
- Tube degradation
- Gastric fistula after removal of PEG tube
- Granulation around site of insertion of PEG

*May be a common occurence, with no serious symptoms.[24]

What are the contraindications to percutaneous endoscopic gastrostomy?

Few absolute contraindications to percutaneous endoscopic gastrostomy exist. Active coagulopathies and thrombocytopenia (platelets <50   10⁹/l) must be corrected before tube insertion. Anything that precludes endoscopy, such as haemodynamic compromise, sepsis, or a perforated viscus, would be an absolute contraindication to gastrostomy insertion. Relative contraindications include acute severe illness, anorexia, previous gastric surgery, peritonitis, ascites, and gastric outlet obstruction. Crohn's disease used to be considered a contraindication to gastrostomy insertion because of concerns about possible fistula formation around the gastrostomy tract, but an observational study has shown percutaneous gastrostomy to be safe and without increased complications in patients with this disease.[w11]

How are complications managed?

The rate of complications after percutaneous endoscopic gastrostomy has been reported as 8-30%.[3][24] Box 2 lists these complications, which may be immediate or delayed. Most gastrostomy insertions are done in hospital, and immediate complications usually occur in hospital. Delayed complications are more often seen in the community setting. If favourable outcomes are to be achieved, prompt decisions should be made as to whether the problem can be managed within the community or whether it requires hospital admission.

What complications can be managed in the community?

Overly granulated stoma sites occur commonly, and we have little evidence to guide management. Cauterisation of the lesion with silver nitrate has been tried, but this may be painful, and cautery may damage the gastrostomy tube. Treating the cause of overgranulation, such as gastric leakage, infection, or a poorly positioned fixation device that is a source of friction, may be more appropriate. Preventive measures combined with a steroid preparation cream, such as 1% hydrocortisone, may reduce granulation. Infections around stoma sites are fairly common and should be suspected if inflammation or discharge are seen around the stoma site, If infection is suspected, swabs from the peristomal area should be sent for culture and antibiotic treatment given either topically or enterally, depending on the sensitivities of the organism.

Blockage of the gastrostomy tube usually occurs secondary to drugs or feed. The obstruction can sometimes be removed by massaging the PEG tube. If this fails, a push-pull method using a syringe on the end of the PEG tube may help to dislodge the blockage. In cases where these mechanisms fail, enzyme preparations or fizzy drinks may be delivered into the tube. Inadvertent removal of the gastrostomy tube occasionally occurs, and the tube should be replaced with a balloon gastrostomy. These temporary tubes can last up to three months and have a balloon inflated with sterile water, which maintains the tube's position within the stoma tract. A delay in recognising a dislodged tube may result in closure of the stoma, which will require hospital admission and endoscopic reinsertion of the tube. A urinary catheter may be used as a holding measure if necessary to prevent closure of the tract, before permanent insertion of a balloon gastrostomy. Feed related peritonitis is possible after reinsertion of a gastrostomy tube. When uncertainty exists about the position of the replacement tube, then water soluble contrast can be used to determine the position before feeding is restarted.

What complications require hospital admission?

Any complication may require hospital admission. We highlight some serious complications that require relatively urgent hospital admission. Any of the immediate complications noted in box 2 should prompt readmission if the patient has been discharged.

The "buried bumper" syndrome is a rare but serious complication that occurs in 1.5-1.9% of patients.[24] The internal bumper migrates from the gastric wall towards the skin, anywhere along the PEG tract, as a consequence of excessive tension between the internal and external bumper. Symptoms may include pain on feeding, retrograde leakage of feed on to the skin, and rarely gastric perforation. Correction is achieved through removing and re-siting the internal bumper endoscopically or by surgical intervention.

Patients who have serious complications such as peritonitis or gastric outlet obstruction may present with symptoms of acute or chronic abdominal pain. Red flag signs that should prompt emergency admission are pain on feeding, external leakage of gastric contents, or bleeding within or around the gastrostomy tube.[25]

What are the ethical and legal considerations in gastrostomy feeding?

PEG feeding raises ethical and legal considerations. Both the Royal College of Physicians and the General Medical Council in the UK have provided guidance on oral feeding and nutrition.[26][27] Artificial feeding is considered a medical treatment in legal terms and requires valid consent before it is started. For consent to be valid the person giving consent must have the capacity to do so voluntarily after being given sufficient information to guide informed choice. When a patient has capacity their wish to consent to or refuse treatment should be upheld, even if that decision may lead

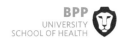

CASE SCENARIO

An 83 year old man with advanced Parkinson's disease was referred to the gastroenterology team for consideration of a percutaneous endoscopic gastrostomy. He had had three episodes of aspiration pneumonia in the previous six months, and his oral intake had declined. The speech and language therapist believed that he had an unsafe swallow and suggested referral for a gastrostomy. The admitting medical team referred him to the nutrition team, who suggested that he might gain no benefits from the procedure, given his frailty, cognitive decline, and comorbidity. Nevertheless, the family was convinced that gastrostomy feeding might benefit him. A limited trial of nasogastric feeding was started, but within four days the patient died.

This case scenario is fictitious.

A PATIENT'S PERSPECTIVE

I am a 64 year old woman who had a percutaneous endoscopic gastrostomy (PEG) inserted in January 2010. I was diagnosed with motor neurone disease nearly a year ago after I started to lose weight and developed problems with my speech. I am now unable to talk and have to write everything down to communicate. The PEG was inserted after I developed problems with swallowing, which led to an episode of pneumonia. When I was told I might need a PEG, neither my husband nor I had a clear understanding of what this entailed. Further information was obtained from a hospital leaflet and a meeting with a PEG specialist nurse. The decision to proceed with a PEG was based on medical opinion and the belief that there really was no alternative.

Four weeks on from my PEG insertion, my husband and I are managing the PEG well. I have had no complications, and my weight is being maintained. I have no regrets about having the procedure, and we have contact details should we encounter any problems. Knowledge about PEG feeding varied among the healthcare professionals we met, and a better understanding of this matter would help patients and carers alike.

advance directives, the patient's prognosis, and the likely benefits of gastrostomy feeding when making decisions. A limited trial of feeding may sometimes be used, but strict criteria regarding what constitutes success should be determined before starting gastrostomy feeding.[28] Where conflicts arise between healthcare professionals or between healthcare professionals and those close to the patient, it may be necessary to seek legal advice or resolution through a local clinical ethics committee.[26]

The National Institute for Health and Clinical Excellence guidelines on dementia highlight the importance of quality of life in advanced dementia and support the role of palliative care in these patients, from diagnosis until death.[29] Best practice in these patients could be to encourage eating and drinking by mouth for as long as tolerated, to use good feeding techniques, to alter the consistencies of food, and to promote good mouth care. When disease progression is such that the patient no longer wants to eat or drink, then rather than inserting a gastrostomy tube, end of life care pathways might be considered. Views held by carers and medical staff may prevent progression to end of life care pathways. A questionnaire survey showed that allied healthcare professionals were more likely than doctors to consider PEG feeding when presented with patient scenarios relating to malnutrition.[30]

Conclusion

Percutaneous endoscopic gastrostomy feeding is an effective way to deliver nutritional support to people who are unable to meet their nutritional requirements orally. Improved nutritional status and survival have been demonstrated in selected subgroups of patients. Careful selection of patients on an individual case basis may improve outcomes.

to death. When a patient lacks capacity, an independent mental capacity advocate should represent that person. The multidisciplinary team caring for the patient is responsible for giving, withholding, or withdrawing treatment, including artificial feeding and hydration, and it should consider any

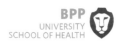

Contributors: MK designed and drafted the article and is the guarantor. MEM and DW revised the article and approved the final manuscript. DSS designed and revised the article and approved the final manuscript.

Funding: No funding received.

Competing interests: DW and DSS are coauthors of the current BSG guidelines on PEG feeding. DSS was a member of the working party of the Royal College of Physicians' publication entitled *Oral Feeding Difficulties and Dilemmas* (2010). DSS is an honorary professor in gastroenterology at the University of Sheffield and chairman of the small bowel and nutrition committee of the British Society of Gastroenterology. These are honorary posts with no financial benefits.

Provenance and peer review: Not commissioned; externally peer reviewed.

Patient consent obtained.

1 Gauderer MW, Ponsky JL, Izant RJ Jr. Gastrostomy without laparotomy: a percutaneous endoscopic technique. *J Pediatr Surg* 1980;15:872-5.
2 Moran BJ, Taylor MB, Johnson CD. Percutaneous endoscopic gastrostomy. *Br J Surg* 1990;77:858-62.
3 Loser C, Aschl G, Hebuterne X, Mathus-Vliegen EM, Muscaritoli M, Niv Y, et al. ESPEN guidelines on artificial enteral nutrition—percutaneous endoscopic gastrostomy (PEG). *Clin Nutr* 2005;24:848-61.
4 National Institute for Health and Clinical Excellence. Nutrition support in adults: oral nutrition support, enteral tube feeding and parenteral nutrition. 2006. www.nice.org.uk/cg32.
5 Senft M, Fietkau R, Iro H, Sailer D, Sauer R. The influence of supportive nutritional therapy via percutaneous endoscopically guided gastrostomy on the quality of life of cancer patients. *Support Care Cancer* 1993;1:272-5.
6 Norton B, Homer-Ward M, Donnelly MT, Long RG, Holmes GK. A randomised prospective comparison of percutaneous endoscopic gastrostomy and nasogastric tube feeding after acute dysphagic stroke. *BMJ* 1996;312:13-6.
7 Dennis MS, Lewis SC, Warlow C; FOOD Trial Collaboration. Effect of timing and method of enteral tube feeding for dysphagic stroke patients (FOOD): a multicentre randomised controlled trial. *Lancet* 2005;365:764-72.
8 NCEPOD. Scoping our practice: the 2004 report of the National Confidential Enquiry into Patient Outcome and Death. 2005.
9 Green CJ. Existence, causes and consequences of disease related malnutrition in the hospital and the community, and the clinical and financial benefits of nutritional intervention. *Clin Nutr* 1999;18(suppl 2):3-38S.
10 Wicks C, Gimson A, Vlavianos P, Lombard M, Panos M, Macmathuna P, et al. Assessment of the percutaneous endoscopic gastrostomy feeding tube as part of an integrated approach to enteral feeding. *Gut* 1992;33:613-6.
11 Wiggenraad RG, Flierman L, Goossens A, Brand R, Verschuur HP, Croll GA, et al. Prophylactic gastrostomy placement and early tube feeding may limit loss of weight during chemoradiotherapy for advanced head and neck cancer, a preliminary study. *Clin Otolaryngol* 2007;32:384-90.
12 Nugent B, Lewis S, O'Sullivan JM. Enteral feeding methods for nutritional management in patients with head and neck cancers being treated with radiotherapy and/or chemotherapy. *Cochrane Database Syst Rev* 2010;3:CD007904.
13 Mekhail TM, Adelstein DJ, Rybicki LA, Larto MA, Saxton JP, Lavertu P. Enteral nutrition during the treatment of head and neck carcinoma: is a percutaneous endoscopic gastrostomy tube preferable to a nasogastric tube? *Cancer* 2001;91:1785-90.
14 Park RH, Allison MC, Lang J, Spence E, Morris AJ, Danesh BJ, et al. Randomised comparison of percutaneous endoscopic gastrostomy and nasogastric tube feeding in patients with persisting neurological dysphagia. *BMJ* 1992;304:1406-9.
15 Norman K, Pichard C, Lochs H, Pirlich M. Prognostic impact of disease-related malnutrition. *Clin Nutr* 2008;27:5-15.
16 McWhirter JP, Pennington CR. Incidence and recognition of malnutrition in hospital. *BMJ* 1994;308:945-8.
17 Jones B. Annual BANS report 2008: artificial nutrition support in the UK, 2000-2007. British artificial nutrition survey 2008. www.bapen.org.uk/pdfs/bans_reports/bans_report_08.pdf.
18 Sampson EL, Candy B, Jones L. Enteral tube feeding for older people with advanced dementia. *Cochrane Database Syst Rev* 2009;2:CD007209.
19 Sanders DS, Carter MJ, D'Silva J, James G, Bolton RP, Bardhan KD. Survival analysis in percutaneous endoscopic gastrostomy feeding: a worse outcome in patients with dementia. *Am J Gastroenterol* 2000;95:1472-5.
20 Mitchell SL, Teno JM, Kiely DK, Shaffer ML, Jones RN, Prigerson HG, et al. The clinical course of advanced dementia. *N Engl J Med* 2009;361:1529-38.
21 Sanders DS, Carter MJ, D'Silva J, James G, Bolton RP, Willemse PJ, et al. Percutaneous endoscopic gastrostomy: a prospective audit of the impact of guidelines in two district general hospitals in the United Kingdom. *Am J Gastroenterol* 2002;97:2239-45.
22 Abuksis G, Mor M, Plaut S, Fraser G, Niv Y. Outcome of percutaneous endoscopic gastrostomy (PEG): comparison of two policies in a 4-year experience. *Clin Nutr* 2004;23:341-6.
23 Monteleoni C, Clark E. Using rapid-cycle quality improvement methodology to reduce feeding tubes in patients with advanced dementia: before and after study. *BMJ* 2004;329:491-4.
24 Schrag SP, Sharma R, Jaik NP, Seamon MJ, Lukaszczyk JJ, Martin ND, et al. Complications related to percutaneous endoscopic gastrostomy (PEG) tubes. A comprehensive clinical review. *J Gastrointest Liver Dis* 2007;16:407-18.
25 National Patient Safety Agency. Early detection of complications after gastrostomy. A rapid response report. www.nrls.npsa.nhs.uk/resources/type/alerts/?entryid45=73457.
26 Royal College of Physicians and British Society of Gastroenterology. Oral feeding difficulties and dilemmas: a guide to practical care, particularly towards the end of life. Royal College of Physicians, 2010.
27 General Medical Council. Withholding and withdrawing life-prolonging treatments: good practice in decision-making. Artificial nutrition and hydration. 2006. www.gmc-uk.org/guidance/current/library/witholding_lifeprolonging_guidance.asp#7.
28 Stroud M, Duncan H, Nightingale J; British Society of Gastroenterology. Guidelines for enteral feeding in adult hospital patients. *Gut* 2003;52:vii,1-12.
29 National Institute for Health and Clinical Excellence. Dementia: supporting people with dementia and their carers in health and social care. 2006. www.nice.org.uk/cg42.
30 Watts DT, Cassel CK, Hickam DH. Nurses' and physicians attitudes toward tube-feeding decisions in long-term care. *J Am Geriatr Soc* 1986;34:607-11.

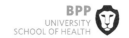

Bariatric surgery for obesity and metabolic conditions in adults

David E Arterburn, associate investigator[1], Anita P Courcoulas, professor of surgery[2]

[1]Group Health Research Institute, Group Health Cooperative, Seattle, WA 98101, USA

[2]University of Pittsburgh Medical Center, Pittsburgh, PA, USA

Correspondence to: D E Arterburn arterburn.d@ghc.org

Cite this as: *BMJ* 2014;349:g3961

DOI: 10.1136/bmj.g3961

http://www.bmj.com/content/349/bmj.g3961

ABSTRACT

This review summarizes recent evidence related to the safety, efficacy, and metabolic outcomes of bariatric surgery to guide clinical decision making. Several short term randomized controlled trials have demonstrated the effectiveness of bariatric procedures for inducing weight loss and initial remission of type 2 diabetes. Observational studies have linked bariatric procedures with long term improvements in body weight, type 2 diabetes, survival, cardiovascular events, incident cancer, and quality of life. Perioperative mortality for the average patient is low but varies greatly across subgroups. The incidence of major complications after surgery also varies widely, and emerging data show that some procedures are associated with a greater risk of substance misuse disorders, suicide, and nutritional deficiencies. More research is needed to enable long term outcomes to be compared across various procedures and subpopulations, and to identify those most likely to benefit from surgical intervention. Given uncertainties about the balance between the risks and benefits of bariatric surgery in the long term, the decision to undergo surgery should be based on a high quality shared decision making process.

Introduction

Although the global pandemic of obesity has continued unabated over the past two decades, little progress has been made in its behavioral and drug treatment, especially in patients with severe obesity. By contrast, the evidence base for bariatric surgical procedures has expanded rapidly over this time, and it has yielded important short term and long term data on the efficacy and safety of surgical treatment for obesity and related metabolic disorders. Because trade-offs between the potential risks and benefits of bariatric surgical procedures exist, this review of the evidence for bariatric surgery aims to guide adult patients and their clinicians through a well informed, shared decision making process.

Prevalence

Nationally representative estimates from 2009 to 2010 indicate that 35.5% of the adult population in the United States is obese (defined as a body mass index (BMI) ≥30).[1] About 15.5% of the US adult population has a BMI of 35 or more and 6.3% are severely obese (BMI ≥40).[1]

Data on the prevalence of severe obesity in other countries is scant, but the health survey of England showed that 1.7% of men and 3.1% of women had a BMI of 40 or more in 2012.[2] In Sweden in 2005, 1.3% of men had a BMI of 35 or more,[3] and in Australia in 2006, 8.1% of adults had a BMI of 35 or more.[4]

The total number of bariatric procedures worldwide was estimated at 340 768 in 2011.[5] The most commonly performed procedures were Roux-en-Y gastric bypass (46.6%), vertical sleeve gastrectomy (27.8%), adjustable gastric banding (17.8%), and biliopancreatic diversion with duodenal switch (2.2%).[5] The largest number of operations were performed in the US and Canada together (101 645), followed by Brazil (65 000), France (27 648), Mexico (19 000), Australia and New Zealand (12 000), and the United Kingdom (10 000). No other nation performed 10 000 or more operations in 2011.[5]

Obesity related complications

Severe obesity (most often defined as a BMI ≥35 with comorbid health conditions or a BMI ≥40 without such conditions) is a highly prevalent chronic disease,[1] which leads to substantial morbidity,[6] premature mortality,[7] impaired quality of life,[8] and excess healthcare expenditures.[9] Severely obese adults are disproportionately affected by chronic health conditions, such as type 2 diabetes (28% of severely obese adults),[10] major depression (7%),[11] coronary heart disease (14-19%),[6] and osteoarthritis (10-17%).[6]

Treatment options

Treatments for severe obesity include lifestyle interventions, pharmacotherapy, and bariatric surgical procedures. Evidence from decades of weight loss research indicates that lifestyle interventions and pharmacotherapy often fail to help severely obese people lose enough weight to improve their health and quality of life in the long term.[12] [13] [14] However, a growing body of evidence indicates that bariatric surgery can induce sustained reductions in weight, improve comorbidities, and prolong survival.[15] [16] [17] [18] [19] [20] [21] [22] [23] [24]

Bariatric procedures were first developed more than 50 years ago. However, in the past 20 years, a dramatic increase in the prevalence of severe obesity combined with improvements in the efficacy and safety of bariatric surgical techniques has led to a 20-fold increase in the number of procedures performed annually in the US.[25] Recent improvements in bariatric safety outcomes have been linked to an increase in the volume of cases performed, a shift to the laparoscopic technique, and an increase in the use of the lower risk adjustable gastric banding procedure.[26] Current US guidelines recommend consideration of bariatric surgery for people who have not responded to non-surgical treatments if they have a BMI of at least 40 or at least 35 if they also have serious diseases related to obesity.[27]

Types of bariatric surgery procedures and mechanisms of weight loss

Bariatric surgical procedures have evolved dramatically over the past 50 years (fig 1). Modern procedures are most often described in anatomic terms according to their presumed mechanical effect, using phrases like "gastric restrictive"

SOURCES AND SELECTION CRITERIA

We based this review on articles found by searching Medline, the Cochrane Collaboration Library, and Clinical Evidence from their inception until September 2013 with the terms "bariatric surgery", "gastric bypass", "gastric banding", "sleeve gastrectomy", and "biliopancreatic diversion". Our search was limited to English language articles. Priority was given to evidence obtained from systematic literature reviews, meta-analyses, and randomized controlled trials when possible.

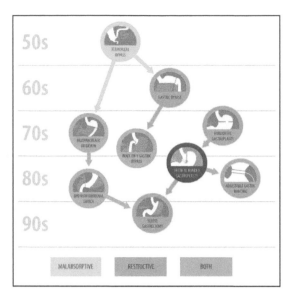

Fig 1 The evolution of bariatric surgery procedures. Use the interactive tool at:http://www.bmj.com/content/349/bmj.g3961/infographic

or "intestinal bypass" for ease of understanding, but recent basic science investigations may soon change this characterization to one based on physiology. In addition, since the 1990s the standard surgical technique has shifted from an open incisional approach to a minimally invasive or laparoscopic approach, almost exclusively.[28]

The first bariatric procedure in wide use was known as the jejunoileal bypass, and it involved an intestinal bypass in which the proximal jejunum was bypassed into the distal ileum. This resulted in extreme weight loss by way of profound malabsorption and was eventually abandoned some years later after many patients developed severe protein-energy malnutrition.[29]

The next major bariatric procedures to be introduced were the horizontal gastroplasty and the vertical banded gastroplasty, which were thought to be purely restrictive procedures made possible through the development of surgical stapling devices. In a horizontal gastroplasty, a pouch was created in the upper stomach by introducing a horizontal suture line with several staples removed (the stoma) to allow for the passage of food (fig 2A). With vertical banded gastroplasty, a vertical staple line was created parallel to the lesser curvature of the stomach and the outlet or stoma was reinforced with a mesh collar to prevent enlargement (fig 2B). Both procedures have now been abandoned owing to the introduction of newer more effective laparoscopic procedures, and because the stomach staple line often separated or the stoma tended to enlarge, leading to weight regain or severe gastroesophageal reflux, or both.[30] [31]

The gastric bypass was originally introduced in 1969 by Mason and Ito,[32] and it was later modified into a Roux-en-Y gastric bypass configuration for drainage of the proximal gastric pouch to avoid bile reflux (fig 2C).[33] Over time, the Roux-en-Y gastric bypass has been refined into its current laparoscopic form. This includes a small proximal gastric pouch of 15-20 mL, a measured and smaller gastric-to-intestinal stoma size (with or without cuff restriction), and a complete staple line transection to avoid staple line separation or failure (fig 2D).[34]

The next major procedure to be introduced was the adjustable form of gastric banding, which has been modified for laparoscopic placement and creates a small superior gastric pouch with an adjustable outlet (fig 2E).[35]

[36] The adjustable gastric band is a silicone belt with an inflatable balloon in the lining that is buckled into a closed ring around the upper stomach. A reservoir port is placed under the skin for adjustments to the stoma size.

Two procedures that use a more extreme intestinal bypass along with some modest gastric reduction are the biliopancreatic diversion and the biliopancreatic diversion with duodenal switch operations, which are most often used for "super" obese patients (usually BMI .50).[37] [38] [39] Biliopancreatic diversion combines a subtotal (2/3rds) distal gastrectomy and a very long Roux-en-Y anastomosis with a short common intestinal channel for nutrient absorption (fig 2F). Biliopancreatic diversion with duodenal switch combines a 70% greater curve gastrectomy with a long intestinal bypass, where the duodenal stump is defunctionalized or "switched" to a gastroileal anastomosis (fig 2G).

Finally, the most recent major bariatric procedure to be introduced is the vertical sleeve gastrectomy, and it is rapidly increasing in popularity.[40] This technique consists of a 70% vertical gastric resection, which creates a long and narrow tubular gastric reservoir with no intestinal bypass component (fig 2H).

Despite the basic "restrictive" and "intestinal bypass" anatomic conceptualizations of bariatric surgical procedures, there is much research ongoing in animal and human models towards understanding their underlying mechanisms of action. These actions may be more physiological (altered gastrointestinal signals) than nutrient restrictive and are likely to be both endocrine and neuronal in nature.[41]

Some of the potential candidates for the mechanisms of action of bariatric procedures include alterations in ghrelin, leptin, glucagon-like peptide-1, cholecystokinin, peptide YY, gut microbiota, and bile acids.[42 43 44 45 46 47 48 49 50 51 52 53 54 55 56 57 58 59] It may be necessary in the future to group bariatric procedures not on the basis of anatomic surgical similarities but on how they affect key physiological variables, which would provide greater mechanistic insight into how the procedures work.[41]

Effectiveness of bariatric surgery compared with non-surgical management

Below we summarize key findings from randomized trials and major long term observational studies that compare bariatric procedures with non-surgical management of obesity. Table 1 provides an overview of the results of these studies in terms of weight change, remission from and incidence of type 2 diabetes, as well as long term survival.

Randomized controlled trials

A recent systematic review and meta-analysis summarized all randomized controlled trials (RCTs) that have compared bariatric surgery with non-surgical treatments for obesity.[21] The review analysed 11 trials comprising 796 people with a BMI of 30-52. These studies generally focused on cohorts with type 2 diabetes with one to two years of follow-up. They provided good evidence of the effectiveness of bariatric procedures, including Roux-en-Y gastric bypass,[60 61 62] adjustable gastric banding,[63 64] biliopancreatic diversion,[61] and vertical sleeve gastrectomy.[62] These procedures resulted in greater short term (1-2 years) weight loss (mean difference 26 kg; 95% confidence interval 31 to 21; P<0.001) and greater remission of type 2 diabetes (complete case analysis relative risk of remission: 22.1, 3.2 to 154.3; P=0.002; conservative analysis: 5.3, 1.8 to 15.8; P=0.003) compared with various non-surgical treatments.[60 61 62 63 64]

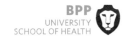
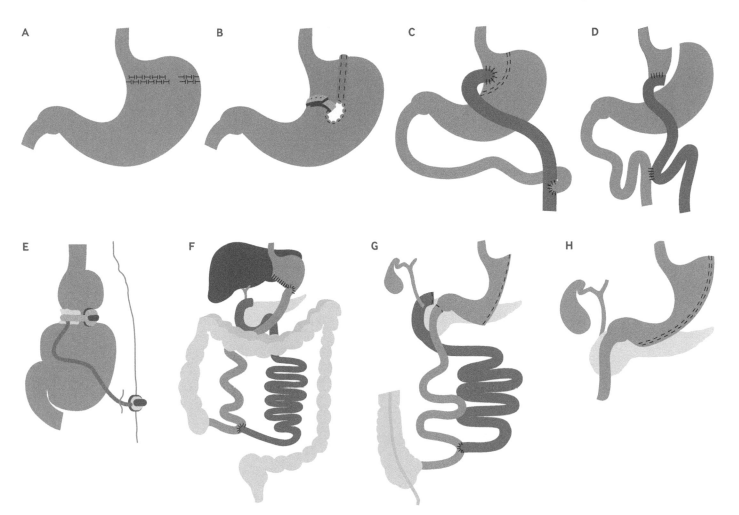

Fig 2 (A) Horizontal gastroplasty; (B) vertical banded gastroplasty; (C) Roux-en-Y gastric bypass; (D) transected Roux-en-Y gastric bypass; (E) laparoscopic adjustable gastric band; (F) biliopancreatic diversion; (G) biliopancreatic diversion with duodenal switch; (H) vertical sleeve gastrectomy

Recently, two additional small RCTs have been published that show similar short term results for both weight loss and type 2 diabetes.[65][66]

In addition, serum triglycerides and high density lipoproteins were significantly reduced by bariatric procedures, but blood pressure and other lipoproteins were not (although some studies showed reduced use of drugs for these conditions).[21] The review also noted a lack of evidence from RCTs beyond two years with respect to mortality, cardiovascular diseases, and adverse events.

Another recent systematic review focused on weight loss and glycemic control in class I obese (BMI 30-34.9) adults with type 2 diabetes and identified three RCTs with results similar to those seen in class II (BMI 35-39.9) and severely obese populations. However, the review also noted a lack of long term studies.[22]

Swedish Obese Subjects study
Given the absence of long term RCTs comparing bariatric procedures with non-surgical treatment of obesity, we must turn to large observational cohort studies to answer important questions about long term outcomes.[18][24][67][68] Much of our current knowledge about the long term results of bariatric surgery come from the Swedish Obese Subjects (SOS) study. This study started in 1987 as a prospective trial of 2010 people undergoing bariatric surgery compared with 2037 usual care controls who were matched on 18 clinical and demographic variables.[24]

The most common bariatric procedure performed in SOS was the vertical banded gastroplasty (68%), followed by gastric banding (19%), and Roux-en-Y gastric bypass (13%). Follow up rates are reported at 99% for some endpoints (including mortality), but physical and laboratory follow-up rates are lower, with imputation techniques used for sensitivity analysis.[24] The SOS investigators have published widely on health outcomes beyond 10 years, including weight loss, mortality, remission from and incidence of type 2 diabetes, cardiovascular events, incident cancer, psychosocial outcomes, and healthcare use and costs.[18][24][68][69][70][71][72]

Weight loss among surgical patients in SOS was greater than in controls (mean changes in body weight at 2, 10, 15, and 20 years were −23%, −17%, −16%, and −18% in the surgery group and 0%, 1%, −1%, and −1% in the control group, respectively).[24] After 15 years, the mean weight loss by procedure type was 27% (standard deviation 12%) for Roux-en-Y gastric bypass, 18% (11%) for vertical banded gastroplasty, and 13% (14%) for gastric banding.[24]

The SOS study also showed major improvements in obesity related comorbidities. In the surgical group there was a 72% remission of type 2 diabetes after two years (odds ratio for remission 8.4, 5.7 to 12.5; P<0.001) and 36% durable remission after 10 years (3.5, 1.6 to 7.3; P<0.001).[69]

In spite of the considerable recurrence of type 2 diabetes over time, bariatric surgery was associated with a lower incidence of myocardial infarction (hazard ratio 0.56, 0.34 to 0.93; P=0.025) and other complications of type 2 diabetes.[68]

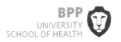

[73] Recently the SOS study showed that bariatric surgery also reduced the risk of developing type 2 diabetes by 96%, 84%, and 78% after two, 10, and 15 years in people without the condition at baseline.[74] This study also found that bariatric surgery was associated with a reduced incidence of fatal or non-fatal cancer in women but not in men (hazard ratio in women 0.58, 0.44 to 0.77; P<0.001; in men 0.97, 0.62 to 1.52; P=0.90).[71] Finally, at 16 years' follow-up, surgery was associated with a 29% lower risk of death from any cause (0.71, 0.54 to 0.92; P=0.01) compared with usual care.[18]

Utah obesity studies

Another important long term observational study performed in Utah from 1984 to 2002 comprised 7925 people who had undergone Roux-en-Y gastric bypass and 7925 weight, age, and sex matched controls. This study showed a 40% reduction in all cause mortality (hazard ratio 0.60, 0.45 to 0.67; P<0.001) and a 49% (0.51, 0.36 to 0.73; P<0.001) and 92% (0.08, 0.01 to 0.47; P=0.005) reduction in death from cardiovascular disease and death related to type 2 diabetes, respectively, at an average of 7.1 years later.[17]

Two other large retrospective observational studies support the findings from the SOS and Utah studies that bariatric surgery is associated with lower mortality than usual care.[75 76] However, another retrospective observational study of US veterans found no significant association between bariatric surgery and survival compared with usual care at a mean 6.7 years of follow-up.[77] The discrepant findings of this last study are probably a result of its focus on a high risk population as well as insufficient power and duration of follow-up.

A separate ongoing prospective Utah Obesity Study looked at more than 400 people who had undergone Roux-en-Y gastric bypass surgery and two non-randomized matched control groups—each with about 400 severely obese subjects. One control group comprised people who had sought surgery but did not undergo the operation; the other was a population based group. The study found that those in the surgery group lost 27.7% of their initial body weight compared with 0.2% weight gain in the surgery seekers and 0% change in the population based group at six years.[67] Diabetes was in remission in 62% of Roux-en-Y gastric bypass group and in only 8% and 6% of the control groups. Incident type 2 diabetes was noted in 2% of the Roux-en-Y gastric bypass group and in 17% and 15% of the control groups at six years.[67]

The LABS-2 study

The Longitudinal Assessment of Bariatric Surgery (LABS-2) study deserves mention, despite not including a non-surgical control group, because it is the largest ongoing prospective multicenter observational bariatric cohort study. LABS-2 will assess weight change and comorbid conditions in 2458 participants (1738 Roux-en-Y gastric bypass surgery, 610 adjustable gastric banding, and 110 other procedures) recruited between 2005 and 2009 who have been followed for three years to date.[78] In the LABS-2 cohort, median weight change was 31.5% for Roux-en-Y gastric bypass and 15.9% for adjustable gastric banding after three years, with much variability in response to each surgical treatment. Remission of type 2 diabetes was noted in 67% and 28% of those who had undergone Roux-en-Y gastric bypass and adjustable gastric banding, respectively. The incidence of type 2 diabetes was 0.9% and 3.2%, respectively, over the three years.[78]

Long term studies of quality of life

Few long term studies have assessed the impact of bariatric surgery on quality of life. However, three studies of six to 10 years' duration suggest that bariatric procedures are associated with greater improvements in generic and obesity specific measures of quality of life than non-surgical care.[72 79 80] Physical functioning domains seem to be more responsive to bariatric procedures than mental health domains, although more research is needed, especially in patients with class I obesity.

Effectiveness of bariatric surgery—comparisons between procedures

In the past 10 years, many systematic reviews of bariatric surgery have attempted to summarize and quantify differences in the efficacy and safety of various procedures.[15 16 19 20 23 81 82 83 84 85 86] A major challenge in summarizing this literature is the fact that no single randomized trial has included all of the most common procedures (Roux-en-Y gastric bypass, adjustable gastric banding, vertical sleeve gastrectomy, and biliopancreatic diversion with duodenal switch). Therefore, inference must be made through pooled analysis of data from many disparate randomized and non-randomized studies of bariatric surgery. In addition, no studies have examined differences in long term survival, incident cardiovascular events, and quality of life across procedures.

One of the most comprehensive systematic reviews analysed 136 studies and 22 094 patients undergoing bariatric surgery.[16] However, only five of the included studies were randomized trials (28 non-RCTs and 101 uncontrolled case series), and the review did not include data on vertical sleeve gastrectomy. The review found a strong trend towards different weight loss outcomes across procedures. Weighted mean percentage of excess weight loss (%EWL) was 50% (32% to 70%) for adjustable gastric banding, 68% (33% to 77%) for Roux-en-Y gastric bypass, 69% (48% to 93%) for vertical banded gastroplasty, and 72% (62% to 75%) for biliopancreatic diversion with duodenal switch. The rate of type 2 diabetes remission also varied greatly across procedures. The rate was 48% (29% to 67%) for adjustable gastric banding, 84% (77% to 90%) for Roux-en-Y gastric bypass, 72% (55% to 88%) for vertical banded gastroplasty, and 99% (97% to 100%) for biliopancreatic diversion with duodenal switch. A similar pattern of disease remission was seen for hypertension, dyslipidemia, and obstructive sleep apnea, with the highest rates of remission seen in patients who had undergone biliopancreatic diversion with duodenal switch, followed by Roux-en-Y gastric bypass, vertical banded gastroplasty, and lastly adjustable gastric banding.[16]

There is an ongoing debate about the comparative effectiveness of two of the most common procedures—adjustable gastric banding and Roux-en-Y gastric bypass—for weight loss and improvement in comorbidity. Consistent with the systematic review presented above, several other systematic reviews have concluded that Roux-en-Y gastric bypass is more effective for weight loss than adjustable gastric banding.[16 81 82 83] However, there have been only two small head to head RCTs (with follow-up at four and five years).[87 88]

Insufficient data are available from RCTs to examine differences between adjustable gastric banding and Roux-en-Y gastric bypass in improvements in comorbidity. However, systematic reviews of non-randomized studies indicate greater remission of type 2 diabetes, hypertension,

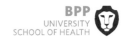

Table 1 Effectiveness of bariatric surgery compared with non-surgical management*

Study	Study details	Weight change	T2DM remission	T2DM incidence	Mortality and survival
Meta-analysis[21]	Meta-analysis of 11 RCTs (n=796); cohorts include RYGB, AGB, BPD, VSG v non-surgical treatments	Bariatric surgery treatment: 1-2 year weight change, mean difference −26 kg, 95% CI −31 to −21; P<0.001 v non-surgical treatment	Bariatric surgery treatment: complete case analysis relative risk 22.1, 3.2 to 154.3; P=0.002; conservative analysis 5.3, 1.8 to 15.8; P=0.003 v non-surgical treatment	Not reported	No cardiovascular events or deaths reported after bariatric surgery or in control populations
Swedish Obese Subjects study[18 24]	Prospective observational with matched controls (n=2010; 68% VBG, 19% banding, 13 % RYGB); 2037 matched controls	Bariatric surgery treatment: 2, 10, 15, 20 year weight change mean −23%, −17%, −16%, and −18%, respectively; matched control treatment: 2, 10, 15, 20 year weight loss mean 0%, 1%, −1%, and −1%, respectively	Bariatric surgery treatment: 2 years 72% remission (odds ratio for remission: 8.4, 5.7 to 12.5; P<0.001); 10 years 36% durable remission (3.5, 1.6 to 7.3; P<0.001)	Bariatric surgery treatment: 2, 10, and 15 years, reduced risk of developing T2DM by 96%, 84%, and 78%, respectively, in people without the condition at baseline	Bariatric surgery treatment: 16 years, 29% lower risk of death from any cause (hazard ratio 0.71, 0.54 to 0.92; P=0.01) v usual care; common causes of death: cancer and myocardial infarction
Utah Mortality study[17]	Retrospective observational with matched controls (7925 RYGB; 7925 weight matched controls)	Not reported	Not reported	Not reported	Bariatric surgery treatment: average 7.1 years post-treatment, 40% (hazard ratio 0.60, 0.45 to 0.67; P<0.001), 49% (0.51, 0.36 to 0.73; P<0.001), and 92% (0.08, 0.01 to 0.47; P=0.005) reduction in all cause mortality, cardiovascular mortality, and T2DM mortality, respectively
Utah Obesity study[67]	Prospective observational with matched controls; 418 RYGB; 417 bariatric surgery seekers who did not undergo surgery (control 1); 321 population based severely obese matched controls (control 2)	6 year weight change: −27.7%, +0.2%, and 0% of initial body weight for bariatric surgery, control 1, and control 2, respectively	6 year remission: 62%, 8%, and 6% for bariatric surgery, control 1, and control 2, respectively	6 year incident T2DM: 2%, 17%, and 15% for bariatric surgery, control 1, and control 2, respectively	Deaths at 6 years: 12 (2.8%), 14 (3.3%), and 3 (0.93%) for bariatric surgery, control 1, and control 2, respectively

* AGB=adjustable gastric banding; BPD=biliopancreatic diversion; LABS=Longitudinal Assessment of Bariatric Surgery study; RCT=randomized controlled trial; RYGB=Roux-en-Y gastric bypass; T2DM=type 2 diabetes; VBG=vertical banded gastroplasty; VSG=vertical sleeve gastrectomy.

dyslipidemia, and sleep apnea with Roux-en-Y gastric bypass versus adjustable gastric banding.[16 81] By contrast, one systematic review of 19 long term observational studies (≥10 years' duration; no RCTs) found a mean %EWL of 54.2% for adjustable gastric banding versus 54.0% for Roux-en-Y gastric bypass.[23] These discrepant data suggest that some very experienced, high volume surgical centers with rigorous programs for long term post-surgical care and follow-up may achieve weight loss results with adjustable gastric banding similar to those achieved with Roux-en-Y gastric bypass. However, data from these types of centers are not often seen in the surgical literature, and more research is needed to identify the optimal requirements of an adjustable gastric banding program.

Two recent systematic reviews compared the outcomes of vertical sleeve gastrectomy with other procedures.[85 86] One review identified 15 RCTs with 1191 patients.[85] The %EWL ranged from 49% to 81% for vertical sleeve gastrectomy, from 62% to 94% for Roux-en-Y gastric bypass, and from 29% to 48% for adjustable gastric banding, with follow-up ranging from six months to three years. The type 2 diabetes remission rate ranged from 27% to 75% for vertical sleeve gastrectomy versus 42% to 93% for Roux-en-Y gastric bypass.[85]

The second review compared only vertical sleeve gastrectomy and Roux-en-Y gastric bypass. It identified six RCTs and two non-randomized controlled studies with follow-up ranging from three months to two years.[86] It found significantly greater improvements in BMI with Roux-en-Y gastric bypass than with vertical sleeve gastrectomy (mean difference in BMI 1.8, 0.5 to 3.2). It also found greater improvements in total cholesterol, high density lipoprotein-cholesterol, and insulin resistance with Roux-en-Y gastric bypass versus vertical sleeve gastrectomy.[86] Longer term comparative effectiveness data on vertical sleeve gastrectomy are clearly needed. However, the effect of vertical sleeve gastrectomy on weight loss and comorbidity improvements seems to be somewhere between those of Roux-en-Y gastric bypass and adjustable gastric banding.[89]

Complications of bariatric surgery
Bariatric surgery is not without risks. Perioperative mortality for the average patient is low (<0.3%) and declining,[88] but it varies greatly across subgroups, with perioperative mortality rates of 2.0% or higher in some patient populations.[90 91 92 93] The incidence of complications in the first 30-180 days after surgery varies widely from 4% to 25% and depends on the definition of complication used, the type of bariatric procedure performed, the duration of follow-up, and individual patient characteristics.[15 26 91 94 95]

Findings from major studies
Among the 11 RCTs (796 patients) that have compared bariatric surgery with non-surgical care, rates of adverse events were higher in patients having surgery, but follow-up was limited to two years.[21] No cardiovascular events or deaths were seen in either group, but the most common adverse events after surgery were iron deficiency anemia (15% with intestinal bypass operations) and reoperations (8%).[21] These RCTs were not large enough to compare safety across procedure types, and most of the comparative data on complications come from larger observational studies.

The first phase of the Longitudinal Assessment of Bariatric Surgery (LABS-1) study prospectively assessed 30 day complications in 4776 severely obese patients who underwent a first bariatric surgical procedure (25% adjustable gastric banding, 62% laparoscopic Roux-en-Y gastric bypass, 9% open Roux-en-Y gastric bypass, and 3% another procedure) between 2005 and 2007.[91] The 30 day mortality rate was 0.3% for all procedures, with a major adverse outcome rate (predefined composite endpoint that included death, venous thromboembolism, reintervention (percutaneous, endoscopic, or operative), or failure to be discharged from

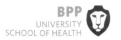

the hospital in 30 days) of 4.1%. Major predictors of an increased risk of complications were a history of venous thromboembolism, a diagnosis of obstructive sleep apnea, impaired functional status (inability to walk 61 m; 1 m=3.28 ft), extreme BMI (≥60), and undergoing Roux-en-Y gastric bypass by the open technique.[91]

Other large observational studies, such as SOS, have shown higher rates of complications, with 14.5% having at least one non-fatal complication over the first 90 days, including (in order of frequency) pulmonary complications, vomiting, wound infection, hemorrhage, and anastomotic leak.[24] However, the SOS included mostly open and vertical banded gastroplasty procedures, which are rarely performed today. Nonetheless, the 90 day mortality rate in SOS was low at 0.25%.

A meta-analysis of 361 studies (97.7% non-randomized observational design) of 85 048 patients reported important differences in mortality up to 30 days across different laparoscopic bariatric procedures. It found 0.06% (0.01% to 0.11%) for adjustable gastric banding, 0.21% (0.00% to 0.48%) for vertical banded gastroplasty, 0.16% (0.09% to 0.23%) for Roux-en-Y gastric bypass, and 1.11% (0.00% to 2.70%) for biliopancreatic diversion with duodenal switch.[90] The review also found significantly higher mortality with open procedures than with laparoscopic procedures.[90] A clinically useful prognostic risk score has been developed and validated in 9382 patients to predict 90 day mortality after Roux-en-Y gastric bypass surgery using five clinical characteristics: BMI 50 or more, male sex, hypertension, known risk factor for pulmonary embolism, and age 45 years or more.[96][97] Patients with four to five of these characteristics are at higher risk of death (4.3%) by 90 days than those with none or one of these characteristics (0.26%).[98]

A systematic review of 15 RCTs of vertical sleeve gastrectomy found no deaths in 795 patients but a 9.2% mean complication rate (range 0-18%).[85] In the American College of Surgeons Bariatric Surgery Network database, mortality 30 days after vertical sleeve gastrectomy was 0.11%, between that for adjustable gastric banding (0.05%) and Roux-en-Y gastric bypass (0.14%).[89] The 30 day complication (morbidity) rate was 5.6% for vertical sleeve gastrectomy, 1.4% for adjustable gastric banding, and 5.9% for Roux-en-Y gastric bypass.

Reoperation
A worrying trend is the relatively frequent rate of reoperation as a result of complications or insufficient weight loss (or both), especially for adjustable gastric banding. In a prospective cohort of 3227 patients who had undergone this procedure, 1116 (35%) patients underwent revisional procedures. These were performed because of proximal enlargement (26%), port and tubing problems (21%), and erosion (3.4%), with no acute band slippages specifically noted. The need for revision because of proximal enlargement of the gastric pouch decreased dramatically over 17 years as the surgical technique evolved, from 40% to 6.4%, and no acute slippages were specifically noted; however, the band was ultimately removed in 5.6% of all people.[23]

Other long term cohorts suggest that adjustable gastric banding removal rates may be as high as 50%.[99][100] In the LABS-2 cohort study, the rate of revision or reoperation was higher for adjustable gastric banding than for Roux-en-Y gastric bypass at three years of follow-up.[101] However, one systematic review of long term studies indicates that the rate of revisional surgery for Roux-en-Y gastric bypass

is similar to that for adjustable gastric banding (22% for Roux-en-Y gastric bypass, range 8-38%; 26% for adjustable gastric banding, 8-60%).[23] Many revisions are probably due to weight regain or failure to lose enough weight, but the specific cause for revision is often not indicated. The higher rates of reoperation with adjustable gastric banding may simply reflect the reversible nature of that surgical procedure compared with other relatively permanent procedures. Overall, more long term data are needed for all procedure types to categorize and understand the cause, nature, and severity of these complications.[102]

Psychosocial risks
Emerging data from observational studies suggest that some bariatric procedures introduce a greater long term risk of substance misuse disorders,[103][104][105] suicide,[106] and nutritional deficiencies.[107] Pharmacokinetic studies indicate that the gastrointestinal anatomy after Roux-en-Y gastric bypass and vertical sleeve gastrectomy leads to more rapid absorption of alcohol and marked increases in blood alcohol concentrations per dose. This may inadvertently increase the frequency of physiological binges and subsequent alcohol misuse disorder.[108][109][110]

In the SOS study, Roux-en-Y gastric bypass was associated with increased alcohol consumption and an increase in alcohol misuse events (hazard ratio 4.9) over 20 years, but more than 90% of patients remained below the World Health Organization cut off for low risk alcohol consumption.[105] Similarly, in the LABS-2 study, alcohol misuse disorders were more common in the second postoperative year (9.6%) in those undergoing Roux-en-Y gastric bypass than at baseline (7.6%).[103]

The risk of suicide may be increased after bariatric surgery, although the cause is unclear. The Utah Mortality study showed a 58% increase in all non-disease causes of death in the Roux-en-Y gastric bypass group compared with the matched control population, including a small but significant increase in suicides, accidental deaths, and poisonings.[17] Similar findings were observed in the second Utah Obesity Study,[67] and another observational study found that suicide rates in post-bariatric surgery patients were significantly higher than age and sex matched rates in the US.[111] Given the paucity of data on preoperative psychological risk assessment and long term follow-up after bariatric surgery, rigorous research is needed to inform future practice guidelines and care standards in this area.

Nutritional deficiencies
Finally, evidence indicates that vitamin and mineral deficiencies, including deficiencies of calcium, vitamin D, iron, zinc, and copper, are common after bariatric surgery.[107] Guidelines suggest screening patients for iron, vitamin B12, folic acid, and vitamin D deficiencies preoperatively. Patients should also be given daily nutritional supplementation postoperatively, including two adult multivitamin plus mineral supplements (each containing iron, folic acid, and thiamine), 1200 to 1500 mg of elemental calcium, at least 3000 IU of vitamin D, and vitamin B12 as needed. In addition, they should receive annual screening for specific deficiencies, including vitamin B12 (table 2).[112] Insufficient evidence is available on optimal dietary and nutritional management after bariatric surgery, including how to manage some of the complications of surgery (such as chronic nausea and vomiting, hypoglycemia, anastomotic ulcers and strictures, and failed weight loss).

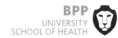
Table 2 Recommended postoperative nutritional monitoring* [112]

Recommendation	AGB	VSG	RYGB	BPD-DS
Bone density (DXA) at 2 years	Yes	Yes	Yes	Yes
24 hour urinary calcium excretion at 6 months and annually	Yes	Yes	Yes	Yes
Vitamin B12 annually (methylmalonic acid and homocysteine optional) then every 3-6 months if supplemented	Yes	Yes	Yes	Yes
Folic acid (red blood cell folic acid optional), iron studies, vitamin D, intact parathyroid hormone	No	No	Yes	Yes
Vitamin A initially and every 6-12 months thereafter	No	No	Optional	Yes
Copper, zinc, and selenium evaluation with specific findings	No	No	Yes	Yes
Thiamine evaluation with specific findings	Yes	Yes	Yes	Yes

*AGB=adjustable gastric banding; BPD-DS=biliopancreatic diversion with duodenal switch; DXA=dual energy X ray absorptiometry; RYGB=Roux-en-Y gastric bypass; VSG=vertical sleeve gastrectomy.

Guideline supported indications for bariatric surgery and their limitations

The first guidelines for patient selection in bariatric surgery were established in 1991 at a National Institutes of Health (NIH) consensus conference and were based on the limited literature available at that time.[113] The initial selection criteria were a BMI of 40 or more, or a BMI of 35.0-39.9 with one or more obesity related comorbidity. In 2004, a Medicare Coverage Advisory Committee concluded that there was enough scientific evidence to support the coverage of open and laparoscopic bariatric surgery for patients who met the NIH criteria, and many private insurers and state Medicaid programs in the US soon followed suit.[114]

Currently, the Centers for Medicare and Medicaid Services (CMS) covers open and laparoscopic Roux-en-Y gastric bypass, laparoscopic adjustable gastric banding, and open and laparoscopic biliopancreatic diversion with duodenal switch for Medicare beneficiaries.[115] In addition, in 2012 the CMS determined that local Medicare administrative contractors may individually determine coverage of laparoscopic vertical sleeve gastrectomy. In 2009, the CMS added a requirement that, for surgery to be reimbursed, it must be performed in "centers of excellence."[115] However, that requirement was removed in 2013 after the CMS determined that it did not improve health outcomes for Medicare beneficiaries. Although the 1991 NIH guidelines continue to be the most widely accepted standards for selecting patients for bariatric surgery,[27] many experts have indicated a need to develop updated guidelines. This is because the criteria do not consider age; race or ethnicity; and, particularly for the lower BMI range, the severity of coexisting comorbidities.[114 116]

In 2007, a 50 member international, multidisciplinary Diabetes Surgery Summit Consensus Conference concluded that strictly BMI based criteria were inadequate for selecting candidates for diabetes surgery. It was proposed that Roux-en-Y gastric bypass surgery could be considered in carefully selected moderately obese patients (BMI 30-35) with type 2 diabetes who were inadequately controlled by conventional medical and behavioral therapies.[117] Consensus was not reached on the use of adjustable gastric banding or other bariatric procedures for this lower BMI population. These recommendations were endorsed by 21 professional and scientific organizations.[112 117 118] However, in 2009, the CMS determined that bariatric procedures in patients with type 2 diabetes and a BMI less than 35 were "not reasonable and necessary" and therefore not covered.[115] Despite the

CMS coverage decision, in 2011, the US Food and Drug Administration approved the use of laparoscopic adjustable gastric banding for adults with a BMI 30-35 and at least one obesity related health condition. The strength of the evidence base for the FDA's decision has been questioned.[119] Finally, in 2013, updated guidelines were released for the perioperative nutritional, metabolic, and non-surgical support of patients who have undergone bariatric surgery.[112]

Costs

The ability of bariatric surgery to reduce expenditures sufficiently to achieve cost savings continues to be debated.[120] In two early observational studies, bariatric surgery seemed to be cost saving over a relatively short period of time.[121 122] More recent observational studies,[70 123] including an analysis of 29 820 Blue Cross Blue Shield Association enrollees, show no evidence of cost savings.[124]

In general, evidence suggests that outpatient costs, including pharmacy costs, are reduced after bariatric surgery. However, long term inpatient costs are increased or unchanged in patients who have undergone bariatric surgery compared with matched non-surgical patients, so no long term net cost benefit is seen. These results from observational cohorts are consistent with previous modeled cost effectiveness evaluations.[19 20 125] Such evaluations have shown that bariatric procedures are likely to be cost effective, but not cost saving, compared with usual medical care or intensive lifestyle interventions for the average patient with severe obesity.

Shared decision making in the management of obesity

Given the considerable trade-offs between the risks, benefits, and uncertainties of the long term effects of bariatric procedures, the decision to undergo surgery should be based on a shared decision making process.[126 127] The essential components of this process are clear communication of the clinician's expert judgment, elicitation of the patient's own values and preferences, and use of a patient decision aid that provides objective information about all clinically appropriate treatment options and encourages the patient to be meaningfully involved in decision making.[128] One RCT showed that use of a video based patient decision aid for bariatric surgery led to greater improvements in patient knowledge, decisional conflict, and outcome expectancies than an educational booklet on bariatric surgery produced by the NIH.[129]

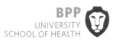

The shared decision making approach was endorsed at the 1991 NIH consensus conference on bariatric surgery.[113] It recommended the following:

- All patients should have an opportunity to explore with the physician any previously unconsidered treatment options and the advantages and disadvantages of each
- The physician must fully discuss with the patient:
  - The probable outcomes of the surgery
  - The probable extent to which surgery will eliminate the patient's problems
  - The compliance that will be needed in the postoperative regimen
  - The possible complications from the surgery, both short term and long term
- The need for lifelong medical surveillance after surgery should be clear
- With all of these considerations, the patient should be helped to arrive at a fully informed independent decision about his or her treatment.[113]

Looking ahead

Several important studies in the area of bariatric surgery are ongoing, including prospective and retrospective observational studies, and RCTs comparing contemporary procedures with non-surgical care of severely obese patients. The previously mentioned LABS-2 study will answer some questions about the comparative efficacy and safety of surgical procedures as well as the durability of weight loss and health improvements.[130] Three year data were recently published, and seven year follow-up is planned.

A parallel Teen-LABS study will answer similar questions in adolescents with severe obesity undergoing bariatric surgery. Seven NIH funded RCTs of bariatric surgery are ongoing or have been recently completed, and at least 13 international RCTs are ongoing. In the next few years, these RCTs will probably provide more definitive answers to questions about the efficacy of bariatric procedures versus usual or intensive medical care or lifestyle interventions in the short term, especially for patients with type 2 diabetes and a BMI of 30.0-39.9. In addition, several of these RCTs are currently planning follow-up for five years or longer, so pooled longer term results will be available.

Ongoing observational studies, including the Utah Obesity Study, the Michigan Bariatric Surgery Collaborative, and cohorts in the Health Maintenance Organization Research Network and US Department of Veterans Affairs, are all likely to yield important information in the next five years on the comparative efficacy, safety, and costs of surgical and non-surgical care. They should also provide data on the durability of weight loss and health improvements, including the impact on incident microvascular disease and cancer.

Conclusion

High quality data from RCTs have clearly established that bariatric procedures are more effective than medical or lifestyle interventions for inducing weight loss and initial remission of type 2 diabetes, even in less obese patients with a BMI between 30.0 and 39.9.[21] Although evidence from randomized trials does not go beyond two years, a few rigorous observational studies have shown encouraging results. These include an improvement in long term survival,[17] [18] a reduced risk of incident cardiovascular disease and diabetes,[68] [74] and more durable improvements in obesity related comorbidities among patients who have

---

FUTURE RESEARCH QUESTIONS

- What are the specific mechanisms of action responsible for weight loss and the type 2 diabetes response to bariatric surgical procedures?
- What patient level factors can predict success (weight loss, health improvements, and cost savings) after bariatric surgical procedures?
- Is bariatric surgery more effective than non-surgical care for the long term treatment of type 2 diabetes in people with less severe obesity (body mass index <35)?
- On implementation of standardized reporting of complications across bariatric studies, what are the long term complication rates after different bariatric procedures?
- What is the effect of bariatric surgery on long term microvascular and macrovascular event rates?

---

undergone bariatric surgery than among matched non-surgical controls.[24] [67]

However, bariatric procedures are not without risks. The perioperative mortality for the average patient is low (<0.3%) and declining,[90] but varies across subgroups, with perioperative mortality rates of 2.0% or higher in some patient populations.[90] [91] [92] [93] The incidence of complications after surgery varies from 4% to 25% and depends on the duration of follow-up, the definition of complication used, the type of bariatric procedure performed, and individual patient characteristics.[15] [26] [91] [94] [95]

Emerging data from observational studies also show that some procedures are associated with a greater long term risk of substance misuse disorders,[103] [104] [105] suicide,[106] and nutritional deficiencies.[107] More research is needed to examine differences in long term outcomes across various procedures and heterogeneous patient populations, and to identify those who are most likely to benefit from surgical intervention. Given the persistent uncertainties about the long term trade-offs between the risks and benefits of bariatric surgery, the decision to undergo surgery should be based on a high quality shared decision making process.

Contributors: Both authors planned, conducted, and prepared for publication all the review work described in this article; they both act as guarantors. Both authors also accept full responsibility for the work and the conduct of the study, had access to the data, and controlled the decision to publish.

Competing interests: We have read and understood BMJ policy on declaration of interests and declare: no support from any organization for the submitted work. DEA reports grants from the National Institutes of Health, grants and non-financial support from Informed Medical Decisions Foundation, grants from Department of Veterans Affairs, and grants from the Agency for Healthcare Research and Quality outside the submitted work. APC reports other funding from J&J Ethicon Scientific, personal fees from J&J Ethicon Scientific, grants from NIH-NIDDK, grants from Covidien, grants from EndoGastric Solutions, and grants from Nutrisystem outside the submitted work.

Provenance and peer review: Commissioned; externally peer reviewed.

1 Flegal KM, Carroll MD, Kit BK, Ogden CL. Prevalence of obesity and trends in the distribution of body mass index among US adults, 1999-2010. *JAMA* 2012;307:491-7.
2 Public Health England. Morbid obesity. 2014. www.noo.org.uk/NOO_about_obesity/Morbid_obesity.
3 Neovius M, Teixeira-Pinto A, Rasmussen F. Shift in the composition of obesity in young adult men in Sweden over a third of a century. *Int J Obes (Lond)* 2008;32:832-6.
4 Howard NJ, Taylor AW, Gill TK, Chittleborough CR. Severe obesity: investigating the socio-demographics within the extremes of body mass index. *Obes Res Clin Pract* 2008;2:I-II.
5 Buchwald H, Oien DM. Metabolic/bariatric surgery worldwide 2011. *Obes Surg* 2013;23:427-36.
6 Must A, Spadano J, Coakley EH, Field AE, Colditz G, Dietz WH. The disease burden associated with overweight and obesity. *JAMA* 1999;282:1523-9.

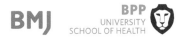

7   Flegal KM, Kit BK, Orpana H, Graubard BI. Association of all-cause mortality with overweight and obesity using standard body mass index categories: a systematic review and meta-analysis. JAMA2013;309:71-82.

8   Sarwer DB, Lavery M, Spitzer JC. A review of the relationships between extreme obesity, quality of life, and sexual function. Obes Surg2012;22:668-76.

9   Arterburn DE, Maciejewski ML, Tsevat J. Impact of morbid obesity on medical expenditures in adults. Int J Obes (Lond)2005;29:334-9.

10 Gregg EW, Cheng YJ, Narayan KM, Thompson TJ, Williamson DF. The relative contributions of different levels of overweight and obesity to the increased prevalence of diabetes in the United States: 1976-2004. Prev Med2007;45:348-52.

11 Ma J, Xiao L. Obesity and depression in US women: results from the 2005-2006 national health and nutritional examination survey. Obesity (Silver Spring)2010;18:347-53.

12 Li Z, Maglione M, Tu W, Mojica W, Arterburn D, Shugarman LR, et al. Meta-analysis: pharmacologic treatment of obesity. Ann Intern Med2005;142:532-46.

13 Look Ahead Research Group; Wing RR, Bolin P, Brancati FL, Bray GA, Clark JM, Coday M, et al. Cardiovascular effects of intensive lifestyle intervention in type 2 diabetes. N Engl J Med2013;369:145-54.

14 Moyer VA; Force US Preventive Services Task Force. Screening for and management of obesity in adults: US Preventive Services Task Force recommendation statement. Ann Intern Med2012;157:373-8.

15 Maggard MA, Shugarman LR, Suttorp M, Maglione M, Sugarman HJ, Livingston EH, et al. Meta-analysis: surgical treatment of obesity. Ann Intern Med2005;142:547-59.

16 Buchwald H, Avidor Y, Braunwald E, Jensen MD, Pories W, Fahrbach K, et al. Bariatric surgery: a systematic review and meta-analysis. JAMA2004;292:1724-37.

17 Adams TD, Gress RE, Smith SC, Halverson RC, Simper SC, Rosamond WD, et al. Long-term mortality after gastric bypass surgery. N Engl J Med 2007;357:753-61.

18 Sjostrom L, Narbro K, Sjostrom CD, Karason K, Larsson B, Wedel H, et al. Effects of bariatric surgery on mortality in Swedish obese subjects. N Engl J Med2007;357:741-52.

19 Picot J, Jones J, Colquitt JL, Gospodarevskaya E, Loveman E, Baxter L, et al. The clinical effectiveness and cost-effectiveness of bariatric (weight loss) surgery for obesity: a systematic review and economic evaluation. Health Technol Assess2009;13:1-190, 215-357, iii-iv.

20 Padwal R, Klarenbach S, Wiebe N, Hazel M, Birch D, Karmali S, et al. Bariatric surgery: a systematic review of the clinical and economic evidence. J Gen Intern Med2011;26:1183-94.

21 Gloy VL, Briel M, Bhatt DL, Kashyap SR, Schauer PR, Mingrone G, et al. Bariatric surgery versus non-surgical treatment for obesity: a systematic review and meta-analysis of randomised controlled trials. BMJ2013;347:f5934.

22 Maggard-Gibbons M, Maglione M, Livhits M, Ewing B, Maher AR, Hu J, et al. Bariatric surgery for weight loss and glycemic control in nonmorbidly obese adults with diabetes: a systematic review. JAMA2013;309:2250-61.

23 O'Brien PE, MacDonald L, Anderson M, Brennan L, Brown WA. Long-term outcomes after bariatric surgery: fifteen-year follow-up of adjustable gastric banding and a systematic review of the bariatric surgical literature. Ann Surg2013;257:87-94.

24 Sjostrom L. Review of the key results from the Swedish Obese Subjects (SOS) trial—a prospective controlled intervention study of bariatric surgery. J Intern Med2013;273:219-34.

25 Buchwald H, Oien DM. Metabolic/bariatric surgery worldwide 2008. Obes Surg2009;19:1605-11.

26 Encinosa WE, Bernard DM, Du D, Steiner CA. Recent improvements in bariatric surgery outcomes. Med Care2009;47:531-5.

27 Pi-Sunyer FX, Becker DM, Bouchard C, Carleton RA, Colditz GA, Dietz WH, et al. Clinical guidelines on the identification, evaluation, and treatment of overweight and obesity in adults: the evidence report. Government Printing Office, 1998. www.nhlbi.nih.gov/guidelines/obesity/ob_gdlns.pdf.

28 Nguyen NT, Masoomi H, Magno CP, Nguyen XM, Laugenour K, Lane J. Trends in use of bariatric surgery, 2003-2008. J Am Coll Surgeons2011;213:261-6.

29 Balsiger BM, Murr MM, Poggio JL, Sarr MG. Bariatric surgery. Surgery for weight control in patients with morbid obesity. Med Clin N Am2000;84:477-89.

30 Goldberg S, Rivers P, Smith K, Homan W. Vertical banded gastroplasty: a treatment for morbid obesity. AORN journal2000;72:988, 91-3, 95-1003; quiz 04-10.

31 Sugerman HJ. Bariatric surgery for severe obesity. J Assoc Acad Minor Phys2001;12:129-36.

32 Mason EE, Ito C. Gastric bypass. Ann Surg1969;170:329-39.

33 Colquitt J, Clegg A, Sidhu M, Royle P. Surgery for morbid obesity. Cochrane Database Syst Rev2003;2:CD003641.

34 Wittgrove AC, Clark GW. Laparoscopic gastric bypass, Roux-en-Y—500 patients: technique and results, with 3-60 month follow-up. Obes Surg2000;10:233-9.

35 Favretti F, Cadiere GB, Segato G, Himpens J, De Luca M, Busetto L, et al. Laparoscopic banding: selection and technique in 830 patients. Obes Surg2002;12:385-90.

36 Weiner R, Blanco-Engert R, Weiner S, Matkowitz R, Schaefer L, Pomhoff I. Outcome after laparoscopic adjustable gastric banding—8 years' experience. Obes Surg2003;13:427-34.

37 Scopinaro N, Marinari GM, Camerini G. Laparoscopic standard biliopancreatic diversion: technique and preliminary results. Obes Surg2002;12:362-5.

38 Baltasar A, Bou R, Miro J, Bengochea M, Serra C, Perez N. Laparoscopic biliopancreatic diversion with duodenal switch: technique and initial experience. Obes Surg2002;12:245-8.

39 Paiva D, Bernardes L, Suretti L. Laparoscopic biliopancreatic diversion: technique and initial results. Obes Surg2002;12:358-61.

40 Nguyen NT, Nguyen B, Gebhart A, Hohmann S. Changes in the makeup of bariatric surgery: a national increase in use of laparoscopic sleeve gastrectomy. J Am Coll Surg2013;216:252-7.

41 Stefater MA, Wilson-Perez HE, Chambers AP, Sandoval DA, Seeley RJ. All bariatric surgeries are not created equal: insights from mechanistic comparisons. Endocr Rev2012;33:595-622.

42 Basso N, Capoccia D, Rizzello M, Abbatini F, Mariani P, Maglio C, et al. First-phase insulin secretion, insulin sensitivity, ghrelin, GLP-1, and PYY changes 72 h after sleeve gastrectomy in obese diabetic patients: the gastric hypothesis. Surg Endosc2011;25:3540-50.

43 Karamanakos SN, Vagenas K, Kalfarentzos F, Alexandrides TK. Weight loss, appetite suppression, and changes in fasting and postprandial ghrelin and peptide-YY levels after Roux-en-Y gastric bypass and sleeve gastrectomy: a prospective, double blind study. Ann Surg2008;247:401-7.

44 Langer FB, Reza Hoda MA, Bohdjalian A, Felberbauer FX, Zacherl J, Wenzl E, et al. Sleeve gastrectomy and gastric banding: effects on plasma ghrelin levels. Obes Surg2005;15:1024-9.

45 Busetto L, Segato G, De Luca M, Foletto M, Pigozzo S, Favretti F, et al. High ghrelin concentration is not a predictor of less weight loss in morbidly obese women treated with laparoscopic adjustable gastric banding. Obes Surg2006;16:1068-74.

46 Tymitz K, Engel A, McDonough S, Hendy MP, Kerlakian G. Changes in ghrelin levels following bariatric surgery: review of the literature. Obes Surg2011;21:125-30.

47 Lee H, Te C, Koshy S, Teixeira JA, Pi-Sunyer FX, Laferrere B. Does ghrelin really matter after bariatric surgery? Surg Obes Relat Dis2006;2:538-48.

48 Woelnerhanssen B, Peterli R, Steinert RE, Peters T, Borbely Y, Beglinger C. Effects of postbariatric surgery weight loss on adipokines and metabolic parameters: comparison of laparoscopic Roux-en-Y gastric bypass and laparoscopic sleeve gastrectomy—a prospective randomized trial. Surg Obes Relat Dis2011;7:561-8.

49 Korner J, Inabnet W, Conwell IM, Taveras C, Daud A, Olivero-Rivera L, et al. Differential effects of gastric bypass and banding on circulating gut hormone and leptin levels. Obesity (Silver Spring)2006;14:1553-61.

50 Le Roux CW, Aylwin SJ, Batterham RL, Borg CM, Coyle F, Prasad V, et al. Gut hormone profiles following bariatric surgery favor an anorectic state, facilitate weight loss, and improve metabolic parameters. Ann Surg2006;243:108-14.

51 Korner J, Bessler M, Inabnet W, Taveras C, Holst JJ. Exaggerated glucagon-like peptide-1 and blunted glucose-dependent insulinotropic peptide secretion are associated with Roux-en-Y gastric bypass but not adjustable gastric banding. Surg Obes Relat Dis2007;3:597-601.

52 Rubino F, Gagner M, Gentileschi P, Kini S, Fukuyama S, Feng J, et al. The early effect of the Roux-en-Y gastric bypass on hormones involved in body weight regulation and glucose metabolism. Ann Surg2004;240:236-42.

53 Kellum JM, Kuemmerle JF, O'Dorisio TM, Rayford P, Martin D, Engle K, et al. Gastrointestinal hormone responses to meals before and after gastric bypass and vertical banded gastroplasty. Ann Surg1990;211:763-70; discussion 70-1.

54 Peterli R, Wolnerhanssen B, Peters T, Devaux N, Kern B, Christoffel-Courtin C, et al. Improvement in glucose metabolism after bariatric surgery: comparison of laparoscopic Roux-en-Y gastric bypass and laparoscopic sleeve gastrectomy: a prospective randomized trial. Ann Surg2009;250:234-41.

55 Liou AP, Paziuk M, Luevano JM Jr, Machineni S, Turnbaugh PJ, Kaplan LM. Conserved shifts in the gut microbiota due to gastric bypass reduce host weight and adiposity. Sci Transl Med2013;5:178ra41.

56 Aron-Wisnewsky J, Dore J, Clement K. The importance of the gut microbiota after bariatric surgery. Nat Rev Gastroenterol Hepatol2012;9:590-8.

57 Nakatani H, Kasama K, Oshiro T, Watanabe M, Hirose H, Itoh H. Serum bile acid along with plasma incretins and serum high-molecular weight adiponectin levels are increased after bariatric surgery. Metabolism2009;58:1400-7.

58 Stefater MA, Sandoval DA, Chambers AP, Wilson-Perez HE, Hofmann SM, Jandacek R, et al. Sleeve gastrectomy in rats improves postprandial lipid clearance by reducing intestinal triglyceride secretion. Gastroenterology2011;141:939-49 e1-4.

59 Patti ME, Houten SM, Bianco AC, Bernier R, Larsen PR, Holst JJ, et al. Serum bile acids are higher in humans with prior gastric bypass: potential contribution to improved glucose and lipid metabolism. Obesity (Silver Spring)2009;17:1671-7.

60 Ikramuddin S, Korner J, Lee WJ, Connett JE, Inabnet WB, Billington CJ, et al. Roux-en-Y gastric bypass vs intensive medical management for the control of type 2 diabetes, hypertension, and hyperlipidemia: the Diabetes Surgery Study randomized clinical trial. JAMA2013;309:2240-9.

61 Mingrone G, Panunzi S, De Gaetano A, Guidone C, Iaconelli A, Leccesi L, et al. Bariatric surgery versus conventional medical therapy for type 2 diabetes. N Engl J Med2012;366:1577-85.

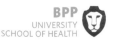

62 Schauer PR, Kashyap SR, Wolski K, Brethauer SA, Kirwan JP, Pothier CE, et al. Bariatric surgery versus intensive medical therapy in obese patients with diabetes. *N Engl J Med* 2012;366:1567-76.

63 Dixon JB, O'Brien PE, Playfair J, Chapman L, Schachter LM, Skinner S, et al. Adjustable gastric banding and conventional therapy for type 2 diabetes: a randomized controlled trial. *JAMA* 2008;299:316-23.

64 O'Brien PE, Dixon JB, Laurie C, Skinner S, Proietto J, McNeil J, et al. Treatment of mild to moderate obesity with laparoscopic adjustable gastric banding or an intensive medical program: a randomized trial. *Ann Intern Med* 2006;144:625-33.

65 Courcoulas AP, Goodpaster BH, Eagleton JK, Belle SH, Kalarchian MA, Lang W, et al. Surgical vs medical treatments for type 2 diabetes mellitus: a randomized clinical trial. *JAMA Surg* 2014; published online 4 Jun.

66 Halperin F, Ding SA, Simonson DC, Panosian J, Goebel-Fabbri A, Wewalka M, et al. Roux-en-Y gastric bypass surgery or lifestyle with intensive medical management in patients with type 2 diabetes: feasibility and 1-year results of a randomized clinical trial. *JAMA Surg* 2014; published online 4 Jun.

67 Adams TD, Davidson LE, Litwin SE, Kolotkin RL, LaMonte MJ, Pendleton RC, et al. Health benefits of gastric bypass surgery after 6 years. *JAMA* 2012;308:1122-31.

68 Sjostrom L, Peltonen M, Jacobson P, Sjostrom CD, Karason K, Wedel H, et al. Bariatric surgery and long-term cardiovascular events. *JAMA* 2012;307:56-65.

69 Sjostrom L, Lindroos AK, Peltonen M, Torgerson J, Bouchard C, Carlsson B, et al. Lifestyle, diabetes, and cardiovascular risk factors 10 years after bariatric surgery. *N Engl J Med* 2004;351:2683-93.

70 Neovius M, Narbro K, Keating C, Peltonen M, Sjoholm K, Agren G, et al. Health care use during 20 years following bariatric surgery. *JAMA* 2012;308:1132-41.

71 Sjostrom L, Gummesson A, Sjostrom CD, Narbro K, Peltonen M, Wedel H, et al. Effects of bariatric surgery on cancer incidence in obese patients in Sweden (Swedish Obese Subjects Study): a prospective, controlled intervention trial. *Lancet Oncol* 2009;10:653-62.

72 Karlsson J, Taft C, Ryden A, Sjostrom L, Sullivan M. Ten-year trends in health-related quality of life after surgical and conventional treatment for severe obesity: the SOS intervention study. *Int J Obes (Lond)* 2007;31:1248-61.

73 Romeo S, Maglio C, Burza MA, Pirazzi C, Sjoholm K, Jacobson P, et al. Cardiovascular events after bariatric surgery in obese subjects with type 2 diabetes. *Diabetes Care* 2012;35:2613-7.

74 Carlsson LM, Peltonen M, Ahlin S, Anveden A, Bouchard C, Carlsson B, et al. Bariatric surgery and prevention of type 2 diabetes in Swedish obese subjects. *N Engl J Med* 2012;367:695-704.

75 Flum DR, Dellinger EP. Impact of gastric bypass operation on survival: a population-based analysis. *J Am Coll Surg* 2004;199:543-51.

76 Christou NV, Sampalis JS, Liberman M, Look D, Auger S, McLean AP, et al. Surgery decreases long-term mortality, morbidity, and health care use in morbidly obese patients. *Ann Surg* 2004;240:416-23; discussion 23-4.

77 Maciejewski ML, Livingston EH, Smith VA, Kavee AL, Kahwati LC, Henderson WG, et al. Survival among high-risk patients after bariatric surgery. *JAMA* 2011;305:2419-26.

78 Courcoulas AP, Christian NJ, Belle SH, Berk PD, Flum DR, Garcia L, et al. Weight change and health outcomes at 3 years after bariatric surgery among individuals with severe obesity. *JAMA* 2013;310:2416-25.

79 Kolotkin RL, Davidson LE, Crosby RD, Hunt SC, Adams TD. Six-year changes in health-related quality of life in gastric bypass patients versus obese comparison groups. *Surg Obes Relat Dis* 2012;8:625-33.

80 Nickel MK, Loew TH, Bachler E. Change in mental symptoms in extreme obesity patients after gastric banding, part II: six-year follow up. *Int J Psychiatry Med* 2007;37:69-79.

81 Tice JA, Karliner L, Walsh J, Petersen AJ, Feldman MD. Gastric banding or bypass? A systematic review comparing the two most popular bariatric procedures. *Am J Med* 2008;121:885-93.

82 Chakravarty PD, McLaughlin E, Whittaker D, Byrne E, Cowan E, Xu K, et al. Comparison of laparoscopic adjustable gastric banding (LAGB) with other bariatric procedures; a systematic review of the randomised controlled trials. *Surgeon* 2012;10:172-82.

83 Padwal R, Klarenbach S, Wiebe N, Birch D, Karmali S, Manns B, et al. Bariatric surgery: a systematic review and network meta-analysis of randomized trials. *Obes Rev* 2011;12:602-21.

84 Delaet D, Schauer D. Obesity in adults. *Clin Evid (Online)* 2011;2011: pii:0604.

85 Trastulli S, Desiderio J, Guarino S, Cirocchi R, Scalercio V, Noya G, et al. Laparoscopic sleeve gastrectomy compared with other bariatric surgical procedures: a systematic review of randomized trials. *Surg Obes Relat Dis* 2013;9:816-29.

86 Yang X, Yang G, Wang W, Chen G, Yang H. A meta-analysis: to compare the clinical results between gastric bypass and sleeve gastrectomy for the obese patients. *Obes Surg* 2013;23:1001-10.

87 Angrisani L, Lorenzo M, Borrelli V. Laparoscopic adjustable gastric banding versus Roux-en-Y gastric bypass: 5-year results of a prospective randomized trial. *Surg Obes Relat Dis* 2007;3:127-32; discussion 32-3.

88 Nguyen NT, Slone JA, Nguyen XM, Hartman JS, Hoyt DB. A prospective randomized trial of laparoscopic gastric bypass versus laparoscopic adjustable gastric banding for the treatment of morbid obesity: outcomes, quality of life, and costs. *Ann Surg* 2009;250:631-41.

89 Hutter MM, Schirmer BD, Jones DB, Ko CY, Cohen ME, Merkow RP, et al. First report from the American College of Surgeons Bariatric Surgery Center Network: laparoscopic sleeve gastrectomy has morbidity and effectiveness positioned between the band and the bypass. *Ann Surg* 2011;254:410-20; discussion 20-2.

90 Buchwald H, Estok R, Fahrbach K, Banel D, Sledge I. Trends in mortality in bariatric surgery: a systematic review and meta-analysis. *Surgery* 2007;142:621-32; discussion 32-5.

91 Longitudinal Assessment of Bariatric Surgery (LABS) Consortium; Flum DR, Belle SH, King WC, Wahed AS, Berk P, Chapman W, et al. Perioperative safety in the longitudinal assessment of bariatric surgery. *N Engl J Med* 2009;361:445-54.

92 Flum DR, Salem L, Elrod JA, Dellinger EP, Cheadle A, Chan L. Early mortality among Medicare beneficiaries undergoing bariatric surgical procedures. *JAMA* 2005;294:1903-8.

93 Livingston EH. Obesity, mortality, and bariatric surgery death rates. *JAMA* 2007;298:2406-8.

94 Birkmeyer NJ, Dimick JB, Share D, Hawasli A, English WJ, Genaw J, et al. Hospital complication rates with bariatric surgery in Michigan. *JAMA* 2010;304:435-42.

95 Finks JF, Kole KL, Yenumula PR, English WJ, Krause KR, Carlin AM, et al. Predicting risk for serious complications with bariatric surgery: results from the Michigan Bariatric Surgery Collaborative. *Ann Surg* 2011;254:633-40.

96 DeMaria EJ, Murr M, Byrne TK, Blackstone R, Grant JP, Budak A, et al. Validation of the obesity surgery mortality risk score in a multicenter study proves it stratifies mortality risk in patients undergoing gastric bypass for morbid obesity. *Ann Surg* 2007;246:578-82; discussion 83-4.

97 DeMaria EJ, Portenier D, Wolfe L. Obesity surgery mortality risk score: proposal for a clinically useful score to predict mortality risk in patients undergoing gastric bypass. *Surg Obes Relat Dis* 2007;3:134-40.

98 Thomas H, Agrawal S. Systematic review of obesity surgery mortality risk score—preoperative risk stratification in bariatric surgery. *Obes Surg* 2012;22:1135-40.

99 Himpens J, Cadiere GB, Bazi M, Vouche M, Cadiere B, Dapri G. Long-term outcomes of laparoscopic adjustable gastric banding. *Arch Surg* 2011;146:802-7.

100 Lanthaler M, Aigner F, Kinzl J, Sieb M, Cakar-Beck F, Nehoda H. Long-term results and complications following adjustable gastric banding. *Obes Surg* 2010;20:1078-85.

101 Courcoulas A, Christian NJ, Belle SH, Berk PD, Flum DR, Garcia L, et al. Weight change and health outcomes at 3 years after bariatric surgery among patients with severe obesity. 2013;310:2416-25.

102 Courcoulas AP, Yanovski SZ, Bonds D, Eggerman TL, Horlick M, Staten MA, et al. Long-term outcomes of bariatric surgery: a National Institutes of Health symposium. *JAMA Surg* (forthcoming).

103 King WC, Chen JY, Mitchell JE, Kalarchian MA, Steffen KJ, Engel SG, et al. Prevalence of alcohol use disorders before and after bariatric surgery. *JAMA* 2012;307:2516-25.

104 Ostlund MP, Backman O, Marsk R, Stockeld D, Lagergren J, Rasmussen F, et al. Increased admission for alcohol dependence after gastric bypass surgery compared with restrictive bariatric surgery. *JAMA Surg* 2013;148:374-7.

105 Svensson PA, Anveden A, Romeo S, Peltonen M, Ahlin S, Burza MA, et al. Alcohol consumption and alcohol problems after bariatric surgery in the Swedish Obese Subjects study. *Obesity (Silver Spring)* 2013;21:2444-5.

106 Peterhansel C, Petroff D, Klinitzke G, Kersting A, Wagner B. Risk of completed suicide after bariatric surgery: a systematic review. *Obes Rev* 2013;14:369-82.

107 Gletsu-Miller N, Wright BN. Mineral malnutrition following bariatric surgery. *Adv Nutr* 2013;4:506-17.

108 Hagedorn JC, Encarnacion B, Brat GA, Morton JM. Does gastric bypass alter alcohol metabolism? *Surg Obes Relat Dis* 2007;3:543-8; discussion 48.

109 Klockhoff H, Naslund I, Jones AW. Faster absorption of ethanol and higher peak concentration in women after gastric bypass surgery. *Br J Clin Pharmacol* 2002;54:587-91.

110 Maluenda F, Csendes A, De Aretxabala X, Poniachik J, Salvo K, Delgado I, et al. Alcohol absorption modification after a laparoscopic sleeve gastrectomy due to obesity. *Obes Surg* 2010;20:744-8.

111 Tindle HA, Omalu B, Courcoulas A, Marcus M, Hammers J, Kuller LH. Risk of suicide after long-term follow-up from bariatric surgery. *Am J Med* 2010;123:1036-42.

112 Mechanick JI, Youdim A, Jones DB, Garvey WT, Hurley DL, McMahon MM, et al. Clinical practice guidelines for the perioperative nutritional, metabolic, and nonsurgical support of the bariatric surgery patient—2013 update: cosponsored by American Association of Clinical Endocrinologists, the Obesity Society, and American Society for Metabolic and Bariatric Surgery. *Obesity (Silver Spring)* 2013;21(suppl 1):S1-27.

113 NIH conference. Gastrointestinal surgery for severe obesity. Consensus development conference panel. *Ann Intern Med* 1991;115:956-61.

114 Pories WJ, Dohm LG, Mansfield CJ. Beyond the BMI: the search for better guidelines for bariatric surgery. *Obesity (Silver Spring)* 2010;18:865-71.

115 Centers for Medicare and Medicaid Services. National coverage determination (NCD) for bariatric surgery for treatment of morbid obesity. 2009. www.cms.gov/medicare-coverage-database/details/ncd-details.aspx?NCDId=57&bc=AgAAQAAAAAAA&ncdver=3.

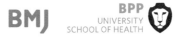

116 Yermilov I, McGory ML, Shekelle PW, Ko CY, Maggard MA. Appropriateness criteria for bariatric surgery: beyond the NIH guidelines. *Obesity (Silver Spring)*2009;17:1521-7.

117 Rubino F, Kaplan LM, Schauer PR, Cummings DE. The Diabetes Surgery Summit consensus conference: recommendations for the evaluation and use of gastrointestinal surgery to treat type 2 diabetes mellitus. *Ann Surg*2010;251:399-405.

118 Zimmet P, Alberti KG, Rubino F, Dixon JB. IDF's view of bariatric surgery in type 2 diabetes. *Lancet*2011;378:108-10.

119 Arterburn D, Maggard MA. Revisiting the 2011 FDA decision on laparoscopic adjustable gastric banding. *Obesity (Silver Spring)*2013;21:2204.

120 Maciejewski ML, Arterburn DE. Cost-effectiveness of bariatric surgery. *JAMA*2013;310:742-3.

121 Cremieux PY, Buchwald H, Shikora SA, Ghosh A, Yang HE, Buessing M. A study on the economic impact of bariatric surgery. *Am J Manag Care*2008;14:589-96.

122 Finkelstein EA, Allaire BT, Burgess SM, Hale BC. Financial implications of coverage for laparoscopic adjustable gastric banding. *Surg Obes Relat Dis*2011;7:295-303.

123 Maciejewski ML, Livingston EH, Smith VA, Kahwati LC, Henderson WG, Arterburn DE. Health expenditures among high-risk patients after gastric bypass and matched controls. *Arch Surg*2012;147:633-40.

124 Weiner JP, Goodwin SM, Chang HY, Bolen SD, Richards TM, Johns RA, et al. Impact of bariatric surgery on health care costs of obese persons: a 6-year follow-up of surgical and comparison cohorts using health plan data. *JAMA Surg*2013;148:555-62.

125 Wang BC, Wong ES, Alfonso-Cristancho R, He H, Flum DR, Arterburn DE, et al. Cost-effectiveness of bariatric surgical procedures for the treatment of severe obesity. *Eur J Health Econ*2014;15:253-63.

126 O'Connor AM, Llewellyn-Thomas HA, Barry A. Modifying unwarranted variations in health care: shared decision making using patient decision aids. *Health Affairs*2004; Suppl Variation:VAR63-72.

127 Keirns CC, Goold SD. Patient-centered care and preference-sensitive decision making. *JAMA*2009;302:1805-6.

128 Weinstein JN, Clay K, Morgan TS. Informed patient choice: patient-centered valuing of surgical risks and benefits. *Health Aff (Millwood)*2007;26:726-30.

129 Arterburn DE, Westbrook EO, Bogart TA, Sepucha KR, Bock SN, Weppner WG. Randomized trial of a video-based patient decision aid for bariatric surgery. *Obesity (Silver Spring)*2011;19:1669-75.

130 Belle SH, Berk PD, Chapman WH, Christian NJ, Courcoulas AP, Dakin GF, et al. Baseline characteristics of participants in the Longitudinal Assessment of Bariatric Surgery-2 (LABS-2) study. *Surg Obes Relat Dis*2013;9:926-35.

Related links

thebmj.com

• Read previous State of the Art reviews

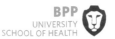

Gallstones

Kurinchi S Gurusamy, lecturer,

Brian R Davidson, professor of hepatopancreatobiliary and liver transplantation surgery

¹Department of Surgery,
9th floor Royal Free Hospital,
Royal Free Campus,
UCL Medical School, London, UK

Correspondence to: K Gurusamy
k.gurusamy@ucl.ac.uk

Cite this as: BMJ 2014;348:g2669

DOI: 10.1136/bmj.g2669

http://www.bmj.com/content/348/
bmj.g2669

Gallstones affect approximately 5-25% of adults in the Western world. It is therefore important to understand the consequences of a diagnosis of gallstones, the associated complications, and treatment to allow patients to be appropriately advised. The purpose of this review is to update clinicians on the diagnosis and management of gallstones.

What are gallstones?

Gallstones are crystalline deposits in the gallbladder (figure).[1] The prevalence of gallstones varies between 5% and 25%, with a higher prevalence in Western countries, women, and older age group.[2] Traditionally, gallstones were classified as cholesterol stones, pigment stones, or mixed stones (a combination of cholesterol and pigment stones) based on their composition,[3] which can only be determined reliably after their removal.[4] Recently, additional types of gallstones have been identified based on their microscopic structure and composition.[1] However, most stones fall under the umbrella of cholesterol (37-86%), pigment (2-27%), calcium (1-17%), or mixed (4-16%).[1] [4] The types of gallstone vary by their cause, the measures attempted to prevent their formation, their appearance on radiographs, and their response to dissolution therapy. The current recommendations for diagnosis and management are, however, the same for all types of gallstone.

Who gets gallstones?

Cholesterol stones are formed because of the alteration in the balance between pronucleating factors and antinucleating factors in the bile. Factors that lead to gallstone formation include excessive bile cholesterol, low bile salt levels, decreased gallbladder motility, and the phosphatidylcholine molecule, which prevents the crystallisation of cholesterol.[5] The main risk factors for cholesterol stone formation include female sex, pregnancy, high dose oestrogen treatment, increasing age, ethnicity (higher prevalence in Native American Indians and lower prevalence in black Americans, Africans, and people from China, Japan, India, and Thailand),

genetic traits, obesity, high serum triglyceride levels, low levels of high density cholesterol, rapid weight loss, high calorific diet, refined carbohydrate diet, lack of physical activity, cirrhosis, Crohn's disease, and gallbladder stasis (for example, as a result of previous gastrectomy or vagotomy).[6] [7] [8] Haemolysis and chronic bacterial or parasitic infections are considered the main risk factors for pigment stones[5] and are preventable causes of gallstones.

Can gallstone formation be prevented?

Although some of the causes of gallstones, such as obesity, rapid weight loss, a high calorific diet, a refined carbohydrate diet, and lack of physical activity are preventable by lifestyle changes, there is currently no evidence that lifestyle modifications can reduce the incidence of gallstones. Haemolysis and infections can be prevented by early recognition of sickle cell disease, taking appropriate measures for prevention of sickling crises, and using prophylactic antibiotics in those who have undergone splenectomy or had splenic infarction. Another way of preventing gallstone formation is to remove the gallbladder in people undergoing anti-obesity operations (as rapid weight loss is one of the risk factors for gallstone formation) and other major abdominal operations to avoid further surgery as a result of the development of symptomatic gallstones. There is currently no evidence to suggest that prophylactic cholecystectomy is indicated in any patient group without gallstones[9] or that any of the above suggested measures of preventing gallstones are effective.

How do gallstones present?

Each year approximately 2-4% of people with gallstones develop symptoms, with biliary colic being the most common symptom (steady right upper quadrant abdominal pain lasting more than half an hour)[10] [11] [12] [13] [14] in the absence of fever. Presence of fever usually indicates acute cholecystitis or cholangitis. Other common symptoms related to gallstones include epigastric pain and intolerance to fried or fatty foods (symptoms such as nausea, bloating, flatulence, frothy and foul smelling stools).[14] The box lists the complications resulting from gallstones, and includes acute cholecystitis (0.3-0.4% annually),[11] [12] [13] [15] acute pancreatitis (0.04-1.5% annually),[15] obstructive jaundice (0.1-0.4% annually),[12] [13] [15] and other rarer complications such as acute cholangitis and intestinal obstruction (gallstone ileus). Of these, acute pancreatitis and cholangitis are life threatening complications, with 3% to 20% mortality after a first attack of acute pancreatitis[16] and 24% mortality after acute cholangitis.[17] Uncomplicated biliary colic often precedes other gallstone related complications.[11] The rates of gallstone related complications are higher in people with a history of uncomplicated biliary colic.[18] Although studies have shown an association between gallstones and cancer of the biliary tract,[19] [20] no causative link has been established and the observed association could be due to the presence of common factors causing gallstones and gallbladder cancer.[21]

SOURCES AND SELECTION CRITERIA

We searched Medline, Embase, the Cochrane Database of Systematic Reviews, and Clinical Evidence online using the search terms "gallstones" or "cholelithiasis", focusing mainly on systematic reviews, meta-analyses, and high quality randomised controlled trials published within the past five years, wherever appropriate and possible.

SUMMARY POINTS

- Gallstones are common in adults
- Currently, treatment is indicated only for symptomatic gallstones
- Pain is the most common symptom related to gallstones
- Occasionally gallstones present with life threatening complications
- Surgery is the only definitive treatment and is recommended for people with symptomatic gallstones who are fit to undergo surgery
- Laparoscopic cholecystectomy is currently the preferred method of surgery and is generally both effective and safe; however, there is a 0.3% risk of serious injury to the bile duct, which may have serious long term consequences

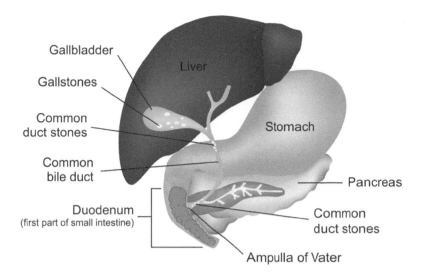

Gallbladder

Gallstones

Common duct stones

Common bile duct

Duodenum (first part of small intestine)

Liver

Stomach

Pancreas

Common duct stones

Ampulla of Vater

Obstruction to the common bile duct by common duct stones may cause jaundice or cholangitis. Obstruction to the pancreatic duct or ampulla of Vater by common duct stones may cause pancreatitis

How should suspected gallstones be investigated?

Ultrasonography is currently the first line method for the diagnosis of gallstones and has a high diagnostic accuracy (90% sensitivity and 88% specificity) even when performed by non-radiologists.[22] Based on the agreement in a consensus conference, the diagnosis of acute cholecystitis is suspected by the presence of local or systemic signs of inflammation, such as Murphy's sign (tenderness in the right upper quadrant below the costal margin on deep inspiration; sensitivity 65% and specificity 87%[23]), fever, increased white cell count or C reactive protein, and confirmed by ultrasonography, computed tomography, or magnetic resonance imaging.[24] Radiological signs of acute cholecystitis include a thickened gallbladder wall (>4 mm), an enlarged gallbladder (long axis diameter >8 cm, short axis diameter >4 cm), or fluid collection around the gallbladder.[24] The diagnosis of pancreatitis is usually suspected by the presence of pain in the epigastric region radiating to the back and confirmed by diffuse abdominal tenderness, increased serum amylase, urine amylase, or serum lipase levels, and is supported by radiological features such as an enlarged pancreas with peripancreatic fluid collections.[25] The consensus conference conducted by the European Association for Endoscopic Surgery concluded that common bile duct stones should be suspected by the presence of clinical features suggestive of obstructive jaundice, such as yellowish discoloration of skin and dark urine supported by an increased serum bilirubin or alkaline phosphatase level and confirmed with magnetic resonance cholangiopancreatography or endoscopic ultrasonography.[26] [27] Fever and rigors in the presence of jaundice should raise the suspicion of cholangitis.

If patients present with symptoms suggestive of gallstones, are systemically well, and do not have features suggestive of acute cholecystitis, acute pancreatitis, obstructive jaundice, or cholangitis, it is reasonable to investigate them by an elective ultrasonography, followed by elective referral to a general surgeon if gallstones are present. If gallstone complications are suspected, urgent referral to the surgeon is warranted because early confirmation of diagnosis and treatment of complications are associated with better outcomes (see section on timing of surgery). Features that suggest the presence of complications include fever, rigors, hypotension, epigastric

pain radiating to the back, dark urine, jaundice, Murphy's sign, diffuse abdominal tenderness, or a positive result for urine bile pigments on urinalysis. Depending on the clinical presentation, further blood tests, such as blood white cell count, levels of serum C reactive protein, serum amylase, serum bilirubin, and serum alkaline phosphatase; urine tests to check levels of urine amylase and urine lipase; and radiological investigations such as ultrasonography, computed tomography, magnetic resonance imaging, magnetic resonance cholangiopancreatography, and endoscopic ultrasonography may be performed to confirm or rule out the presence of gallstones and complications.

How is gallstone disease treated?

Asymptomatic gallstones

The distinction between symptomatic and asymptomatic gallstones can be difficult as symptoms can be mild and varied. While gallstone complications can be diagnosed using one or more of the criteria described, in patients presenting with vague upper abdominal pain or dyspeptic symptoms it can be difficult to discern whether the symptoms are related to gallstones. In one study, 90% of patients with classic biliary colic had high rates of symptom relief after cholecystectomy, suggesting that biliary colic is a fairly reliable indicator of symptomatic gallstones.[28] Around 70% of patients with upper abdominal pain with no further restriction by intensity or duration of pain had symptom relief after cholecystectomy. Only 55% of patients with dyspeptic symptoms had symptom relief, suggesting that in a major proportion of people vague upper abdominal pain or dyspepsia may not be related to gallstones.[28] There is currently no evidence that lifestyle modifications such as decreasing fatty food intake or increasing exercise decreases or prevents the incidence of symptoms in people with asymptomatic gallstones. No treatment is currently recommended for patients with asymptomatic gallstones (irrespective of whether these are cholesterol, pigment, or mixed stones) except for patients with porcelain gallbladders (which is usually identified by ultrasonography), owing to the association with gallbladder cancer.[29] The reason for advising against surgery for asymptomatic gallstones is because of the complications associated with surgical intervention, although this is a topic of ongoing debate.

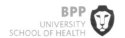
COMPLICATIONS OF GALLSTONES

- Acute cholecystitis
- Choledocholithiasis
- Acute cholangitis
- Acute pancreatitis
- Mucocele of gallbladder
- Empyema of gallbladder
- Gangrenous gallbladder
- Biliary peritonitis
- Porcelain gallbladder
- Gallbladder cancer

In patients with asymptomatic gallstones undergoing major abdominal surgery, it seems reasonable to offer cholecystectomy, as adhesions related to a major operation may make further minimal access surgeries difficult or impossible. There is, however, no evidence from randomised controlled trials or systematic reviews to support this statement.

Symptomatic gallstones

Cholecystectomy (removal of the gallbladder) is the preferred option in the treatment of gallstones, irrespective of whether the gallstones are cholesterol, pigment, or mixed stones. Evidence from randomised controlled trials, systematic reviews, and cohort studies show that extracorporeal shock wave lithotripsy or bile acid dissolution therapy with ursodeoxycholic acid has a low rate of cure, with only 27% of patients having dissolution of stones after treatment with ursodeoxycholic acid and only 55% of carefully selected patients being stone free after extracorporeal shock wave lithotripsy. The rate of recurrent gallstones is also high; more than 40% of patients have recurrence of gallstones within four years after complete dissolution of stones or extracorporeal shock wave lithotripsy. Over three months, only 26% of people remained colic free after treatment with ursodeoxycholic acid compared with 33% after placebo, and about 2% of people had gallstone complications after treatment with ursodeoxycholic acid, which is similar to the annual rate of complications in those not taking the drug.[15][30][31][32][33][34] In patients who are not suitable for cholecystectomy because of their general medical condition, percutaneous cholecystostomy (temporary external drainage of the gallbladder contents through a tube inserted under radiological guidance) may be considered in an emergency situation, although a systematic review revealed that the role of percutaneous cholecystostomy in the management of such patients was not clear.[35] When the patient's condition has improved, cholecystectomy may be reconsidered. Based on evidence from randomised controlled trials, watchful observation may be a suitable alternative to surgery in a small proportion of people who do not get recurrent symptoms.[36][37] It is, however, not possible to predict those patients who will get recurrence of symptoms.

Cholecystectomy: the risks and benefits

Although cholecystectomy is a relatively safe procedure with few serious complications, bile duct injury resulting from surgery is a serious complication, with potential long term consequences.[38] The overall short term mortality after surgery varies between 0% and 0.3%.[9] Although traditionally less than 0.5% of people undergoing cholecystectomy are believed to have bile duct injury,[9] a study of more than 50 000 unselected patients from the Swedish Registry for Gallstone Surgery and ERCP, GallRiks, revealed that 1.5% of patients undergoing cholecystectomy between 2005 and 2010 developed a bile duct injury, although only a fifth of these injuries (0.3%) involved partial or complete transection of the bile duct.[38] The patients with bile duct injury had a significantly higher one year mortality compared with those without such an injury.[38]

Cholecystectomy is generally performed by key hole operation (laparoscopic cholecystectomy)[39] because of the shorter length of hospital stay, decreased pain, earlier return to work, and better cosmesis. Laparoscopic cholecystectomy can be performed as a day procedure and generally involves four incisions measuring less than 1 cm each. Fat intolerance may develop in a small proportion of people after cholecystectomy, and a low fat diet is recommended in these patients. However, there is currently no strong evidence to support the usefulness of such a diet.

In patients with symptomatic gallbladder stones and common bile duct stones, the treatment options include open cholecystectomy with open exploration of the common bile duct, laparoscopic cholecystectomy with laparoscopic exploration of the common bile duct, and laparoscopic cholecystectomy with endoscopic sphincterotomy (performed preoperatively, intraoperatively, or postoperatively).[40] Evidence from a systematic review of randomised controlled trials shows that there is no evidence of difference in the morbidity or incidence of retained stones between endoscopic sphincterotomy and laparoscopic exploration of the common bile duct and inconsistency as to whether there is any difference in the length of hospital stay between the two approaches.[40]

When is the optimum time for surgery?

The timing of surgery for various indications is controversial. In patients with biliary colic there is no medical reason to delay surgery, the delays being caused only by the availability of resources (although surgery can be delayed by surgeons recommending weight reduction for particular patients). Evidence from a randomised controlled trial, which compared early surgery within 24 hours of hospital admission versus delayed surgery with an average wait of about four months on the waiting list, showed that delaying surgery increased complications (0% in early group versus 22.5% in the delayed group) and hospital stay (an average of one additional day).[41] The timing of cholecystectomy in patients with acute cholecystitis is also controversial. Although the traditional belief was to allow the inflammation to settle and perform laparoscopic cholecystectomy after a period of at least six weeks, a systematic review on this topic has shown that early laparoscopic cholecystectomy performed within one week of onset of symptoms can avoid further complications from gallstones while waiting for surgery.[42] Early laparoscopic cholecystectomy can also decrease hospital stay by about four days without increasing surgical complications (approximately 5-6% in each group) or the proportion of people requiring conversion from laparoscopic to open surgery (approximately 20% in each group).[42] Although most of the gallbladder related complications during the waiting time in the delayed group in the studies included in the systematic review were recurrence or non-resolution of acute cholecystitis, there is potential for further episodes of pain, pancreatitis, or obstructive jaundice while waiting. Evidence from a randomised controlled trial showed that morbidity after laparoscopic cholecystectomy between seven and 45 days was approximately two or three times that of surgery

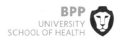

performed early; hence surgery within this timeframe is not recommended.[43] For timing of surgery in patients with mild acute pancreatitis (no organ failure or local complications), evidence from a systematic review that included only one small randomised controlled trial showed that performing surgery as early as possible (rather than waiting until symptoms settle and for blood test results to return to normal levels) decreased the hospital stay by one day,[44] although experts have expressed concerns that the severity of pancreatitis may not be evident until 48 hours and surgery in patients with severe pancreatitis (organ failure or local complications) within 48 hours can be harmful.[45] Delaying surgery for 48 hours overcomes this concern. The two circumstances where early cholecystectomy may not be appropriate are in patients with severe acute pancreatitis and those presenting during pregnancy.[9 44] Further trials are necessary to resolve these problems.

What is the impact of gallstone disease on health services and society?

In 2004 in the United States, a total of 1.8 million outpatient visits were related to gallstones.[46] Each year, more than 0.5 million cholecystectomies are performed in the United States[47] and 70 000 in England.[48] The cost of cholecystectomy and loss of working time because of symptoms related to gallstones, and their treatment has an important impact on health services and society.

The illustration was produced by Rakhee Bashar from UCL Medical Illustration in collaboration with the authors.

Contributors: KG performed the literature search, wrote the article, and is the guarantor. BRD critically commented on the article.

Competing interests: We have read and understood the BMJ Group policy on declaration of interests and declare the following interests: BRD acts as an expert witness in court proceedings related to gallstone management but this has no influence on the submitted work.

Provenance and peer review: Commissioned; externally peer reviewed.

1   Qiao T, Ma RH, Luo XB, Yang LQ, Luo ZL, Zheng PM. The systematic classification of gallbladder stones. PLoS One2013;8:e74887.

2   Kratzer W, Mason RA, Kachele V. Prevalence of gallstones in sonographic surveys worldwide. J Clin Ultrasound1999;27:1-7.

3   Trotman BW, Soloway RD. Pigment vs cholesterol cholelithiasis: clinical and epidemiological aspects. Am J Dig Dis1975;20:735-40.

4   Schafmayer C, Hartleb J, Tepel J, Albers S, Freitag S, Volzke H, et al. Predictors of gallstone composition in 1025 symptomatic gallstones from Northern Germany. BMC Gastroenterol2006;6:36.

5   Van Erpecum KJ. Pathogenesis of cholesterol and pigment gallstones: an update. Clin Res Hepatol Gastroenterol2011;35:281-7.

6   Stinton LM, Myers RP, Shaffer EA. Epidemiology of gallstones. Gastroenterol Clin North Am2010;39:157-69, vii.

7   Shaffer EA. Epidemiology and risk factors for gallstone disease: has the paradigm changed in the 21st century? Curr Gastroenterol Rep2005;7:132-40.

8   Banim PJ, Luben RN, Bulluck H, Sharp SJ, Wareham NJ, Khaw KT, et al. The aetiology of symptomatic gallstones quantification of the effects of obesity, alcohol and serum lipids on risk. Epidemiological and biomarker data from a UK prospective cohort study (EPIC-Norfolk). Eur J Gastroenterol Hepatol2011;23:733-40.

9   Gurusamy KS, Davidson BR. Surgical treatment of gallstones. Gastroenterol Clin North Am2010;39:229-44, viii.

10 Berger MY, van der Velden JJIM, Lijmer JG, de Kort H, Prins A, Bohnen AM. Abdominal symptoms: do they predict gallstones? A systematic review. Scand J Gastroenterol2000;35:70-6.

11 Attili AF, De Santis A, Capri R, Repice AM, Maselli S. The natural history of gallstones: the GREPCO experience. The GREPCO Group. Hepatology1995;21:655-60.

12 Del Favero G, Caroli A, Meggiato T, Volpi A, Scalon P, Puglisi A, et al. Natural history of gallstones in non-insulin-dependent diabetes mellitus. A prospective 5-year follow-up. Dig Dis Sci1994;39:1704-7.

13 Halldestam I, Enell EL, Kullman E, Borch K. Development of symptoms and complications in individuals with asymptomatic gallstones. Br J Surg2004;91:734-8.

14 Portincasa P, Moschetta A, Petruzzelli M, Palasciano G, Di Ciaula A, Pezzolla A. Gallstone disease: symptoms and diagnosis of gallbladder stones. Best Pract Res Clin Gastroenterol2006;20:1017-29..

15 Venneman NG, van Erpecum KJ. Gallstone disease: primary and secondary prevention. Best Pract Res Clin Gastroenterol2006;20:1063-73.

16 Yadav D, Lowenfels AB. Trends in the epidemiology of the first attack of acute pancreatitis: a systematic review. Pancreas2006;33:323-30.

17 Salek J, Livote E, Sideridis K, Bank S. Analysis of risk factors predictive of early mortality and urgent ERCP in acute cholangitis. J Clin Gastroenterol2009;43:171-5.

18 Rutledge D, Jones D, Rege R. Consequences of delay in surgical treatment of biliary disease. Am J Surg2000;180:466-9.

19 Hsing AW, Gao YT, Han TQ, Rashid A, Deng J, Chen J, et al. Gallstones and the risk of biliary tract cancer: a population-based study in China. Br J Cancer2007;97:1577-82.

20 Ishiguro S, Inoue M, Kurahashi N, Iwasaki M, Sasazuki S, Tsugane S. Risk factors of biliary tract cancer in a large-scale population-based cohort study in Japan (JPHC study): with special focus on cholelithiasis, body mass index, and their effect modification. Cancer Causes Control2008;19:33-41.

21 Shebl FM, Andreotti G, Meyer TE, Gao YT, Rashid A, Yu K, et al. Metabolic syndrome and insulin resistance in relation to biliary tract cancer and stone risks: a population-based study in Shanghai, China. Br J Cancer2011;105:1424-9.

22 Ross M, Brown M, McLaughlin K, Atkinson P, Thompson J, Powelson S, et al. Emergency physician-performed ultrasound to diagnose cholelithiasis: a systematic review. Acad Emerg Med2011;18:227-35.

23 Trowbridge RL, Rutkowski NK, Shojania KG. Does this patient have acute cholecystitis? JAMA2003;289:80-6.

24 Mayumi T, Takada T, Kawarada Y, Nimura Y, Yoshida M, Sekimoto M, et al. Results of the Tokyo consensus meeting Tokyo guidelines. J Hepatobiliary Pancreat Surg2007;14:114-21.

25 Sunamura M, Lozonschi L, Takeda K, Kobari M, Matsuno S. Criteria for diagnosis of acute pancreatitis in Japan and clinical implications. Pancreas1998;16:243-9.

26 Williams EJ, Green J, Beckingham I, Parks R, Martin D, Lombard M, et al. Guidelines on the management of common bile duct stones (CBDS). Gut2008;57:1004-21.

27 Scientific Committee of the European Association for Endoscopic Surgery. Diagnosis and treatment of common bile duct stones (CBDS). Results of a consensus development conference. Surg Endosc1998;12:856-64.

28 Berger MY, Olde Hartman TC, Bohnen AM. Abdominal symptoms: do they disappear after cholecystectomy? Surg Endosc2003;17:1723-8.

29 Gurusamy KS, Samraj K. Cholecystectomy versus no cholecystectomy in patients with silent gallstones. Cochrane Database Syst Rev2007;1:CD006230.

30 Strasberg SM, Clavien PA. Overview of therapeutic modalities for the treatment of gallstone diseases. Am J Surg1993;165:420-6.

31 Venneman NG, Besselink MG, Keulemans YC, Vanberge-Henegouwen GP, Boermeester MA, Broeders IA, et al. Ursodeoxycholic acid exerts no beneficial effect in patients with symptomatic gallstones awaiting cholecystectomy. Hepatology2006;43:1276-83.

32 May GR, Sutherland LR, Shaffer EA. Efficacy of bile acid therapy for gallstone dissolution: a meta-analysis of randomized trials. Aliment Pharmacol Ther1993;7:139-48.

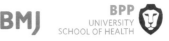

33 Carrilho-Ribeiro L, Pinto-Correia A, Velosa J, Carneiro De Moura M. A ten-year prospective study on gallbladder stone recurrence after successful extracorporeal shock-wave lithotripsy. *Scand J Gastroenterol* 2006;41:338-42.

34 O'Donnell LD, Heaton KW. Recurrence and re-recurrence of gall stones after medical dissolution: a longterm follow up. *Gut* 1988;29:655-8.

35 Gurusamy KS, Rossi M, Davidson BR. Percutaneous cholecystostomy for high-risk surgical patients with acute calculous cholecystitis. *Cochrane Database Syst Rev* 2013;8:CD007088.

36 Schmidt M, Sondenaa K, Vetrhus M, Berhane T, Eide GE. A randomized controlled study of uncomplicated gallstone disease with a 14-year follow-up showed that operation was the preferred treatment. *Dig Surg* 2011;28:270-6.

37 Schmidt M, Sondenaa K, Vetrhus M, Berhane T, Eide GE. Long-term follow-up of a randomized controlled trial of observation versus surgery for acute cholecystitis: non-operative management is an option in some patients. *Scand J Gastroenterol* 2011;46:1257-62.

38 Tornqvist B, Stromberg C, Persson G, Nilsson M. Effect of intended intraoperative cholangiography and early detection of bile duct injury on survival after cholecystectomy: population based cohort study. *BMJ* 2012;345:e6457.

39 Department of Health. NHS reference costs 2012 to 2013. www.gov.uk/government/publications/nhs-reference-costs-2012-to-2013.

40 Dasari BV, Tan CJ, Gurusamy KS, Martin DJ, Kirk G, McKie L, et al. Surgical versus endoscopic treatment of bile duct stones. *Cochrane Database Syst Rev* 2013;12:CD003327.

41 Salman B, Yuksel O, Irkorucu O, Akyurek N, Tezcaner T, Dogan I, et al. Urgent laparoscopic cholecystectomy is the best management for biliary colic. A prospective randomized study of 75 cases. *Dig Surg* 2005;22:95-9.

42 Gurusamy KS, Davidson C, Gluud C, Davidson BR. Early versus delayed laparoscopic cholecystectomy for people with acute cholecystitis. *Cochrane Database Syst Rev* 2013;6:CD005440.

43 Gutt CN, Encke J, Koninger J, Harnoss JC, Weigand K, Kipfmuller K, et al. Acute cholecystitis: early versus delayed cholecystectomy, a multicenter randomized trial (ACDC study, NCT00447304). *Ann Surg* 2013;258:385-93.

44 Gurusamy KS, Nagendran M, Davidson BR. Early versus delayed laparoscopic cholecystectomy for acute gallstone pancreatitis. *Cochrane Database Syst Rev* 2013;9:CD010326.

45 Bouwense SA, Bakker OJ, van Santvoort HC, Boerma D, van Ramshorst B, Gooszen HG, et al. Safety of cholecystectomy in the first 48 hours after admission for gallstone pancreatitis not yet proven. *Ann Surg* 2011;253:1053-4; author reply 54-5.

46 Everhart J. The burden of digestive diseases in the United States. 2008. www3.niddk.nih.gov/Burden_of_Digestive_Diseases/.

47 Centers for Disease Control and Prevention. Discharges with at least one procedure in nonfederal short-stay hospitals, by sex, age, and selected procedures: United States, selected years 1990 through 2009-2010. www.cdc.gov/nchs/hus/contents2012.htm#098.

48 Health and Social Care Information Centre. Hospital episode statistics, Admitted patient care, England—2012-13. www.hscic.gov.uk/catalogue/PUB12566/hosp-epis-stat-admi-proc-2012-13-tab.xlsx.

Related links

bmj.com/archive

Previous articles in this series

- Management of psychosis and schizophrenia in adults (BMJ 2014;348:g1173)
- Early management of head injury: summary of updated NICE guidance (BMJ 2014;348:g104)
- Intravenous fluid therapy for adults in hospital: summary of NICE guidance (BMJ 2013;347:f7073)
- Secondary prevention for patients after a myocardial infarction: summary of updated NICE guidance (BMJ 2013;347:f6544)
- Management of urinary incontinence in women: summary of updated NICE guidance (BMJ 2013;347:f5170)

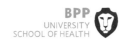

Acute pancreatitis

C D Johnson, professor of surgical sciences[1],
M G Besselink, hepatopancreatobiliary surgeon[2],
R Carter, consultant pancreatic surgeon[3]

[1]University Surgery, University Hospital Southampton, SO16 6YD, UK

[2]Dutch Pancreatitis Study Group, Academic Medical Center Amsterdam, Netherlands

[3]West of Scotland Pancreatic Unit, Glasgow Royal infirmary, Glasgow, UK

Correspondence to: C D Johnson cdj@soton.ac.uk

Cite this as: BMJ 2014;349:g4859

DOI: 10.1136/bmj.g4859

http://www.bmj.com/content/349/bmj.g4859

Acute pancreatitis is a common cause of emergency admission to hospital. Most hospitals in the United Kingdom serving a population of 300 000-400 000 people admit about 100 cases each year. We review up to date evidence for the assessment, diagnosis, and management of acute pancreatitis.

What is acute pancreatitis?

Acute pancreatitis is inflammation of the pancreas; it is sometimes associated with a systemic inflammatory response that can impair the function of other organs or systems. The inflammation may settle spontaneously or may progress to necrosis of the pancreas or surrounding fatty tissue. The distant organ or system dysfunction may resolve or may progress to organ failure. Thus there is a wide spectrum of disease from mild (80%), where patients recover within a few days, to severe (20%) with prolonged hospital stay, the need for critical care support, and a 15-20% risk of death.[3] If patients have organ failure during the first week in hospital, it is usually already present on the first day in hospital.[1] This early organ failure may resolve in response to treatment. The diagnosis of severe acute pancreatitis depends on the presence of persistent organ failure (>48 hours) either during the first week or at a later stage, and also on the presence of local complications (usually apparent after the first week).

What are the risk factors and potential causes of acute pancreatitis?

Acute pancreatitis has many causes, the commonest in most European and North American studies being gallstones (50%) and alcohol (25%). Rare causes (<5%) include drugs (for example, valproate, steroids, azathioprine), endoscopic retrograde cholangiopancreatography, hypertriglyceridaemia or lipoprotein lipase deficiency, hypercalcaemia, pancreas divisum, and some viral infections (mumps, coxsackie B4). About 10% of patients have idiopathic pancreatitis, where no cause is found.

How does acute pancreatitis present?

Acute pancreatitis presents as an emergency, requiring acute admission to hospital. Patients almost always mention severe constant abdominal pain (resembling peritonitis), usually of sudden onset and, in 80% of cases, associated with vomiting. The pain may radiate to the back, usually the lower thoracic area. Most patients present to hospital within 12-24 hours of onset of symptoms. Abdominal examination shows epigastric tenderness, with guarding. Differential diagnoses to consider include perforated peptic ulcer, myocardial infarction, and cholecystitis.

How is the diagnosis confirmed?

Biochemical tests

The diagnosis is based on abdominal pain and vomiting, associated with increases in serum amylase or lipase levels at least more than three times the upper limit of normal.[2][3] In the United Kingdom, amylase testing is widely available, although estimation of lipase is preferred by some because lipase levels remain increased for longer than amylase levels after the onset of acute pancreatitis. In about 5% of patients, enzyme levels may be normal at the time of admission to hospital.

Imaging

In cases where there is diagnostic doubt, either because the biochemical tests are not conclusive (enzyme levels may decrease during delayed presentation to hospital) or because the severity of clinical presentation raises the possibility of other intra-abdominal conditions such as perforation of the gastrointestinal tract, contrast enhanced computed tomography may be needed to make the diagnosis.[2][3][4] International consensus is that acute pancreatitis is diagnosed when two of three criteria are present: typical abdominal pain, raised enzyme levels, or appearances of pancreatitis on computer tomography. Computed tomography also has a role in the assessment of the severity of acute pancreatitis if the illness fails to resolve within one week.

What other diagnostic tests are required?

Once acute pancreatitis has been diagnosed, the cause needs to be sought. In most cases this will be determined from a combination of careful clinical evaluation and initial investigations. When taking a history, it is important to ask about alcohol consumption, drug use, symptoms of viral illness, and a family or personal history of genetic disease. Blood tests may reveal hypercalcaemia and hypertriglyceridaemia. Abdominal ultrasonography may identify gallstones. No evident cause will be found in 10-20% of patients[3]; these people may require further investigation, especially if they have experienced more than one acute attack.

SOURCES AND SELECTION CRITERIA

We have drawn heavily on three recent evidence based guidelines[1][2][3] that we helped to write and we reviewed the Cochrane Library for relevant clinical trials. In December 2013 we again reviewed the Cochrane Library to identify any systematic review or update relevant to acute pancreatitis.

SUMMARY POINTS

- All patients with acute pancreatitis should have liver function tests and abdominal ultrasonography within 24 hours of admission to look for gallstones
- Severe acute pancreatitis is characterised by persistent (>48 hours) organ failure; these patients have a >30% mortality rate
- If symptoms persist for more than seven days computed tomography is required to assess pancreatic and peripancreatic necrosis
- Initial management includes adequate fluid resuscitation and supplemental oxygen
- If gallstones are found, definitive treatment (by cholecystectomy or sphincterotomy) should be given within two weeks of resolution of symptoms
- Necrotising pancreatitis should be managed by a specialist team including surgeons, endoscopists, interventional radiologists, and intensivists

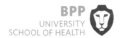

Ultrasonography

Gallstones are found in about half of patients with acute pancreatitis, so in every case abdominal ultrasonography should be performed within 24 hours of admission to look for gallstones in the gallbladder.[3] [5] Early detection helps plan the definitive management of gallstones (usually by cholecystectomy) to prevent further attacks of pancreatitis.

Liver function tests

In addition to ultrasonography, increased liver enzymes levels provide supportive evidence for gallstones as the cause of the acute pancreatitis. Two large observational studies with 139 and 464 patients of whom 101 and 84 had gallstones found that an alanine transaminase (ALT) level >150 U/L has a positive predictive value of 85% for gallstones.[4] [5] [6] These tests should be done in all patients within 24 hours of admission.

Endoscopic ultrasonography

A systematic review of five studies in patients with apparently idiopathic pancreatitis after initial assessment reported a diagnostic yield of up to 88% with endoscopic ultrasonography, with detection of biliary sludge, common bile duct stones, or chronic pancreatitis.[7]

Magnetic resonance cholangiopancreatography

Expert opinion also recommends magnetic resonance cholangiopancreatography to elucidate rare anatomical causes of acute pancreatitis.[2] The sensitivity of this investigation is improved by the addition of secretin stimulation.

Endoscopic ultrasonography and magnetic resonance cholangiopancreatography are usually requested only after patients have recovered from the acute phase and after a detailed history and repeat ultrasonography have failed to identify a cause.

How is the severity of acute pancreatitis assessed?

Eighty per cent of patients with acute pancreatitis respond to initial support with intravenous fluid, oxygen supplements, and analgesia, and they can be discharged home within a week or so. About 20% of patients, however, do not recover during the first few days and may need transfer to a specialist unit.[8]

The Atlanta classification is a useful framework for assessing the severity of acute pancreatitis.[9] The current classification recognises three levels of severity: mild, where patients recover with good supportive care within a week without complication; moderately severe, in which there is transient organ failure that resolves within 48 hours, or a local complication (that is, peripancreatic fluid collections) without organ failure; and severe acute pancreatitis, in which there is persistent organ failure for more than 48 hours. This classification enables non-specialist clinicians to identify those patients who require treatment by, or in consultation with, a specialist centre (box 1). Persistent organ failure during the first week is associated with a 1 in 3 risk of mortality.[10] [11]

Patients who have local complications and organ failure with infection of the pancreas or extrapancreatic necrosis are at extremely high risk of death.[12] This subgroup of patients should be managed in a specialist centre.

Markers of severity in the first week

Markers of systemic inflammatory response syndrome help to identify those patients who may develop persistent organ failure. Several observational studies have shown a strong association between persistent systemic inflammatory response syndrome (>48 hours) and subsequent persistent organ failure (box 2).[11] [13]

There are many different predictive scoring systems for severity based on physiological variables or single biochemical markers, but none of these has shown clear superiority.

The acute physiology and chronic health evaluation (APACHE)-II score can be assessed within 24 hours of admission to hospital and is a useful positive predictor of severe pancreatitis if scored 8 or more.[14] The early warning score (or a modified EWS) is widely used for recording clinical observations (pulse, blood pressure, respiratory rate, and urine output) in hospitals in the United Kingdom and has a similar accuracy for prediction of severe pancreatitis.[15] Scoring systems have limited day to day value in the management of patients and perform best for the description of patient groups in clinical trials and other research studies.

Computed tomography

Computed tomography should be performed to look for local complications in those with signs or symptoms of systemic disturbance, particularly persistent organ failure that lasts for more than one week. As described in the revised Atlanta criteria,[9] local complications include peripancreatic fluid collections, or necrosis (hypoperfusion) of pancreatic or peripancreatic tissue (necrotising pancreatitis). Fluid collections and areas of necrosis may be identified early (<4 weeks) or late (>4 weeks) (box 3 and figure).

Evidence from a descriptive study with 88 patients[16] and the UK guidelines[3] recommend that the first computed tomography scan for assessment of severity should be performed 6-10 days after admission in patients with persistent systemic inflammatory response syndrome or organ failure. Computed tomography scoring systems do not outperform clinical scoring systems for prediction of severity and evidence suggests that early (inappropriate) computed tomography increases length of hospital stay with no improvement in clinical outcome.[2]

BOX 1: REVISED ATLANTA CLASSIFICATION OF ACUTE PANCREATITIS[9]: DEFINITIONS OF SEVERITY

Mild
- No organ failure
- No local or systemic complications

Moderately severe
- Organ failure that resolves within 48 hours (transient organ failure)
- Local or systemic complications (sterile or infected) without persistent organ failure
- A patient with moderately severe pancreatitis may have one or both of these features

Severe
- Persistent organ failure (>48 hours): single organ or multiple organ failure

Definitions of organ failure: thresholds for organ failure
- Respiratory: arterial oxygen pressure/fractional inspired oxygen ≥300
- Circulatory: systolic blood pressure <90 mm Hg and not fluid responsive
- Renal: plasma creatinine concentration ≥170 µmol/L

BOX 2: FEATURES OF SYSTEMIC INFLAMMATORY RESPONSE SYNDROME (SIRS)*
- Core body temperature >38°C or <36°C
- Heart rate >90 bmp
- Respiratory rate >20/min (or arterial carbon dioxide pressure <32 mm Hg)
- White cell count >12×10⁹/L or <4×10⁹/L

*If SIRS is present for >48 hours the patient is likely to have severe pancreatitis

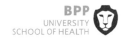

BOX 3: REVISED DEFINITIONS OF TYPES AND GRADES OF SEVERITY OF ACUTE PANCREATITIS[9]

Interstitial oedematous pancreatitis

- Acute inflammation of pancreatic parenchyma and peripancreatic tissues, but without recognisable tissue necrosis

Necrotising pancreatitis

- Pancreatic parenchymal necrosis or peripancreatic necrosis, or both

Acute peripancreatic fluid collection

- Peripancreatic fluid with interstitial edematous pancreatitis but no necrosis (this term applies only within the first 4 weeks after onset of interstitial edematous pancreatitis and without features of a pseudocyst)

Pancreatic pseudocyst

- Encapsulated collection of fluid with a well defined inflammatory wall usually outside pancreas with minimal or no necrosis (usually occurs > 4 weeks after onset of pancreatitis)

Acute necrotic collection

- Fluid and necrosis associated with necrotising pancreatitis affecting pancreas or peripancreatic tissues, or both

Walled-off necrosis

- Mature, encapsulated collection of pancreatic or peripancreatic necrosis with an inflammatory wall, or both (walled-off necrosis usually occurs >4 weeks after onset of necrotising pancreatitis)

How is acute pancreatitis managed?

Fluid management

Two small randomised studies with 40 and 41 patients investigated the effect of different types of fluid on outcomes. These showed benefit for Ringer's lactate compared with other types of fluid, in that fewer patients had systemic inflammatory response syndrome, and C reactive protein levels were lower although clinical outcomes did not differ.[17][18] Guidelines by the International Association of Pancreatology[2] recommend the use of Ringer's lactate; in the United Kingdom, Hartmann's solution is a widely used alternative.

Infusion rates during the first 24 hours in hospital should be sufficient to restore circulating volume and urine output.[4] Consensus opinion is that 2.5-4 litres in 24 hours will be sufficient for most patients, but that volumes infused should be determined by the clinical response. Two randomised studies with a total of 191 patients[19][20] showed that more aggressive fluid replacement increased the requirement for mechanical ventilation and rates of sepsis and death. In these studies the control groups received 2.5-4.8 litres of crystalloid daily in the first 48 hours, whereas the treatment groups received 4.0-5.8 litres daily. Restoration of circulating volume while maintaining haematocrit above 0.35 was associated with a better outcome. However, further prospective data are needed to clarify whether patients deteriorate because of inadequate fluid replacement or because of the severity of illness despite large volumes.

Consensus opinion is that response to fluid resuscitation should be assessed by non-invasive response monitoring (heart rate <120 bpm, mean arterial pressure 65-85 mm Hg, urine output 0.5-1 mL/kg/h). However, a recent large three arm randomised trial[21] with 64-68 patients per arm compared non-invasive monitoring with invasive monitoring in patients with severe acute pancreatitis admitted to an intensive care unit within 24 hours of onset of the disease. All the patients received saline and colloid (hydroxyethyl starch), and one group received fresh frozen plasma in addition. Rates of infusion were regulated by vital signs, urine output, and haematocrit over the first 24 hours in the control group. The other two groups had invasive monitoring. The patients who received early goal directed treatment with invasive monitoring had fewer days of ventilator support or intensive care unit stay and lower rates of abdominal compartment syndrome, organ failure, and death. This carefully monitored approach to rapid fluid resuscitation is rational and requires further evaluation.

Early antibiotic treatment

A Cochrane review[22] of seven evaluable studies with 404 patients found no statistically significant effect of early antibiotics on reduction of mortality. Rates of infected necrotising pancreatitis were similar (treatment 19.7%, controls 24.4%) and rates of non-pancreatic infection were

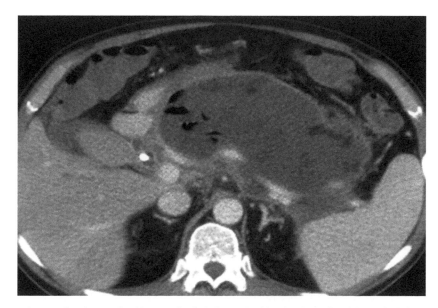

Body of pancreas and surrounding tissue replaced by area of walled-off necrosis with enhancing wall, which contains bubbles of gas (black areas), clearly different from heterogeneous variations in density elsewhere and diagnostic of infection

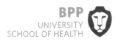
not affected by early antibiotic treatment. The authors concluded that antibiotics had no benefit in preventing infection of necrosis or death. None of the included studies was adequately powered, but a separate analysis showed an inverse relation between the study quality and effect size.[23]

At present there is no indication for early antibiotics to prevent infection of (presumed or existing) pancreatic necrosis.[4] If infection is clinically suspected or found, antibiotic treatment should be guided by sensitivity of cultured organisms when available and by the duration and severity of septic symptoms.

Pain relief

The main symptom of acute pancreatitis is pain, and respiratory function may be impaired by restriction of abdominal wall movement. Providing effective analgesia may require the use of opioids. There are some theoretical risks of exacerbation of pancreatitis by morphine, which can increase pressure in the sphincter of Oddi, but there is little good evidence that this is clinically significant and no evidence exists about the comparative effectiveness of different opioids in acute pancreatitis.

Nutrition

Pancreatic endotoxin absorption is thought to be a potent stimulus of the systemic inflammatory response syndrome and contributes to a cycle of events that leads to organ failure in acute pancreatitis. It is assumed that enteral nutrition may help maintain the gut mucosal barrier and so reduce the absorption of endotoxin. However, these theoretical advantages have not been supported by clinical trials.

Mild pancreatitis

Three randomised trials with a total of 413 patients have shown that early oral nutrition in patients with mild pancreatitis does not increase the rate of complications. Enteral tube feeding shows no benefit in patients with mild pancreatitis, and such patients can resume oral intake as soon as they feel able.[2]

Severe pancreatitis

A Cochrane review[24] of enteral versus parenteral nutrition in patients with (predicted) severe acute pancreatitis identified eight trials that showed a substantial reduction in mortality and complications with early enteral nutrition. It is possible that the difference between enteral and parenteral nutrition is an excess of complications such as line sepsis and other infections in the parenteral group.

One small randomised trial[25] showed no difference between enteral nutrition and no support. A recent large multicentre trial in the Netherlands randomised 101 patients to early nasojejunal tube feeding started within 24 hours of admission and 104 to a control group with starvation for 72 hours followed by an oral diet with on-demand nasoenteral feeding whenever oral intake was insufficient. Preliminary data[26] showed no difference in outcome. Therefore no evidence supports the use of enteral nutrition as prophylaxis for complications. Most specialist units in the United Kingdom refrain from early enteral nutrition and allow oral intake as tolerated.

Route of enteral nutrition

If enteral nutrition is required, it is usually delivered by tube feeding. Two randomised trials with 50 and 31 patients[27] [28] suggest that at least 80% of patients can tolerate the nasogastric route, avoiding the need for nasojejunal intubation. Nasogastric intubation is a ward based procedure and does not require specialist techniques such as radiological screening or endoscopic placement; nasojejunal tubes require these resources, and in practice the tube often becomes displaced back into the stomach. The patient experience of the two types of tube is similar.

Enteral nutritional supplements

The type of nutritional supplement used for tube feeding seems to have no effect on outcome in severe acute pancreatitis. A meta-analysis of 20 randomised trials concluded that no specific enteral nutrition supplement or immunonutrition formulation had any advantage.[29]

What is the best time for cholecystectomy after gallstone pancreatitis?

Expert consensus is that the best time to operate to deal definitively with gallstones is during the index admission with acute pancreatitis, after the initial symptoms have resolved. The risk of recurrent pancreatitis is directly related to the interval between first attack and cholecystectomy.[30] Any recommended time limit is arbitrary, but the shorter the interval the lower the risk.

Whereas after mild biliary pancreatitis, cholecystectomy must be undertaken as soon as possible, the patient who has had a severe attack may be debilitated and may have ongoing intra-abdominal inflammatory changes. Further interventions within the abdomen may be needed. All of these considerations affect the timing of cholecystectomy, which should probably be delayed at least six weeks after discharge from hospital to allow resolution of inflammatory changes. No evidence supports this expert consensus.

How is necrotising pancreatitis managed?

Necrotising pancreatitis is suspected when there are persistent signs of systemic inflammation for more than 7-10 days after the onset of pancreatitis.

It is now widely accepted that intervention in the first two weeks of severe acute pancreatitis should be avoided if possible because of high mortality. Rare exceptions to the non-intervention approach include intra-abdominal haemorrhage or necrosis of bowel. In either case, it is better if possible not to disturb the pancreatic inflammatory mass at this time.

There is consensus that pancreatic intervention should be delayed until walled-off necrosis has developed, typically 3-5 weeks after the onset of symptoms. Indications for intervention include confirmed (or strongly suspected) infection of necrosis and persistent organ failure for several weeks with a walled-off collection. Patients who might require intervention—that is, anyone with a hospital stay of more than 14 days after the onset of symptoms—should be managed by, or in consultation with, a specialist pancreatic team.

A randomised trial of 88 patients compared primary open necrosectomy with a "step-up" approach of percutaneous drainage, followed by minimally invasive surgical necrosectomy if needed.[31] The step-up approach reduced major morbidity by 43%. Of the patients assigned to this approach, 35% were treated with percutaneous drainage only. Based on this trial and other studies, including a systematic review,[32] the consensus is that the initial step should be catheter drainage,[2] but there is no consensus on the best intervention for necrotising pancreatitis.

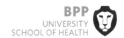

Pancreatic exocrine insufficiency (PEI) and diabetes after acute pancreatitis in participants of two small observational studies

Study		All participants		Mild PEI		Severe PEI	
	No of patients	No (%) with PEI	No with diabetes	No of patients	No affected	No of patients	No affected
Symersky et al[35]	34	22	12	22	12	12	10
Boreham et al[36]	23	8	4	16	2	7	6
Total	57	30	16	38	14	19	16

ADDITIONAL EDUCATIONAL RESOURCES

Information for healthcare professionals

- References 1-4 contain detailed literature reviews of the clinical management of patients with acute pancreatitis
- Cochrane Library (www.thecochranelibrary.com/details/browseReviews/578409/Acute.html)—contains several Cochrane reviews on aspects of pancreatitis

Information for patients

- NHS UK (www.nhs.uk/Conditions/Pancreatitis/Pages/Introduction.aspx)—provides information for patients on the causes, symptoms, and treatment of acute pancreatitis
- Patient.co.uk (www.patient.co.uk/health/acute-pancreatitis)—has information about the causes, symptoms, and treatment of acute pancreatitis

What treatment is required after discharge following severe acute pancreatitis?

After severe acute pancreatitis, patients need general supportive measures and some specific treatments. In addition, the cause of the pancreatitis should be identified and treated if possible, most often by treatment of gallstones. Many pancreatic specialists recommend avoidance of alcohol for 6-12 months whatever the cause or severity of the pancreatitis. There is evidence from a randomised trial that interventions to manage alcoholism may reduce recurrent attacks of pancreatitis in those with high alcohol intake.[33 34]

This review will not consider the needs of patients who have spent a considerable period in intensive care with a serious illness, apart from pancreatitis specific problems. Most patients recovering from severe acute pancreatitis will have had weight loss during their illness, and at the time of discharge from hospital may have ongoing anorexia, which impairs their ability to regain weight. Such patients therefore benefit from nutritional supplements, which may need to be varied to improve acceptability. In specialist centres a dietitian is often available to advise on nutritional support during this recovery phase.

After severe acute pancreatitis, patients often have impaired pancreatic exocrine and endocrine function. Hyperglycaemia may be absent initially if nutritional intake is low, and blood glucose should be tested in the weeks after discharge as intake improves.

Pancreatic exocrine insufficiency is under-recognised in the recovery phase after severe acute pancreatitis. In two small observational studies with 57 patients, 53% overall (and 84% after severe pancreatitis) had pancreatic exocrine insufficiency (table) and were thought to possibly benefit from pancreatic enzyme supplements.[35 36] These should be given for at least six months, after which exocrine function can be tested by measuring faecal elastase levels. Endocrine insufficiency (diabetes) was less common but should also be considered. Functional recovery may continue for up to 12 months after the onset of pancreatitis, but further recovery after this time is unlikely. Most patients gain some additional useful exocrine function, but those with necrosis of a substantial proportion of pancreas may require supplements indefinitely.

Contributors: All authors contributed to the design and planning of this manuscript, edited drafts, and approved the final version. CDJ wrote the manuscript and amended it in line with comments from the other authors. CDJ is the guarantor.

Competing interests: We have read and understood the BMJ Group policy on declaration of interests and declare the following interests: each author has recently contributed to evidence based reviews of diagnosis and management of acute pancreatitis. CDJ has conducted an evidence based review of the diagnosis and management of acute pancreatitis, and contributed to an international consensus on definitions and classification of the disease. MGB was the lead for development of guidelines for the management of acute pancreatitis for the International Association of Pancreatology and the American Pancreatic Association. RC is the joint lead of a working group of the United Kingdom and Ireland Pancreatic Guidelines Development Group.

Provenance and peer review: Commissioned; externally peer reviewed.

1. Johnson CD, Kingsnorth AN, Imrie CW, McMahon MJ, Neoptolemos JP, McKay C, et al. Double blind, randomised, placebo controlled study of a platelet activating factor antagonist, lexipafant, in the treatment and prevention of organ failure in predicted severe acute pancreatitis. *Gut*2001;48:62-9.
2. Working Group IAP/APA Acute Pancreatitis Guidelines. IAP/APA evidence-based guidelines for the management of acute pancreatitis. *Pancreatology*2013;13(4 Suppl 2):e1-15.
3. Working Party of the British Society of Gastroenterology; Association of Surgeons of Great Britain and Ireland; Pancreatic Society of Great Britain and Ireland; Association of Upper GI Surgeons of Great Britain and Ireland, UK guidelines for the management of acute pancreatitis. *Gut*2005;54(Suppl 3):pp iii1-9.
4. Tenner S, Baillie J, DeWitt J, Vege SS, American College of Gastroenterology. American College of Gastroenterology guideline: management of acute pancreatitis. *Am J Gastroenterol*2013;1081400-15;1416.
5. Liu CL, Fan ST, Lo CM, Tso WK, Wong Y, Poon RT, et al. Clinico-biochemical prediction of biliary cause of acute pancreatitis in the era of endoscopic ultrasonography. *Aliment Pharmacol Ther*2005;22:423-31.
6. Moolla Z, Anderson F, Thomson SR. Use of amylase and alanine transaminase to predict acute gallstone pancreatitis in a population with high HIV prevalence. *World J Surg*2013;37:156-61.
7. Wilcox CM, Varadarajulu S, Eloubeidi M. Role of endoscopic evaluation in idiopathic pancreatitis: a systematic review. *Gastrointest Endosc*2006;63:1037-45.
8. Gislason H, Horn A, Hoem D, Andren-Sandberg A, Imsland AK, Soreide O, et al. Acute pancreatitis in Bergen, Norway. A study on incidence, etiology and severity. *Scand J Surg*2004;93:29-33.
9. Banks PA, Bollen TL, Dervenis C, Gooszen HG, Johnson CD, Sarr MG, et al. Classification of acute pancreatitis—2012: revision of the Atlanta classification and definitions by international consensus. *Gut*2013;62:102-11.
10. Johnson CD, Abu-Hilal M. Persistent organ failure during the first week as a marker of fatal outcome in acute pancreatitis. *Gut*2004;53:1340-4.
11. Mofidi R, Duff MD, Wigmore SJ, Madhavan KK, Garden OJ, Parks RW. Association between early systemic inflammatory response, severity of multiorgan dysfunction and death in acute pancreatitis. *Br J Surg*2006;93:738-44.
12. Dellinger EP, Forsmark CE, Layer P, Levy P, Maravi-Poma E, Petrov MS, et al. Determinant-based classification of acute pancreatitis severity: an international multidisciplinary consultation. *Ann Surg*2012;256:875-80.
13. Singh VK, Wu BU, Bollen TL, Repas K, Maurer R, Mortele KJ, et al. Early systemic inflammatory response syndrome is associated with severe acute pancreatitis. *Clin Gastroenterol Hepatol*2009;7:1247-51.
14. Larvin M. Assessment of severity and prognosis in acute pancreatitis. *Eur J Gastroenterol Hepatol*1997;9:122-30.
15. Garcea G, Gouda M, Hebbes C, Ong SL, Neal CP, Dennison AR, et al. Predictors of severity and survival in acute pancreatitis: validation of the efficacy of early warning scores. *Pancreas*2008;37:e54-61.
16. Balthazar EJ, Robinson DL, Megibow AJ, Ranson JH. Acute pancreatitis: value of CT in establishing prognosis. *Radiology*1990;174:331-6.
17. Du XJ, Hu WM, Xia Q, Huang ZW, Chen GY, Jin XD, et al. Hydroxyethyl starch resuscitation reduces the risk of intra-abdominal hypertension in severe acute pancreatitis. *Pancreas*2011;40:1220-5.
18. Wu BU, Hwang JQ, Gardner TH, Repas K, Delee R, Yu S, et al. Lactated Ringer's solution reduces systemic inflammation compared with saline in patients with acute pancreatitis. *Clin Gastroenterol Hepatol*2011;9:710-7,e1.

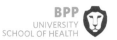

19 Mao EQ, Fei J, Peng YB, Huang J, Tang YQ, Zhang SD. Rapid hemodilution is associated with increased sepsis and mortality among patients with severe acute pancreatitis. *Chin Med J (Engl)*2010;123:1639-44.

20 Mao EQ, Tang YQ, Fei J, Qin S, Wu J, Li L, et al. Fluid therapy for severe acute pancreatitis in acute response stage. *Chin Med J (Engl)*2009;122:169-73.

21 Wang MD, Ji Y, Xu J, Jiang DH, Luo L, Huang SW. Early goal-directed fluid therapy with fresh frozen plasma reduces severe acute pancreatitis mortality in the intensive care unit. *Chin Med J (Engl)*2013;126:1987-8.

22 Villatoro E, Mulla M, Larvin M. Antibiotic therapy for prophylaxis against infection of pancreatic necrosis in acute pancreatitis. *Cochrane Database Syst Rev*2010 12;5:CD002941.

23 De Vries AC, Besselink MG, Buskens E, Ridwan BU, Schipper M, van Erpecum KJ, et al. Randomized controlled trials of antibiotic prophylaxis in severe acute pancreatitis: relationship between methodological quality and outcome. *Pancreatology*2007;7:531-8.

24 Al-Omran M, AlBalawi ZH, Tashkandi MF, Al-Ansary LA. Enteral versus parenteral nutrition for acute pancreatitis. *Cochrane Database Syst Rev*2010;1:CD002837.

25 Powell JJ, Murchison JT, Fearon KC, Ross JA, Siriwardena AK. Randomized controlled trial of the effect of early enteral nutrition on markers of the inflammatory response in predicted severe acute pancreatitis. *Br J Surg*2000;87:1375-81.

26 Bakker OJ and the Dutch Pancreatitis Study Group. Early versus on-demand nasoenteral feeding in severe pancreatitis: a multicenter randomised controlled trial. *United European Gastroenterol J*2013;1:A1.

27 Eatock FC, Chong P, Menezes N, Murray L, McKay CJ, Carter CR, et al. A randomized study of early nasogastric versus nasojejunal feeding in severe acute pancreatitis. *Am J Gastroenterol*2005;100:432-9.

28 Kumar A, Singh N, Prakash S, Saraya A, Joshi YK. Early enteral nutrition in severe acute pancreatitis: a prospective randomized controlled trial comparing nasojejunal and nasogastric routes. *J Clin Gastroenterol*2006;40:431-4.

29 Petrov MS, Loveday BP, Pylypchuk RD, McIlroy K, Phillips AR, Windsor JA. Systematic review and meta-analysis of enteral nutrition formulations in acute pancreatitis. *Br J Surg*2009;96:1243-52.

30 Van Baal MC, Besselink MG, Bakker OJ, van Santvoort HC, Schaapherder AF, Nieuwenhuijs VB, et al. Timing of cholecystectomy after mild biliary pancreatitis: a systematic review. *Ann Surg*2012;255:860-6.

31 Van Santvoort HC, Besselink MG, Bakker OJ, Hofker HS, Boermeester MA, Dejong CH, et al. A step-up approach or open necrosectomy for necrotizing pancreatitis. *N Engl J Med*2010;362:1491-502.

32 Van Baal MC, van Santvoort HC, Bollen TL, Bakker OJ, Besselink MG, Gooszen HG. Systematic review of percutaneous catheter drainage as primary treatment for necrotizing pancreatitis. *Br J Surg*2011;98:18-27.

33 Nikkola J, Raty S, Laukkarinen J, Seppanen H, Lappalainen-Lehto R, Jarvinen S, et al. Abstinence after first acute alcohol-associated pancreatitis protects against recurrent pancreatitis and minimizes the risk of pancreatic dysfunction. *Alcohol Alcohol*2013;48:483-6.

34 Nordback I, Pelli H, Lappalainen-Lehto R, Jarvinen S, Raty S, Sand J. The recurrence of acute alcohol-associated pancreatitis can be reduced: a randomized controlled trial. *Gastroenterology*2009;136:848-55.

35 Boreham B, Ammori BJ. A prospective evaluation of pancreatic exocrine function in patients with acute pancreatitis: correlation with extent of necrosis and pancreatic endocrine insufficiency. *Pancreatology*2003;3:303-8.

36 Symersky T, van Hoorn B, Masclee AA. The outcome of a long-term follow-up of pancreatic function after recovery from acute pancreatitis. *JOP*2006;7:447-53.

Related links

bmj.com/archive

- The management of spasticity in adults (*BMJ* 2014;349:g4737)
- Non-alcoholic fatty liver disease (**BMJ** 2014;349:g4596)
- Diagnosis and management of heritable thrombophilias (*BMJ* 2014;348:g4387)
- HIV testing and management of newly diagnosed HIV (*BMJ* 2014;349:g4275)
- Allergic rhinitis in children (*BMJ* 2014;348:g4153)

thebmj.com

- Get CME/CPD points for this article

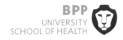

Pancreatic adenocarcinoma

Giles Bond-Smith, general and hepatopancreatic-biliary surgical registrar[1],

Neal Banga, general and transplant surgical registrar[1],

Toby M Hammond, general and colorectal surgical registrar[2],

Charles J Imber, consultant hepatopancreatic-biliary and liver transplant surgeon[1]

[1]Hepatopancreatic-biliary Surgery and Liver Transplant Unit, Royal Free Hospital, London NW3 2QG, UK

[2]Department of Surgery, St Mark's Hospital, Harrow, Middlesex

Correspondence to: G Bond-Smith
gelsmith@yahoo.co.uk

Cite this as: BMJ 2012;344:e2476

DOI: 10.1136/bmj.e2476

http://www.bmj.com/content/344/bmj.e2476

In 2008, an estimated 217 000 new cases of pancreatic cancer were diagnosed worldwide, and in the UK 8000 new cases of pancreatic cancer are reported every year.[4] [5] [6] Worldwide, pancreatic cancer is 13th in incidence but 8th in terms of cancer death.[4] In the UK, pancreatic cancer is the 5th most common cause of cancer death in both sexes, despite being only the 11th most common cancer overall.[7] This is largely due to red flag symptoms usually appearing only once the disease has progressed to involve other structures. Consequently, only 10-20% of patients will have resectable pancreatic cancer at presentation.[7]

The term pancreatic cancer encompasses both exocrine and endocrine tumours (see box 1), of which over 80% are adenocarcinomas. The aim of this review is to update the non-specialist clinician on the cause, clinical presentation, and current management of so called curable and incurable pancreatic adenocarcinomas. The main surgical options available to the patient are discussed, including the decision making process involved in considering patients for curative surgery. The potential complications and morbidity of current treatment regimes, and their management, is covered.

How does pancreatic cancer present?

Almost 50% of cases of pancreatic cancer are diagnosed on attending an emergency department for non-specific abdominal pain or jaundice or both. Only 13% are diagnosed via the two week wait pathway utilised by general practitioners in the UK.[8]

The peak incidence for pancreatic cancer is in the seventh and eighth decades of life. There is no difference in incidence between the sexes.[2] Courvoisier's sign, described as a palpable gallbladder in the presence of painless jaundice, occurs in less than 25% of patients. The majority of patients present with non-specific symptoms. Those presenting late frequently have symptoms secondary to metastatic spread. Approximately 80% of patients have unresectable disease at the time of diagnosis.[2]

Abdominal pain and jaundice are the most common presenting complaints. Abdominal pain predominantly features in up to two thirds of patients, and is typically located in the epigastric region, radiating through to the back, but can present as simple back pain. This can usually be attributed to direct invasion of the celiac plexus or secondary to pancreatitis. Thirteen per cent of patients will

SOURCES AND SELECTION CRITERIA

We searched PubMed to identify peer reviewed original research articles, meta-analyses, and reviews. Search terms were pancreatic cancer, pancreatic adenocarcinoma, pancreatic neoplasia or neoplasm. Only papers written in English were considered.

present with painless jaundice, and 46% will present with both pain and jaundice.[9] It is reported that those patients presenting with painless jaundice have a better prognosis than those patients that present with pain alone.[10] Pancreatic cancer should be considered in the differential diagnosis of any elderly patient presenting for the first time with acute pancreatitis, particularly in the absence of known precipitating factors such as gallstones or alcohol abuse.

Unexplained weight loss may occur as a result of anorexia, or malabsorption due to pancreatic exocrine insufficiency. This is usually secondary to a blocked pancreatic duct, and often manifests as steatorrhoea. Patients describe foul smelling, oily stools that are difficult to flush away. Peripancreatic oedema or a large tumour may compress the duodenum or the stomach, causing gastric outlet obstruction or delayed gastric emptying, with associated nausea and early satiety.

Development of any of the above symptoms in the presence of late onset diabetes should strongly alert the physician to the possibility of pancreatic cancer. Patients over the age of 50 years with late onset diabetes have an eightfold increased risk of developing pancreatic cancer within three years of the diagnosis compared to the general population (see box 2 for other risk factors).[11]

The clinician should be alert to a potential diagnosis of pancreatic cancer with patients over 50 years old who present with unexplained weight loss, persistent abdominal or back pain, dyspepsia, vomiting, or change of bowel function. Currently there is no specific diagnostic algorithm for pancreatic cancer within the National Institute for Health and Clinical Excellence guidelines for cancer referral. If pancreatic cancer is suspected, patients should be referred to a high volume specialist pancreatic centre. In the UK, this can be performed via the suspected upper gastrointestinal cancer two week wait referral pathway.

What is the pathology of pancreatic cancer?

Ninety five per cent of pancreatic cancers originate from the exocrine portion of the gland. A proposed mechanism for the development of invasive pancreatic adenocarcinoma is a stepwise progression through genetically and histologically well defined non-invasive precursor lesions, called pancreatic intraepithelial neoplasias (PanINs). They are microscopic lesions in small (less than 5 mm) pancreatic ducts, and are classified into three grades (see box 3). The understanding of molecular alterations in PanINs has provided rational candidates for the development of early detection biomarkers and therapeutic targets.[12]

SUMMARY POINTS

- Pancreatic cancer can present with non-specific symptoms, such as abdominal or back pain, dyspepsia, and unexplained weight loss, as well as the classic presentation of painless jaundice
- The majority of pancreatic cancer is incurable at presentation[1] [2]
- Whether or not pancreatic cancer is deemed curable, current surgical, endoscopic, and oncological management regimes can significantly improve quality of life
- Trials are currently ongoing to improve outcomes in pancreatic cancer[3]

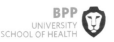

BOX 1 TYPES OF PANCREATIC CANCER

Pancreatic exocrine cancers

- Adenocarcinoma
- Acinar cell carcinoma
- Adenosquamous carcinoma
- Giant cell tumour
- Intraductal papillary mucinous neoplasm (IPMN)
- Mucinous cystadenocarcinoma
- Pancreatoblastoma
- Serous cystadenocarcinoma
- Solid and pseudopapillary tumours

Pancreatic endocrine cancers (pancreatic neuroendocrine tumours)

- Gastrinoma
- Glucagonoma
- Insulinoma
- Nonfunctional islet cell tumour
- Somatostatinoma
- Vasoactive intestinal peptide releasing tumour (VIPoma)

BOX 2 RISK FACTORS FOR PANCREATIC CANCER

Risk factors

- Smoking
- Alcohol
- Increased BMI
- Diabetes mellitus
- Chronic pancreatitis
- Family history of pancreatic cancer

Familial cancer syndromes

- BRCA1, BRCA2
- Familial adenomatous polyposis (FAP)
- Peutz-Jeghers syndrome
- Familial atypical multiple mole melanoma syndrome (FAMMM)
- Lynch syndrome
- von Hippel-Lindau syndrome
- Multiple endocrine neoplasia type 1
- Gardner syndrome

Other medical conditions

- Inflammatory bowel disease
- Periodontal disease
- Peptic ulcer disease

BOX 3 TYPES OF PANCREATIC INTRAEPITHELIAL NEOPLASIA (PANIN)

PanIN 1 (low grade)

- Minimal degree of atypia
- Subclassified into PanIN 1A: absence of micropapillary infoldings of the epithelium; and 1B, presence of micropapillary infoldings of the epithelium

PanIN 2 (intermediate grade)

- Moderate degree of atypia, including loss of polarity, nuclear crowding, enlarged nuclei, pseudostratification, and hyperchromatism
- Mitoses are rarely seen

PanIN 3 (high grade/carcinoma in situ)

- Severe atypia, with varying degrees of cribriforming, luminal necrosis, and atypical mitoses
- Contained within the basement membrane

How do we investigate and diagnose suspected pancreatic cancer?

The most important investigative tool for the diagnosis of pancreatic cancer is computed tomography. However, certain blood tests help guide further management and can be performed while the patient is awaiting specialist review.

Blood tests and tumour markers

A full blood count may reveal a normochromic anaemia or thrombocytosis or both. Those presenting with obstructive jaundice will have significant elevations in serum bilirubin (conjugated and total), alkaline phosphatase, and -glutamyltransferase. Serum aspartate aminotransferase (AST) and serum alanine aminotransferase (ALT) may also be raised, but usually to a lesser extent. Liver metastases alone are not frequently associated with clinically evident jaundice, but may result in relatively low grade elevations of serum alkaline phosphatase and transaminase levels.

Carbohydrate 19-9 (CA19-9), also known as sialylated Lewis (a) antigen, was first identified in pancreatic cancer patients in 1981.[13] It is now one of the most widely used serum tumour markers. CA19-9 is normally found in the cells of the biliary tract, and therefore any disease affecting these cells can cause serum elevations, including pancreatitis, cirrhosis, and cholangitis. Five per cent of the population lack the Lewis (a) antigen, and are not able to produce CA19-9, resulting in a sensitivity of 80% and specificity of 73% for pancreatic cancer.[14] As such, it is not currently recommended as a screening tool. CA19-9 does, however, have a role to play in assessing response to surgery and chemoradiotherapy, and as a surveillance tool following treatment.

With the advancement of high throughput techniques (DNA arrays and proteomics), a number of other potential molecular markers for pancreatic cancer have been identified, but to date these have not been found to be any more discriminating than CA19-9.

Imaging

Imaging is not only the most important diagnostic tool for pancreatic cancer, but will also guide the multidisciplinary team in determining whether the disease is surgically curable.

Abdominal ultrasound is safe, non-invasive, and inexpensive. Its main role is in formulating a differential diagnosis among the possible causes of obstructive jaundice. Bile duct dilation (>7 mm, or >10 mm if previous cholecystectomy) with pancreatic duct dilation (>2 mm) can be an indirect sign of pancreatic cancer (the so called double duct sign). Abdominal ultrasound is not as sensitive as computed tomography in imaging the pancreas, and small tumours (less than 3 cm) will frequently be missed.[15] Liver metastases and ascites are important findings in the work-up of a patient with suspected pancreatic cancer and can normally be visualised by ultrasound.

Triple phase computed tomography, preceded by non-contrast computed tomography, is currently the best technique for detecting pancreatic neoplasms and assessing resectability. It is performed in the arterial, pancreatic parenchymal, and portal venous phase (pancreas protocol computed tomography). Multidetector computed tomography is up to 90% effective at predicting the resectability of a pancreatic cancer.[16] There are reports that computed tomography can only reliably detect lesions larger than 3 cm.[14]

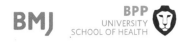

Endoscopic ultrasound (EUS) is becoming an increasingly important imaging modality. A recent meta-analysis showed that it had a sensitivity of 96% (range 85-100%) for diagnosing pancreatic cancer.[17] In comparison to computed tomography, diagnostic sensitivities were significantly in favour of endoscopic ultrasound, especially for small (<3cm) tumours.[12] Endoscopic ultrasound can also accurately detect the involvement of loco-regional lymph nodes.[18] It is further employed to guide fine needle aspiration (FNA) for cytological evaluation of lesions in which there is diagnostic uncertainty. The sensitivity of endoscopic ultrasound guided FNA ranges from 85% to 90% with a false negative rate of up to 15%.[19] Routine endoscopic ultrasound guided FNA of all pancreatic masses is therefore controversial. In a patient with resectable disease who is deemed physiologically fit for surgery, it is arguable whether an FNA is required, as a negative result would not rule out neoplasia, and could delay a potentially curable procedure. The benefit of FNA is mainly in those patients with unresectable disease, as the results may guide further oncological management, or in those patients with significant comorbidities in whom the risk to benefit ratio of surgical intervention is less clear.

The role of MRI (magnetic resonance imaging) remains uncertain at present. Its use in detecting small lesions and determining resectability is increasing as new, faster MRI techniques enable imaging of the pancreas with higher resolution. In a comparative study to determine the diagnostic role of endoscopic ultrasound, computed tomography, and MRI in patients suspected of having pancreatic cancer, the respective sensitivities were 94%, 69%, and 83%.[20]

Positron emission tomography (PET) scanning uses ^{18}F-fluorodeoxyglucose (FDG) to image the primary tumour and establish the presence of metastatic disease. When combined with simultaneous computed tomography scanning (PET-CT), it is more sensitive than conventional imaging for the detection of pancreatic cancer and extrahepatic metastases. Its role in the staging of disease is, however, yet to be fully ascertained.

Similar to endoscopic ultrasound, endoscopic retrograde cholangiopancreatography with brush cytology or forceps biopsy is an effective way (90-95% sensitivity) to confirm the diagnosis of pancreatic adenocarcinoma. Endoscopic retrograde cholangiopancreatography is, however, an invasive procedure that carries a 5-10% risk of significant complications including pancreatitis, and gastrointestinal or biliary perforation, and is therefore usually reserved as a therapeutic procedure for biliary obstruction or for the diagnosis of unusual pancreatic neoplasms.

Staging and treatment of pancreatic adenocarcinoma

The classification of pancreatic adenocarcinoma is shown in table 1, and how it relates to disease stage and prognosis are shown in table 2.[21] [22] At present, surgical resection is the only curative treatment for pancreatic adenocarcinoma. Surgery with curative intent has a five year survival of 10-15%, and median survival of 11 to 18 months. For patients unwilling or not medically fit enough to undergo major pancreatic surgery, alternatives include systemic chemotherapy, chemoradiotherapy, image guided stereotactic radiosurgical systems (such as CyberKnife), surgical bypass, ablative therapies, and endoscopic biliary and gastrointestinal stenting. These are palliative procedures that can improve patients' quality of life by alleviating tumour related symptoms (such as pain and pruritus).

The role of the multidisciplinary team is to determine which patients are suitable to undergo curative surgery, if there is a role for preoperative (neoadjuvant) or postoperative (adjuvant) therapy, or to decide on the most appropriate mode of palliation.

What is resectable and unresectable pancreatic cancer?

The absolute contraindications to pancreatic resection are liver, peritoneal, or distant lymph node metastases, or the patient being deemed medically unfit for major surgery. The age of the patient, size of the tumour, local lymph node metastases, and continuous invasion of the stomach or duodenum are not contraindications to resection.

Advances in surgical techniques and perioperative care mean that tumour involvement of the major vessels around the pancreas is no longer an absolute contraindication to curative resection,[23] although encasement of the hepatic artery, superior mesenteric artery, and coeliac axis means surgery is unlikely to confer any survival benefit. Pancreaticoduodenectomy with resection of the portal and/or superior mesenteric vein is safe and feasible, with a similar mortality and morbidity to pancreaticoduodenectomy without vascular resection.[24] It should, however, only be performed if a disease-free (R0) resection margin can be achieved. If an R0 resection can be obtained, median survival is vastly improved compared to resections with tumour positive margins (13 versus 6 months; p=0.0002).[25]

Table 1 TNM classification of pancreatic adenocarcinoma

Tumour (T)	
TX	Primary tumour cannot be assessed
T0	No evidence of primary tumour
Tis	Carcinoma in situ
T1	Tumour limited to the pancreas, 2 cm or smaller in greatest dimension
T2	Tumour limited to the pancreas, larger than 2 cm in greatest diameter
T3	Tumour extension beyond the pancreas but not involving the coeliac axis or superior mesenteric artery
T4	Tumour involves the coeliac axis or superior mesenteric artery
Regional lymph nodes (N)	
NX	Regional lymph nodes cannot be assessed
N0	No regional lymph node metastasis
N1	Regional lymph node metastasis
Distant metastasis (M)	
MX	Distant metastasis cannot be assessed
M0	No distant metastasis
M1	Distant metastasis

Table 2 Staging and TNM (tumour, lymph node, metastasis) classification related to incidence, treatment, and prognosis

Stage	TNM classification	Clinical classification	Incidence at diagnosis (%)	5-year survival rate (%)
0	Tis, N0, M0	Resectable	7.5	15.2
IA	T1, N0, M0	—	—	—
IB	T2, N0, M0	—	—	—
IIA	T3, N0, M0	—	—	—
IIB	T1-3, N1, M0	Locally advanced	29.3	6.3
III	T4, any N, M0	—	—	—
IV	Any T, any N, M1	Metastatic	47.2	1.6

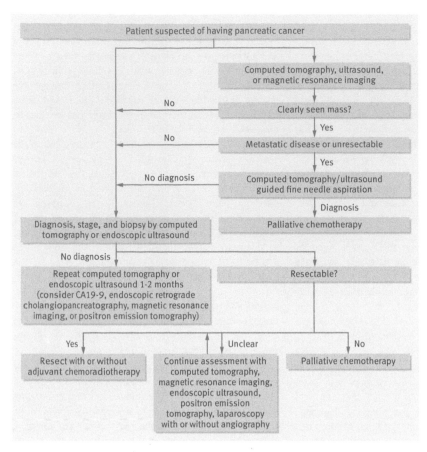

Fig 1 Clinical management pathway

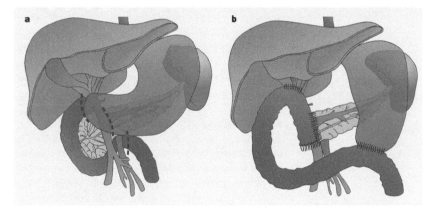

Fig 2 A: Normal anatomy of liver, stomach, duodenum, and pancreas. Dotted lines indicate resection margins at pancreaticoduodenectomy. B: Surgical anastomoses to restore gastrointestinal continuity following a pancreaticoduodenectomy, include a gastrojejunostomy, choledochojejunostomy, and pancreaticojejunostomy (diagram not to scale)

Table 3 Mortality following pancreatic resection in high, medium, and low volume centres[21]

Centre	No. of resections per year	30 day mortality (%)
High volume	>18	2.4
Medium volume	5-18	5.9
Low volume	<5	9.2

Neoadjuvant chemotherapy and chemoradiation

The rationale for neoadjuvant therapy is to increase the incidence of R0 resections, downstage borderline resectable disease to allow resection, and reduce loco-regional recurrence. However, there are no large multicentre randomised controlled trials of neoadjuvant therapy for pancreatic cancer. Meta-analysis of the available data shows that one third of patients with locally advanced disease without distant metastases can achieve a significant oncological response to neoadjuvant treatment increasing the chances of a achieving a R0 resection,[26] thereby reducing local recurrence and potentially improving disease-free survival.

Curative resection

Pancreaticoduodenectomy

The majority of pancreatic adenocarcinomas (78%) are associated with the head, neck, and uncinate process of the pancreas, and require a pancreaticoduodenectomy.[27] First described in the 1930s, it involves resection of the proximal pancreas, along with the distal stomach, duodenum, distal bile duct, and gallbladder as an en bloc specimen.[28] Intestinal continuity is restored via a gastrojejunostomy, choledochojejunostomy, pancreaticojejunostomy (figs 2A and B), or pancreaticogastrostomy.

Morbidity following pancreaticoduodenectomy can be as high as 40%; the most common complications being delayed gastric emptying, pancreatic fistula formation, and pancreatic insufficiency.[29] The operation has wide ranging, 30 day mortality, partly dependent on the surgical volume of the centre where the procedure is performed (see table 3).[30]

Distal pancreatectomy

This procedure is performed for tumours of the body and tail of the pancreas, and carries a morbidity and mortality of 28.1% and 1.2% respectively.[31] The most common major complication is pancreatic fistula formation, due to leakage of pancreatic fluid from the pancreatic duct at the resection margin.[32] Laparoscopic distal pancreatectomy can be safely performed in high volume centres with experience in laparoscopic and pancreatic surgery, and results in less intra-operative blood loss, a shorter time to oral intake, and a shorter postoperative hospital stay than open surgery.[33] Centres that have developed expertise in laparoscopic distal pancreatectomy are now also performing laparoscopic pancreaticoduodenectomy, although this remains rare.

Adjuvant chemotherapy and chemoradiation after curative resection

Treatment regimes have previously employed 5-fluorouracil and radiotherapy.[34] The ESPAC-1 trial in 2004 showed a clear advantage for adjuvant chemotherapy in patients with resected pancreatic cancer over chemoradiotherapy, which had a deleterious impact on survival.[35] ESPAC-3 showed there was no difference between 5-flurouracil/folinic acid and gemcitabine, which is now the most commonly used chemotherapy agent.[36] The ESPAC-4 trial is currently in phase 3, and compares gemcitabine alone against combination therapy of gemcitabine plus capecitabine in patients within one year of a potentially curative resection.

Palliative treatment

Biliary tract or duodenal obstruction can be relieved by surgical, endoscopic, or radiological techniques. Palliative chemotherapy usually involves gemcitabine based regimes. Monoclonal antibodies and the telomerase vaccine GV1001 (the TeloVac trial) are currently under investigation to prolong survival in patients with unresectable or metastatic pancreatic cancer.[3]

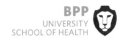

ADDITIONAL EDUCATIONAL RESOURCES

Resources for healthcare professionals

- Hruban RH, Adsay NV, Albores-Saavedra J, Compton C, Garrett ES, Goodman SN, et al. Pancreatic intraepithelial neoplasia: a new nomenclature and classification system for pancreatic duct lesions. *Am J Surg Pathol* 2001;25:579-86—describes a new classification system for pancreatic cancer

- Safi F, Roscher R, Beger HG. Tumour markers in pancreatic cancer. Sensitivity and specificity of CA 19-9. *Hepatogastroenterology* 1989;36:419-23—summarises the role of CA19-9 in pancreatic cancer

- Yeo CJ, Cameron JL, Lillemoe KD, Sohn TA, Campbell KA, Sauter PK, et al. Panctreaticoduodenectomy with or without distal gastrectomy and extended retroperitoneal lymphadenectomy for periampullary adenocarcinoma, part 2: randomized controlled trial evaluating survival, morbidity and mortality. *Ann Surg* 2002;236:355-66—report of a trial showing no benefit for extended lymphadenectomy at the time of pancreaticoduodenectomy for pancreatic cancer

- Zavoral M, Minarikova P, Zavada F, Salek C, Minarik M. Molecular biology of pancreatic cancer. *World J Gastroenterol* 2011;17:2897-908—review of molecular biology of pancreatic cancer

- Hruban RH, Canto MI, Goggins M, Schulick R, Klein AP. Update on familial pancreatic cancer. *Adv Surg* 2010;44:293-311—introduction to familial pancreatic cancer

- Dieterich S, Gibbs IC. The CyberKnife in clinical use: current roles, future expectations. *Front Radiat Ther Oncol* 2011;43:181-94.

Resources for patients

- Pancreatic Cancer UK (www.pancreaticcancer.org.uk)
- Cancer Research UK (www.cancerresearchuk.org)
- Pancreatic Cancer Action (www.pancreaticcanceraction.org)
- Macmillan Cancer Support (www.macmillan.org.uk)
- Patient.co.uk (www.patient.co.uk)
- HPB London (www.hpblondon.com)

TIPS FOR NON-SPECIALISTS

- Patients in the UK with suspected pancreatic cancer should be referred to a specialist pancreatic centre via the two week wait pathway

- Pancreatic cancer should always be considered in the differential diagnosis of an elderly patient with unexplained weight loss, even in the absence of abdominal pain or jaundice

- Multidetector computed tomography is the initial investigation of choice

- All patients with pancreatic cancer should be assessed and managed in a high volume specialist pancreatic centre

How are common postoperative and palliative problems managed?

Locally advanced disease and pancreatic surgery can lead to exocrine insufficiency causing fat malabsorption, which tends to present as excess flatulence, diarrhoea, fatty and offensive smelling stools, or progressive weight loss. These symptoms can be significantly improved by prescribing supplemental pancreatic enzymes (pancreatin). Pancreatin is inactivated by gastric acid and therefore works best when taken with food. There is no linear relationship between the dose of pancreatic enzymes and the symptoms of exocrine insufficiency, so there is no definitive starting dose. Normally the pancreatin preparation is started at a dose of 25 000 to 40 000 units per meal and titrated according to effect on the individual patient.[15]

ONGOING RESEARCH

- **ESPAC 4 trial:** Phase III trial to investigate whether combination adjuvant chemotherapy (gemcitabine and capecitabine) in patients who have undergone resection of pancreatic cancer improves survival when compared to adjuvant chemotherapy (gemcitabine) alone

- **PanGen-EU study:** A large European case control study involving the collection of epidemiological, clinical, and biological information on pancreatic cancer, which aims to validate previous findings as well as explore developmental and progression mechanisms for pancreatic cancer

- **TeloVac trial:** Phase III trial comparing combination chemotherapy (gemcitabine and capecitabine) with concurrent and sequential immunotherapy using the telomerase vaccine (GV1001) in locally advanced and metastatic pancreatic cancer. It is closed to recruitment and the results are expected soon

Delayed gastric emptying is common, causes considerable discomfort, and can prolong the patient's hospital stay. General treatment measures include long term nasogastric drainage, correction of fluid and electrolyte abnormalities, commencement of a proton pump inhibitor or an H2 antagonist, and nutritional supplementation. Prokinetic medications (such as metoclopramide) to improve gastric emptying can also be considered.[15] The onset of delayed gastric emptying shortly after surgery (or an episode of pancreatitis), can indicate an intra-abdominal fluid collection and should be investigated by either ultrasound or computed tomography.

Pancreatic fistulas can result following an anastomotic leak. This is a difficult problem to resolve, with a reported incidence of 0-25%.[37] Early recognition is crucial as a pancreatic fistula may be associated with intra-abdominal sepsis, pseudoaneurysm formation, and possible haemorrhage. If haemorrhage occurs, often preceded by a so called herald bleed, then urgent angiographic imaging is needed to identify and control the source of bleeding, via coil embolisation. The management of simple pancreatic fistulation is still debated. Some advocate conservative management, which includes treatment of sepsis, drainage of intra-abdominal collections, nasogastric suction, total parenteral nutrition, and reducing pancreatic secretions, whereas others favour reoperation.

Contributors: GB-S and NB performed the literature search and wrote the initial draft of the manuscript. TMH and CJI edited and rewrote the manuscript. The original concept for the article was devised by TMH. CJI is guarantor.

Competing interests: All authors have completed the ICMJE uniform disclosure form at www.icmje.org/coi_disclosure.pdf (available on request from the corresponding author) and declare: no support from any organisation for the submitted work; no financial relationships with any organisations that might have an interest in the submitted work in the previous three years; and no other relationships or activities that could appear to have influenced the submitted work.

Provenance and peer review: Not commissioned; externally peer reviewed.

1   Singh SM, Longmire WP Jr, Reber HA. Surgical palliation for pancreatic cancer. The UCLA experience. *Ann Surg* 1990;212:132-9.
2   Singh SM, Reber HA. Surgical palliation for pancreatic cancer. *Surg Clin North Am* 1989;69:599-611.
3   Bernhardt SL, Gjertsen MK, Trachsel S, Møller M, Eriksen JA, Meo M, et al. Telomerase peptide vaccination of patients with non-resectable pancreatic cancer: a dose escalating phase I/II study. *Br J Cancer* 2006;95:1474-82.
4   Anderson K, Mack TM, Silverman DT. Cancer of the pancreas. In: Schottenfeld D, Fraumeni JF Jr, eds. Cancer epidemiology and prevention. 3rd ed. Oxford University Press, 2006.
5   Cancer Research UK. Cancer mortality: UK statistics. 2009. http://info.cancerresearchuk.org/cancerstats/mortality.
6   Hariharan D, Saied A, Kocher HM. Analysis of mortality rates for pancreatic cancer across the world. *HPB (Oxford)* 2008;10:58-62.

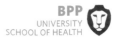

7   Cancer Research UK. Pancreatic cancer: UK incidence statistics. 2011. http://info.cancerresearchuk.org/cancerstats/types/pancreas/incidence.

8   Elliss-Brookes L. Routes to diagnosis. National Cancer Intelligence Network, 2010. www.ncin.org.uk/publications/data_briefings/routes_to_diagnosis.aspx.

9   Gullo L, Tomassetti P, Migliori M, Casadei R, Marrano D. Do early symptoms of pancreatic cancer exist that can allow an earlier diagnosis? *Pancreas*2001;22:210-3.

10 Watanabe I, Sasaki S, Konishi M, Nakagohri T, Inoue K, Oda T, et al. Onset symptoms and tumor locations as prognostic factors of pancreatic cancer. *Pancreas*2004;28:160-5.

11 Chari ST, Leibson CL, Rabe KG, Ransom J, de Andrade M, Petersen GM. Probability of pancreatic cancer following diabetes: a population-based study. *Gastroenterology*2005;129:504-11.

12 Maitra A, Adsay NV, Argani P, Iacobuzio-Donahue C, De Marzo A, Cameron JL, et al. Multicomponent analysis of the pancreatic adenocarcinoma progression model using a pancreatic intraepithelial neoplasia tissue microarray. *Mod Pathol*2003;16:902-12.

13 Koprowski H, Herlyn M, Steplewski Z, Sears HF. Specific antigen in serum of patients with colon carcinoma. *Science*1981;212:53-5.

14 Valls C, Andía E, Sanchez A, Fabregat J, Pozuelo O, Quintero JC, et al. Dual-phase helical CT of pancreatic adenocarcinoma: assessment of resectability before surgery. *AJR Am J Roentgenol*2002;178:821-6.

15 Shrikhande, S, Freiss H, Buchler M, eds. Surgery of pancreatic tumors. BI Publications Pvt Ltd, 2008.

16 Tabuchi T, Itoh K, Ohshio G, Kojima N, Maetani Y, Shibata T, et al. Tumor staging of pancreatic adenocarcinoma using early- and late-phase helical CT. *AJR Am J Roentgenol*1999;173:375-80.

17 Iglesias Garcia J, Lariño Noia J, Domínguez Muñoz JE. Endoscopic ultrasound in the diagnosis and staging of pancreatic cancer. *Rev Esp Enferm Dig*2009;101:631-8.

18 Kahl S, Malfertheiner P. Role of endoscopic ultrasound in the diagnosis of patients with solid pancreatic masses. *Dig Dis*2004;22:26-31.

19 Chang KJ, Nguyen P, Erickson RA, Durbin TE, Katz KD. The clinical utility of endoscopic ultrasound-guided fine needle aspiration in the diagnosis and staging of pancreatic adenocarcinoma. *Gastrointest Endosc*1997;45:387-93.

20 Müller MF, Meyenberger C, Bertschinger P, Schaer R, Marincek B. Pancreatic tumors: evaluation with endoscopic US, CT, and MR imaging. *Radiology*1994;190:745-51.

21 American Joint Committee on Cancer. AJCC cancer staging manual. 6th ed. Springer, 2002.

22 Jemal A, Clegg LX, Ward E, Ries LA, Wu X, Jamison PM, et al. Annual report to the nation on the status of cancer 1975-2001, with a special feature regarding survival. *Cancer*2004;101:3-27.

23 Reddy SK, Tyler DS, Pappas TN, Clary BM. Extended resection for pancreatic adenocarcinoma. *Oncologist*2007;12:654-63.

24 Ramacciato G, Mercantini P, Petrucciani N, Giaccaglia V, Nigri G, Ravaioli M, et al. Does portal-superior mesenteric vein invasion still indicate irresectability for pancreatic carcinoma? *Ann Surg Oncol*2009;16:817-25.

25 Evans DB, Farnell MB, Lillemoe KD, Vollmer C Jr, Strasberg SM, Schulick RD. Surgical treatment of resectable and borderline resectable pancreas cancer: expert consensus statement. *Ann Surg Oncol*2009;16:1736-44.

26 Chua T, Saxena A. Extended pancreaticoduodenectomy with vascular resection for pancreatic cancer: a systematic review. *J Gastrointest Surg*2010;14:1442-52.

27 Gillen S, Schuster T, Meyer Zum Büschenfelde C, Friess H, Kleeff J. Preoperative/neoadjuvant therapy in pancreatic cancer: a systematic review and meta-analysis of response and resection percentages. *PLoS Med*2010;7:e1000267.

28 Whipple AO, Parsons WB, Mullins CR. Treatment of carcinoma of the ampulla of vater. *Ann Surg*1935;102:763-79.

29 Yeo CJ, Cameron JL, Sohn TA, Lillemoe KD, Pitt HA, Talamini MA, et al. Six hundred fifty consecutive pancreaticoduodenectomies in the 1990s: pathology, complications, and outcomes. *Ann Surg*1997;226:248-60.

30 McPhee JT, Hill JS, Whalen GF, Zayaruzny M, Litwin DE, Sullivan ME, et al. Perioperative mortality for pancreatectomy: a national perspective. *Ann Surg*2007;246:246-53.

31 Kelly KJ, Greenblatt DY, Wan Y, Rettammel RJ, Winslow E, Cho CS, et al. Risk stratification for distal pancreatectomy utilizing ACS-NSQIP: preoperative factors predict morbidity and mortality. *J Gastrointest Surg*2011;15:250-61.

32 Zhou W, Lv R, Wang X, Mou Y, Cai X, Herr I. Stapler vs suture closure of pancreatic remnant after distal pancreatectomy: a meta-analysis. *Am J Surg*2010;200:529-36.

33 Briggs CD, Mann CD, Irving GR, Neal CP, Peterson M, Cameron IC, et al. Systematic review of minimally invasive pancreatic resection. *J Gastrointest Surg*2009;13:1129-37.

34 Kalser MH, Ellenberg SS. Pancreatic cancer. Adjuvant combined radiation and chemotherapy following curative resection. *Arch Surg*1985;120:899-903.

35 Neoptolemos JP, Stocken DD, Friess H, Bassi C, Dunn JA, Hickey H, et al. A randomized trial of chemoradiotherapy and chemotherapy after resection of pancreatic cancer. *N Engl J Med*2004;350:1200-10.

36 Neoptolemos JP, Stocken DD, Bassi C, Ghaneh P, Cunningham D, Goldstein D, et al. Adjuvant chemotherapy with fluorouracil plus folinic acid vs gemcitabine following pancreatic cancer resection: a randomized controlled trial. *JAMA*2010;304:1073-81.

37 Yang YM, Tian XD, Zhuang Y, Wang WM, Wan YL, Huang YT. Risk factors of pancreatic leakage after pancreaticoduodenectomy. *World J Gastroenterol*2005;11:2456-61.

Related links

bmj.com
- Get CME credits for this article

bmj.com/archive
Previous articles in this series
- The modern management of incisional hernias (2012;344:e2843)
- Diagnosis and management of bone stress injuries of the lower limb in athletes (2012;344:e2511)
- The management of overactive bladder syndrome (2012;344:e2365)
- Cluster headache (2012;344:e2407)

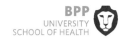

Crohn's disease

Rahul Kalla, clinical research fellow, Nicholas T Ventham, clinical research fellow, Jack Satsangi, professor of gastroenterology, Ian D R Arnott, consultant gastroenterologist

¹Gastrointestinal Unit, Centre for Molecular Medicine, Institute of Genetics and Molecular Medicine, Western General Hospital, Edinburgh EH4 2XU, UK

Correspondence to: I D R Arnott ian.arnott@nhslothian.scot.nhs.uk

Cite this as: BMJ 2014;349:g6670

DOI: 10.1136/bmj.g6670

http://www.bmj.com/content/349/bmj.g6670

Crohn's disease is a chronic inflammatory disorder that can affect any part of the gastrointestinal tract. Although the disease most commonly presents at a young age, it can affect people of all ages. Patients often present with persistent diarrhoea, abdominal pain, and weight loss. Crohn's disease has a global impact on patients' education, work, and social and family life. High quality multidisciplinary care, of which primary care is a key aspect, can attenuate relapse, prevent long term complications, and improve quality of life. In this review we provide a practical approach to the diagnosis, management, and long term care of patients with Crohn's disease.

How common is it?

Crohn's disease is an idiopathic, chronic relapsing immune mediated disease, the pathogenesis of which remains incompletely understood, although the condition is thought to arise from environmental priming and triggering events in a genetically susceptible patient.[1] The incidence and prevalence of Crohn's disease is increasing worldwide, with a recent systematic review reporting the highest incidence in Australia (29.3 per 100 000), Canada (20.2 per 100 000 population), and northern Europe (10.6 per 100 000).[2] Crohn's disease is more likely in those with a strong family history (first degree relatives) of the condition and often presents in the second to fourth decades of life, affecting both sexes equally.[2][3] Crohn's disease is associated with excess mortality compared with the general population, with a standardised mortality ratio of 1.38 (95% confidence interval 1.23 to 1.55).[4]

What are the clinical features?

Diagnosing Crohn's disease can be a challenge because of its widespread and often cryptic manifestations. The clinical features vary according to disease location (table 1) but include chronic diarrhoea (>4 weeks with or without blood and mucus),[5] abdominal pain, and weight loss; patients presenting with this triad of symptoms should initially have blood tests (fig 1). Nocturnal defecation often occurs; this

SOURCES AND SELECTION CRITERIA

We carried out an electronic search of PubMed, the Cochrane Library, and Ovid databases for articles using the term "Crohn's disease". We limited studies to those in adults and focused on high quality randomised control trials, meta-analyses, and systematic reviews.

symptom is not a feature of irritable bowel syndrome and indicates the need for urgent investigations. Non-specific symptoms such as malaise, fever, and anorexia commonly occur and some patients may present with extraintestinal manifestations (fig 2). The presence of aphthous mouth ulcers, pyoderma gangrenosum, or erythema nodosum can be especially suggestive of inflammatory bowel diseases. The course of Crohn's disease is typified by periods of relapse and remission with recurrent cycles of inflammation leading to development of complications such as strictures and fistulas. Distinguishing Crohn's disease from irritable bowel syndrome can be difficult. The prodromal period is often considerable and can be up to 10 years before the diagnosis is established.[6]

How is it diagnosed?

Crohn's disease is diagnosed by a combination of clinical, laboratory, radiological, endoscopic, and histological findings (fig 1). Initial blood tests include a full blood count, haematinics, inflammatory markers, and vitamin D level. Typical findings suggestive of Crohn's disease include increased levels of inflammatory markers (C reactive protein and erythrocyte sedimentation rate), iron deficiency anaemia, and nutritional deficiencies such as low vitamin B12 and folate levels. These tests can help differentiate inflammatory bowel diseasses from irritable bowel syndrome. Stool cultures should be performed for Clostridium difficile, parasites or their ova, and in all patients presenting with diarrhoea.

Faecal calprotectin, a neutrophil cytosolic protein, is an effective marker for the presence of intestinal inflammation. A meta-analysis of six studies (670 adults) found that the faecal calprotectin test had a pooled sensitivity of 0.93 (95% confidence interval 0.85 to 0.97) and a pooled specificity of 0.96 (95% confidence interval 0.79 to 0.99) for inflammatory bowel diseases.[8] The test is a simple and cost effective way of identifying those with probable inflammatory bowel diseases that require urgent investigation. In the United Kingdom, the National Institute for Health and Care Excellence provides guidelines on the use of faecal calprotectin testing in primary care,[9] but this test is not always available. As classic features of Crohn's disease are not always present and blood test results can be normal, referral should be considered in those who have persisting symptoms atypical for irritable bowel syndrome.[10]

Any patients with a suspected diagnosis of inflammatory bowel disease should be referred urgently to specialist services for further investigation.

THE BOTTOM LINE

- The incidence and prevalence of Crohn's disease is increasing worldwide
- Crohn's disease can have a major impact on patients' education, work, and social and family life
- To induce early remission and prevent long term complications, early diagnosis of Crohn's disease is a priority
- Adequate clinical and biochemical (for example, faecal calprotectin level) or endoscopic assessment of disease activity is needed to guide further decisions about treatment
- Drugs such as thiopurines, methotrexate, and anti-tumour necrosis factor are often used to maintain remission in patients with Crohn's disease
- Adverse pregnancy outcomes are associated with active Crohn's disease, and disease flares should be treated aggressively in pregnancy
- A systematic programme of surveillance to monitor long term sequelae should be in place to ensure the best outcomes for patients with Crohn's disease

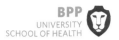

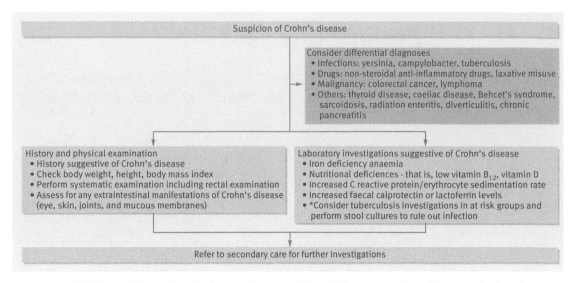

Fig 1 Key clinical features, laboratory investigations, risk factors, and differential diagnoses in patients with suspected Crohn's disease

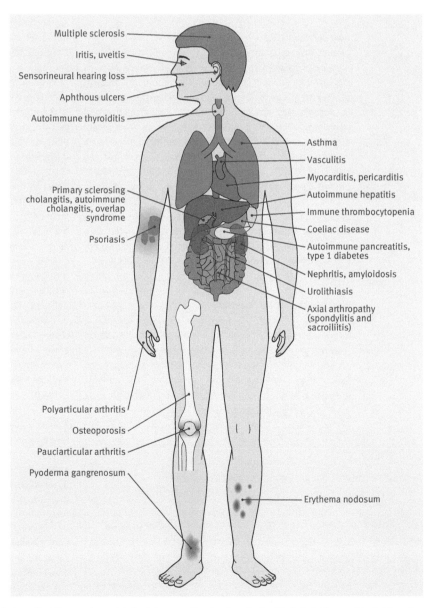

Fig 2 Extraintestinal manifestations and associated autoimmune disorders in patients with Crohn's disease. Adapted from Baumgart and Sandborn[7]

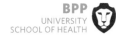

Table 1 Clinical presentation as per Montreal classification in Crohn's disease

Disease location	Montreal classification	Clinical manifestations
Ileal	L1	Malabsorption and nutritional deficiencies; abdominal pain and weight loss; diarrhoea may be absent; acute terminal ileum disease can mimic acute appendicitis
Colonic	L2	Bloody diarrhoea; can mimic acute severe ulcerative colitis; obstruction due to stricturing disease
Ileocolonic	L3	Right sided abdominal pain, diarrhoea, weight loss; obstructive or pseudo-obstructive symptoms due to stricturing disease
Upper gastrointestinal	L4	Can mimic peptic ulcer disease; can present as chronic gastric outlet obstruction
Perianal	P	Recurrent perianal abscesses; perianal fistulas; anal skin tags

In secondary care, ileocolonoscopy and biopsies are desirable when diagnosing Crohn's disease. Findings include discontinuous colonic or ileal inflammation or ulceration, a "cobblestone" appearance, and rectal sparing. Characteristic histology shows focal or patchy chronic inflammation, focal crypt irregularity, and granulomas.[11] In 5% of cases it can be difficult to differentiate histologically between Crohn's disease and ulcerative colitis, and the term inflammatory bowel disease type-unclassified is used.[12] Although a diagnosis based on histology is preferred, this can be challenging when Crohn's disease affects the small bowel. Magnetic resonance imaging of the small bowel is becoming the preferred imaging modality for such cases, and specific sequences can give information on the presence of active complications. Other investigations include computed tomography for extraluminal complications such as abscesses and fistulas, small bowel ultrasonography in specialist centres, and small bowel capsule endoscopy. Small bowel enteroscopy, including double balloon enteroscopy, is often used in those in whom a histological diagnosis is important.[13]

How is it managed?

Crohn's disease has a global impact on patients' health. To ensure the best outcomes for patients, a multidisciplinary approach is important. Patients with active disease often have a poor quality of life and may experience repeat hospital admissions, multiple operations, poor nutrition, and malignancy. Therefore early diagnosis and regular and objective assessment of disease activity is essential to support continued wellbeing. Local services responsive to the needs of patients are vital. Key features are the provision of telephone access to specialist care, expedited review in the event of a relapse, rigorous monitoring of treatment, and a systematic programme of disease surveillance. A range of follow-up options, such as nurse led clinics and guided self management has also been implemented.

Patients should undergo nutritional screening that assesses body mass index and unplanned weight loss, such as the Malnutrition Universal Screening Tool (MUST), which can be completed by all healthcare professionals.[14] Those at high risk of malnutrition require appropriate dietician review. Micronutrient assessment must also be undertaken such as for vitamin B12, folate, iron, calcium, and vitamin D, and patients should receive supplementation where appropriate. Smoking cessation can be as effective as immunomodulatory therapy and can reduce the risk of relapse by 65% compared with continued smoking.[15 16 17 18] Patients should be offered the full remit of smoking cessation services. Non-steroidal anti-inflammatory drugs should be discontinued.[19 20]

The choice of drug treatment is influenced by factors such as efficacy, the need for inducing or maintaining remission, side effect profile, long term risks, and patient choice (table 2). Patients with predictors of a severe disease phenotype (box) should be targeted for early, arguably combined, immunosuppressive therapy.[29 30 31]

Treatment of disease flare

Induction of remission

Crohn's disease is characterised by cycles of inflammation that cause disease flares, with periods of relapse and remission in between. Symptoms of flare vary by disease location (fig 1). Management depends on the severity of symptoms (fig 3). If patients are systemically unwell, doctors should consider seeking urgent specialist advice and arranging hospital admission. Patients without systemic problems should be seen in specialist clinics. While awaiting clinic review, primary care doctors can consider initiating a tapered course of corticosteroids once infection is definitively ruled out, with reassessment before and after treatment. Steroid initiation in primary care should be avoided in patients taking dual immunomodulators or anti-tumour necrosis factor agents.

Corticosteroids—Two randomised controlled trials showed the efficacy of corticosteroids at inducing remission in 60-83% of patients with active Crohn's disease compared with placebo (NNT 3).[26 27] For disease flares, guidelines recommend 30-40 mg of prednisolone or 9 mg of budesonide, tapered over 6-8 weeks.[12] Steroids should not be used to maintain remission and are associated with important short term and long term side effects.[26 32 33] Budesonide acts locally in the gut and consequently has fewer side effects. It is indicated in patients with mild to moderate disease confined to the small bowel or the proximal colon, but it is ineffective in maintaining remission.[34]

Biological treatments—Anti-tumour necrosis factor alpha monoclonal antibodies are effective at inducing remission in patients with moderate to severe Crohn's disease compared with placebo (remission rates of 81% v 17%, respectively at week 4 for infliximab, 35.5% v 12% at week 4 for adalimumab)[22 35] and for treating perianal disease (response in 68% v 26% with infliximab median 12 weeks; 33% v 13% at week 56 for adalimumab).[22 36] Early use of anti-tumour necrosis factor alpha agents (top-down approach) is associated with increased remission rates over three years of treatment.[37 38 39] NICE guidelines recommend the step-up approach: using anti-tumour necrosis factor agents for patients in whom conventional immunomodulatory therapies have failed.[40] A rapid step-up therapy in those with predictors of a severe phenotype should be considered (box).[29 30 31]

Enteral nutrition—In adults, guidelines recommend exclusive enteral nutrition as an adjunct to improve nutritional status or as the preferred treatment in those who decline conventional drugs.[11] A Cochrane review of six randomised controlled trials that included 196 adults treated with exclusive enteral nutrition for active Crohn's disease concluded that corticosteroid treatment was superior to exclusive enteral nutrition in inducing remission (odds ratio 0.33, 95% confidence interval 0.21 to 0.53).[41]

Maintenance of remission

Once patients are in remission, maintenance treatment should be considered, aiming to avoid repeated use of corticosteroids and reduce long term complications.[11 12] Symptoms can be a poor guide to the attainment of complete remission, and clinical, biochemical (including faecal calprotectin test), and endoscopic findings should be used to determine deep remission and guide further treatment decisions.[42]

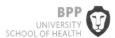

Table 2 Drugs used for induction and maintenance of remission in Crohn's disease[11 12 22-28]

Treatment	Indications and contraindications	Pretest initiation and monitoring	Common side effects	Long term risk	Monitoring	Pregnancy	Numbers needed to treat
Induction of remission:							
Steroids	Induction of remission—luminal disease; contraindicated in glaucoma, fractures, infection	None	Easy bruising; cushingoid facies; weight gain; myopathy; cataracts	Osteoporosis; hypertension; adrenal insufficiency; steroid induced diabetes	Blood glucose where appropriate	Can be used under specialist supervision	2-3
Biologics (infliximab, adalimumab)	Induction of remission—luminal and perianal disease; contraindicated in cancers, active sepsis, tuberculosis, demyelinating disease, congestive heart failure	Live vaccinations before start of treatment*; up to date inactivated vaccines†	Anaphylaxis; myalgia; malaise; rash; infections; rarely neutropenia	Rare: lymphoproliferative disorders; malignancy; reactivation of tuberculosis; opportunistic infections	Full blood count, liver function tests, urea and electrolytes before every infusion	Available data suggest safe in pregnancy, but no long term data available	3-4
Exclusive nutritional therapy	Induction of remission, especially in children; no contraindications	Ensure any electrolyte abnormalities corrected to prevent refeeding syndrome	Poorly tolerated	Steatohepatitis	Urea and electrolytes, magnesium, bone profile testing during initiation of treatment (to monitor for refeeding syndrome)	No contraindications	Not known
Maintenance of remission:							
Thiopurines (azathioprine, mercaptopurine)	Maintains remission, principally in luminal disease; contraindicated in cancers, active sepsis, tuberculosis	Thiopurines-methyltransferase before initiation; live vaccinations before initiation*; up to date inactivated vaccines†; thiopurine metabolites to guide dosing	Nausea and vomiting; hair loss; myalgia; rash; pancreatitis; neutropenia; deranged liver function test results	Rare: non-melanoma skin cancer and lymphoma	Full blood count, liver function tests; every 2 weeks on initiation followed by every 2-3 months once dosing regimen is stable	Can be used under specialist supervision if benefits outweigh harms	4-6
Methotrexate	Maintains remission; contraindicated in pregnancy, liver disease, blood dyscrasias, active sepsis, tuberculosis	Full blood count, liver function tests, urea and electrolytes; chest radiography; live vaccines before initiation*; up to date inactivated vaccines†	Nausea and vomiting; diarrhoea; stomatitis; neutropenia; deranged liver function test results	Hepatotoxicity; pneumonitis	Full blood count, liver function tests; every 2 weeks on initiation followed by every 2-3 months once dosing regimen stable	Contraindicated in pregnancy; discontinue 3-6 months before conception	4-5

*Varicella zoster; BCG (tuberculosis); yellow fever; measles, mumps, and rubella; rotavirus; oral polio; and live attenuated influenza.

†Hepatitis B; pneumococcus; influenza (except intranasal), polio (inactivated poliovirus vaccine); tetanus+diphtheria (combined diphtheria, tetanus, and pertussis vaccine); rabies, and human papillomavirus.

Immunomodulators—Immunomodulatory drugs used to treat Crohn's disease include the thiopurines (azathioprine, mercaptopurine) and methotrexate. These drugs are effective at maintaining remission in patients with moderate to severe Crohn's disease and in those who are steroid dependent. The odds ratio for maintenance of remission with azathioprine was 2.32 (95% confidence interval 1.55 to 3.49, number needed to treat (NNT) 6) and for mercaptopurine was 3.32 (40 to 7.87, NNT 4).[23] The onset of action of the thiopurines is slow (up to 17 weeks) and induction treatments (corticosteroids or anti-tumour necrosis factor agents) are often needed.[11] Methotrexate is also effective at maintaining remission in Crohn's disease compared with placebo (65% v 39%, NNT 4)[24]; however, it is teratogenic, often poorly tolerated, and guidelines recommend its use only in patients who are intolerant or refractory to thiopurines or anti-tumour necrosis factor agents.[12 43] The optimal time for drug withdrawal has been debated, although expert opinion suggests discontinuation once patients have been in clinical remission for four years.[44] Such decisions are often made on an individual basis, taking into account the risk of relapse against the long term risks of treatment.[45]

Biological treatment—Anti-tumour necrosis factor agents are effective at maintaining remission in patients with Crohn's disease.[22 25] They can be used as monotherapy or as combination therapy with immunomodulators. Combination therapy is superior to monotherapy in maintaining steroid-free clinical remission (56.8% v 30%, P<0.001), with evidence of better mucosal healing (43.9% v 16.5%, P<0.001).[45 46] Compared with monotherapy, combination therapy carries the risks of non-melanoma skin cancer and other cancers: standardised incidence ratio 3.46 (95% confidence interval 1.08 to 11.06) and 2.82 (1.07 to 7.44), respectively.[47]

The optimal time for withdrawal of anti-tumour necrosis factor agents is currently unknown, but an expert panel review identified low risk groups where timed withdrawal may be considered.[44 48]

When should surgery be considered?

Failure of medical treatment is the most common reason for resectional surgery.[49] This includes treatment of fibrostenotic disease and penetrating disease (perforation, intra-abdominal abscess, abdominal fistulas). Crohn's disease with perianal involvement may require surgery either to drain sepsis or to control fistulas. Ileocaecal resection can be first line treatment for discrete terminal ileal disease,[50 51 52] although anastomotic recurrence remains common. The role of medical treatment to prevent postoperative recurrence is currently being investigated by the Trial of Prevention of Postoperative Crohn's disease (ISRCTN89489788), Postoperative Crohn's Endoscopic Recurrence (NCT00989560) study, and infliximab (NCT01190839) trial.

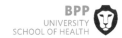

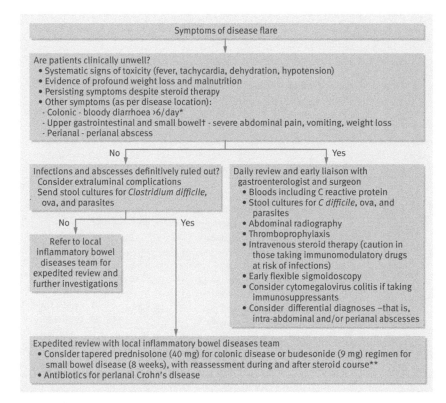

Fig 3 Management of disease flares in Crohn's disease. Although no defined criteria exist for hospital admission of patients, the figure shows the signs and symptoms that should prompt doctors to consider admission. Presentations can vary and often clinical judgment is necessary; particularly in immunosuppressed patients, who are at risk of opportunistic infections. *Colonic Crohn's disease can mimic presentations of acute severe colitis and although the Truelove Witt criteria are validated for ulcerative colitis,[26] These criteria can help guide general practitioners when assessing patients with acute Crohn's disease colitis. †Patients may present with obstructive or pseudo-obstructive symptoms and in some cases. **Steroids should be avoided in patients on dual immunosuppression or those on anti-tumour necrosis factor therapies and expedited specialist review should be sought. See the supplementary figure for a summary of the more pertinent aspects of Crohn's disease along with details on, for example, remission, screening tools, and colorectal cancer surveillance guidelines

The main principle of surgery is to preserve bowel length to avoid short bowel syndrome and intestinal failure. Stricturoplasty can effectively treat strictures without the need for resection. Ileorectal anastomosis is not often indicated owing to the high risk of disease recurrence In proximal small bowel and the risk of anastomotic leaks.[52] [53]

What is the long term care for patients with Crohn's disease?

A complete vaccination history is vital before starting immunomodulator therapy in patients with Crohn's disease. Ensuring adequate titres of antihepatitis B surface antigen, that antivaricella zoster virus antibodies are present, and screening for latent tuberculosis is essential. Patients who are carriers of hepatitis B virus are at risk of hepatic failure, whereas those with latent tuberculosis are at risk of reactivation if exposed to immunomodulatory therapies. Live vaccines should only be administered before the start of treatment. Table 2 provides a summary of live, inactivated, and conjugate vaccines. Patients receiving immunomodulatory therapy are at an increased risk of severe influenza and pneumococcal infections and should be vaccinated against these pathogens every year and every five years, respectively.[54] Patients receiving triple immunosuppression are at an increased risk of *Pneumocystis jivoreci* pneumonia and should be given cotrimoxazole prophylaxis.[54]

Fertility

Infertility in men and women with inflammatory bowel diseases is common and often due to voluntary childlessness based on inaccurate beliefs about pregnancy outcomes in Crohn's disease.[55] Fertility in patients with inactive Crohn's disease is similar to that in those without Crohn's disease but is lower in those with active disease. Preconception planning to minimise disease activity is important to ensure the best possible pregnancy outcomes.[56]

Patients who have had pelvic surgery are at a threefold increased risk of infertility and may benefit from fertility counselling.[57] Patients taking methotrexate should be informed of the risk of teratogenicity and offered detailed contraception counselling, and should stop treatment for 6-9 months before conception.[12]

Pregnancy and breast feeding

Inflammatory bowel diseases often affect people of childbearing age, and patients should be counselled about the risks and benefits of treatment during pregnancy. The risk of flares is similar between pregnant and non-pregnant women and disease activity at conception influences the disease course during pregnancy.[58] [59] Only a third of women will achieve remission during pregnancy if Crohn's disease was active at conception.[60] [61] Adverse pregnancy outcomes are associated with active disease and flares should be treated aggressively to reduce fetal and maternal complications. Neonates born to mothers receiving immunosuppressive and anti-tumour necrosis factor drugs are considered to be immunosuppressed and

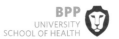

RISK FACTORS FOR A SEVERE CROHN'S DISEASE PHENOTYPE[29] [30] [31]

- Younger age of onset (<40 years)
- Perianal disease
- Stricturing, and penetrating disease (perforation, intra-abdominal abscess, abdominal fistulas)
- Presence of upper gastrointestinal lesions
- Need for steroids for treating first flare
- Female sex

ADDITIONAL EDUCATIONAL RESOURCES

Resources for healthcare professionals
- British Society of Gastroenterology guidelines (www.bsg.org.uk)—Provides evidence based guidelines on the diagnosis and management of Crohn's disease
- European Crohn's and Colitis Organisation. Inflammatory bowel diseases (www.ecco-ibd.eu)—Provides European evidence based guidelines on the diagnosis and management of Crohn's disease
- Inflammatory Bowel Disease Standards (www.ibdstandards.org.uk)—National UK standards for the care of patients with inflammatory bowel diseases
- National Institute for Health and Care Excellence. Crohn's disease: management in adults, children and young people (www.nice.org.uk/guidance/cg152)
- InnovAiT CD review (http://ino.sagepub.com/content/7/1/43.full)—A review on the diagnosis and management of Crohn's disease tailored for general practitioners
- BAPEN: Malnutrition Universal Screening Tool (MUST) (www.bapen.org.uk/must/)—A nutritional screening tool for healthcare professionals to assess patients at risk of malnutrition

Resources for patients
- Crohn's and Colitis UK (www.crohnsandcolitis.org.uk) and Crohn's and Colitis Foundation of America (www.ccfa.org)—UK and US based charities that raise awareness of inflammatory bowel diseases and provide information and support for patients and fund research into the diseases
- CORE: fighting gut and liver disease (www.corecharityorg.uk)—A UK based charity that raises awareness and funds research in gut and liver diseases
- EFCCA: the European Federation of Ulcerative colitis and Crohn's Associations (hwww.efcca.org)—An umbrella organisation representing 28 national patients' associations from 27 European countries
- IA: The ileostomy and internal pouch Support Group (www.iasupport.org) and UOAA: United Ostomy Associations of America (www.ostomy.org)—UK and US based support groups for patients with ileostomy and internal pouch

QUESTIONS FOR FUTURE RESEARCH

- Can new stool, tissue, blood, and serum biomarkers be identified to allow the early diagnosis and risk stratification of the course of inflammatory bowel diseases?
- Can genetic analysis and gene expression profiling allow us to better prognosticate for patients and to personalise treatments?
- How effective will be new treatments such as "biosimilars" and novel drugs that target specific immunological pathways, such as tofacitinib (Jak 1/3 antagonist) and ustekinumab (targets interleukin 12/23)?

should not receive live vaccines for at least six months after exposure.[54] Women who have undergone pelvic surgery or have extensive perianal disease should be scheduled for elective caesarean to limit potential anal sphincter damage.

Cancer
Patients with Crohn's disease have an increased risk of small bowel (standard incidence ratio 40.6, 95% confidence interval 8.4 to 118) and colorectal malignancy (1.9, 0.7 to 4.1).[62] Surveillance usually begins 10 years after the diagnosis of inflammatory bowel disease, and patients are risk stratified to determine the frequency of ongoing surveillance. Patients with concurrent primary sclerosing cholangitis are at greatest risk and should undergo annual surveillance after diagnosis. The American Society of Gastrointestinal Endoscopy has also produced guidelines for surveillance of colorectal cancer.[63]

Patients receiving thiopurines are at a slightly increased risk of non-melanoma skin cancer (0.66 per 1000 patient years) and B cell lymphoma (0.9 per 1000 patient years) and should undergo dermatological surveillance and use protection, such as clothing and sunscreens against ultraviolet A light to minimise the risk of skin cancer.[64] [65] Treatments with anti-tumour necrosis factor carry a small risk of B cell lymphoma and a rare, often fatal hepatosplenic T cell lymphoma.[66] [67] In contrast, the use of thiopurines is associated with a lower risk of colorectal cancer (relative risk 0.71, 95% confidence interval 0.54 to 0.94; P=0.017).[68] The aforementioned findings may be overwhelming for some patients and the appropriate information should be provided to facilitate an informed decision.

Osteoporosis
Patients with Crohn's disease are at risk of osteoporosis from intermittent steroid use and altered micronutrient absorption. Calcium and vitamin D supplementation during steroid treatment is beneficial. The British Society of Gastroenterology has produced guidelines for the management of osteoporosis risk,[69] including the recommendation that all patients taking steroids for more than three months should have a bone mineral density scan. The guidelines also recommend that patients aged less than 65 with a T score of less than 1.5 should start bisphosphonates, as should those aged more than 65 who take corticosteroids.

Psychosocial health
Depression is an independent risk factor for a poor health related quality of life and is associated with adverse outcomes in patients with Crohn's disease.[70] [71] [72] A study found that the incidence of depression was higher in a cohort with inflammatory bowel diseases than in a control population (odds ratio 2.2, 95% confidence interval 1.64 to 2.95).[73] The fear of incontinence and its impact seems to inhibit social interaction and can lead to missed life events.[74] Doctors must be alert to the psychosocial burden of Crohn's disease and provide support for patients. Patient groups may be a useful source of support.

Contributors: RK wrote the initial draft of the manuscript. All authors amended the manuscript and approved the final version.

Competing interests: We have read and understood the BMJ policy on declaration of interests and declare the following interests: none.

Provenance and peer review: Commissioned; externally peer reviewed.

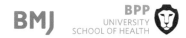

1. Xavier RJ, Podolsky DK. Unravelling the pathogenesis of inflammatory bowel disease. *Nature*2007;448:427-34.

2. Molodecky NA, Soon IS, Rabi DM, Ghali WA, Ferris M, Chernoff G, et al. Increasing incidence and prevalence of the inflammatory bowel diseases with time, based on systematic review. *Gastroenterology*2012;142:46-54.e42; quiz e30.

3. Orholm M, Munkholm P, Langholz E, Nielsen OH, Sørensen TI, Binder V. Familial occurrence of inflammatory bowel disease. *N Engl J Med*1991;324:84-8.

4. Bewtra M, Kaiser LM, TenHave T, Lewis JD. Crohn's disease and ulcerative colitis are associated with elevated standardized mortality ratios: a meta-analysis. *Inflamm Bowel Dis*2013;19:599-613.

5. Fine KD, Schiller LR. AGA technical review on the evaluation and management of chronic diarrhea. *Gastroenterology*1999;116:1464-86.

6. Pimentel M, Chang M, Chow EJ, Tabibzadeh S, Kirit-Kiriak V, Targan SR, et al. Identification of a prodromal period in Crohn's disease but not ulcerative colitis. *Am J Gastroenterol*2000;95:3458-62.

7. Baumgart DC, Sandborn WJ. Crohn's disease. *Lancet*2012;380:1590-605.

8. Van Rheenen PF, Van de Vijver E, Fidler V. Faecal calprotectin for screening of patients with suspected inflammatory bowel disease: diagnostic meta-analysis. *BMJ*2010;341:c3369.

9. National Institute for Health and Care Excellence. Faecal calprotectin diagnostic tests for inflammatory diseases of the bowel (DG11). NICE, 2013. www.nice.org.uk/guidance/dg11/chapter/5-outcomes.

10. National Institute of Health and Care Excellence. Inflammatory bowel disease: quality standard (GID-QSD70). NICE, 2014. www.nice.org.uk/guidance/indevelopment/gid-qsd70/documents.

11. Dignass A, Van Assche G, Lindsay JO, Lémann M, Söderholm J, Colombel JF, et al. The second European evidence-based consensus on the diagnosis and management of Crohn's disease: current management. *J Crohns Colitis*2010;4:28-62.

12. Mowat C, Cole A, Windsor A, Ahmad T, Arnott I, Driscoll R, et al. Guidelines for the management of inflammatory bowel disease in adults. *Gut*2011;60:571-607.

13. Sidhu R, Sanders DS, Morris AJ, McAlindon ME. Guidelines on small bowel enteroscopy and capsule endoscopy in adults. *Gut*2008;57:125-36.

14. Screening for Malnutrition A Multidisciplinary Responsibility. Development and USe of the Malnutrition Universal Screening Tool (MUST) for Adults. Malnutrition Advisory Group (MAG) BAPEN.

15. Seksik P, Nion-Larmurier I, Sokol H, Beaugerie L, Cosnes J. Effects of light smoking consumption on the clinical course of Crohn's disease. *Inflamm Bowel Dis*2009;15:734-41.

16. Johnson GJ, Cosnes J, Mansfield JC. Review article: smoking cessation as primary therapy to modify the course of Crohn's disease. *Aliment Pharmacol Ther*2005;21:921-31.

17. Dam AN, Berg AM, Farraye FA. Environmental influences on the onset and clinical course of Crohn's disease-part 1: an overview of external risk factors. *Gastroenterol Hepatol (N Y)*2013;9:711-7.

18. Mahid SS, Minor KS, Soto RE, Hornung CA, Galandiuk S. Smoking and inflammatory bowel disease: a meta-analysis. *Mayo Clin Proc*2006;81:1462-71.

19. Takeuchi K, Smale S, Premchand P, Maiden L, Sherwood R, Thjodleifsson B, et al. Prevalence and mechanism of nonsteroidal anti-inflammatory drug-induced clinical relapse in patients with inflammatory bowel disease. *Clin Gastroenterol Hepatol*2006;4:196-202.

20. Meyer AM, Ramzan NN, Heigh RI, Leighton JA. Relapse of inflammatory bowel disease associated with use of nonsteroidal anti-inflammatory drugs. *Dig Dis Sci*2006;51:168-72.

21. Evans JM, McMahon AD, Murray FE, McDevitt DG, MacDonald TM. Non-steroidal anti-inflammatory drugs are associated with emergency admission to hospital for colitis due to inflammatory bowel disease. *Gut*1997;40:619-22.

22. Hanauer SB, Sandborn WJ, Rutgeerts P, Fedorak RN, Lukas M, MacIntosh D, et al. Human anti-tumor necrosis factor monoclonal antibody (adalimumab) in Crohn's disease: the CLASSIC-I trial. *Gastroenterology*2006;130:323-33; quiz 591.

23. Prefontaine E, Sutherland LR, Macdonald JK, Cepoiu M. Azathioprine or 6-mercaptopurine for maintenance of remission in Crohn's disease. *Cochrane Database Syst Rev*2009;1:CD000067.

24. Patel V, Wang Y, MacDonald JK, McDonald JWD, Chande N. Methotrexate for maintenance of remission in Crohn's disease. *Cochrane Database Syst Rev*2014;8:CD006884.

25. Hanauer SB, Feagan BG, Lichtenstein GR, Mayer LF, Schreiber S, Colombel JF, et al. Maintenance infliximab for Crohn's disease: the ACCENT I randomised trial. *Lancet*2002;359:1541-9.

26. Truelove SC, Willoughby CP, Lee EG, Kettlewell MG. Further experience in the treatment of severe attacks of ulcerative colitis. *Lancet*1978;2:1086-8.

27. Malchow H, Ewe K, Brandes JW, Goebell H, Ehms H, Sommer H, et al. European Cooperative Crohn's Disease Study (ECCDS): results of drug treatment. *Gastroenterology*1984;86:249-66.

28. Van der Woude CJ, Kolacek S, Dotan I, Oresland T, Vermeire S, Munkholm P, et al. European evidenced-based consensus on reproduction in inflammatory bowel disease. *J Crohns Colitis*2010;4:493-510.

29. Beaugerie L, Sokol H. Clinical, serological and genetic predictors of inflammatory bowel disease course. *World J Gastroenterol*2012;18:3806-13.

30. Travis SPL, Stange EF, Lémann M, Oresland T, Chowers Y, Forbes A, et al. European evidence based consensus on the diagnosis and management of Crohn's disease: current management. *Gut*2006;55(Suppl 1):i16-35.

31. Blonski W, Buchner AM, Lichtenstein GR. Clinical predictors of aggressive/disabling disease: ulcerative colitis and crohn disease. *Gastroenterol Clin North Am*2012;41:443-62.

32. Lichtenstein GR, Feagan BG, Cohen RD, Salzberg BA, Diamond RH, Price S, et al. Serious infection and mortality in patients with Crohn's disease: more than 5 years of follow-up in the TREATTM registry. *Am J Gastroenterol*2012;107:1409-22.

33. Summers RW, Switz DM, Sessions JT, Becktel JM, Best WR, Kern F, et al. National Cooperative Crohn's Disease Study: results of drug treatment. *Gastroenterology*1979;77:847-69.

34. Benchimol EI, Seow CH, Otley AR, Steinhart AH. Budesonide for maintenance of remission in Crohn's disease. *Cochrane Database Syst Rev*2009;1:CD002913.

35. Targan SR, Hanauer SB, van Deventer SJ, Mayer L, Present DH, Braakman T, et al. A short-term study of chimeric monoclonal antibody cA2 to tumor necrosis factor alpha for Crohn's disease. Crohn's Disease cA2 Study Group. *N Engl J Med*1997;337:1029-35.

36. Present DH, Rutgeerts P, Targan S, Hanauer SB, Mayer L, van Hogezand RA, et al. Infliximab for the treatment of fistulas in patients with Crohn's disease. *N Engl J Med*1999;340:1398-405.

37. Schreiber S, Reinisch W, Colombel JF, Sandborn WJ, Hommes DW, Robinson AM, et al. Subgroup analysis of the placebo-controlled CHARM trial: increased remission rates through 3 years for adalimumab-treated patients with early Crohn's disease. *J Crohns Colitis*2013;7:213-21.

38. D'Haens G, Baert F, van Assche G, Caenepeel P, Vergauwe P, Tuynman H, et al. Early combined immunosuppression or conventional management in patients with newly diagnosed Crohn's disease: an open randomised trial. *Lancet*2008;371:660-7.

39. Schreiber S, Colombel J-F, Bloomfield R, Nikolaus S, Schölmerich J, Panés J, et al. Increased response and remission rates in short-duration Crohn's disease with subcutaneous certolizumab pegol: an analysis of PRECiSE 2 randomized maintenance trial data. *Am J Gastroenterol* 2010;105:1574-82.

40. Infliximab (review) and adalimumab for the treatment of Crohn's disease. Guidance and guidelines. NICE. 2014. www.nice.org.uk/guidance/TA187.

41. Zachos M, Tondeur M, Griffiths AM. Enteral nutritional therapy for induction of remission in Crohn's disease. *Cochrane Database Syst Rev*2007;1:CD000542.

42. Sandborn WJ, Hanauer S, Van Assche G, Panés J, Wilson S, Petersson J, et al. Treating beyond symptoms with a view to improving patient outcomes in inflammatory bowel diseases. *J Crohns Colitis*2014;8:927-35.

43. Fraser AG. Methotrexate: first-line or second-line immunomodulator? *Eur J Gastroenterol Hepatol*2003;15:225-31.

44. Pittet V, Froehlich F, Maillard MH, Mottet C, Gonvers J-J, Felley C, et al. When do we dare to stop biological or immunomodulatory therapy for Crohn's disease? Results of a multidisciplinary European expert panel. *J Crohns Colitis*2013;7:820-6.

45. Bressler B, Siegel CA. Beware of the swinging pendulum: anti-tumor necrosis factor monotherapy vs combination therapy for inflammatory bowel disease. *Gastroenterology*2014;146:884-7.

46. Colombel JF, Sandborn WJ, Reinisch W, Mantzaris GJ, Kornbluth A, Rachmilewitz D, et al. Infliximab, azathioprine, or combination therapy for Crohn's disease. *N Engl J Med*2010;362:1383-95.

47. Osterman MT, Sandborn WJ, Colombel J-F, Robinson AM, Lau W, Huang B, et al. Increased risk of malignancy with adalimumab combination therapy, compared with monotherapy, for Crohn's disease. *Gastroenterology*2014;146:941-9.

48. Louis E, Mary J-Y, Vernier-Massouille G, Grimaud J-C, Bouhnik Y, Laharie D, et al. Maintenance of remission among patients with Crohn's disease on antimetabolite therapy after infliximab therapy is stopped. *Gastroenterology*2012;142:63-70.e5; quiz e31.

49. UK IBD Audit Steering Group. National audits of the Organisation of Adult and Paediatric IBD services in the UK. 2012. www.rcplondon.ac.uk/projects/ibdauditround3.

50. Tilney HS, Constantinides VA, Heriot AG, Nicolaou M, Athanasiou T, Ziprin P, et al. Comparison of laparoscopic and open ileocecal resection for Crohn's disease: a metaanalysis. *Surg Endosc*2006;20:1036-44.

51. Kim NK, Senagore AJ, Luchtefeld MA, MacKeigan JM, Mazier WP, Belknap K, et al. Long-term outcome after ileocecal resection for Crohn's disease. *Am Surg*1997;63:627-33.

52. Yamamoto T, Watanabe T. Surgery for luminal Crohn's disease. *World J Gastroenterol*2014;20:78-90.

53. Cattan P, Bonhomme N, Panis Y, Lémann M, Coffin B, Bouhnik Y, et al. Fate of the rectum in patients undergoing total colectomy for Crohn's disease. *Br J Surg*2002;89:454-9.

54. Rahier JF, Ben-Horin S, Chowers Y, Conlon C, De Munter P, D'Haens G, et al. European evidence-based Consensus on the prevention, diagnosis and management of opportunistic infections in inflammatory bowel disease. *J Crohns Colitis*2009;3:47-91.

55. Tavernier N, Fumery M, Peyrin-Biroulet L, Colombel J-F, Gower-Rousseau C. Systematic review: fertility in non-surgically treated inflammatory bowel disease. *Aliment Pharmacol Ther*2013;38:847-53.

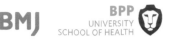

56   Vermeire S, Carbonnel F, Coulie PG, Geenen V, Hazes JMW, Masson PL, et al. Management of inflammatory bowel disease in pregnancy. *J Crohns Colitis*2012;6:811-23.

57   Waljee A, Waljee J, Morris AM, Higgins PDR. Threefold increased risk of infertility: a meta-analysis of infertility after ileal pouch anal anastomosis in ulcerative colitis. *Gut*2006;55:1575-80.

58   Nielsen OH, Andreasson B, Bondesen S, Jacobsen O, Jarnum S. Pregnancy in Crohn's disease. *Scand J Gastroenterol*1984;19:724-32.

59   Mahadevan U, Sandborn WJ, Li D-K, Hakimian S, Kane S, Corley DA. Pregnancy outcomes in women with inflammatory bowel disease: a large community-based study from Northern California. *Gastroenterology*2007;133:1106-12.

60   Khosla R, Willoughby CP, Jewell DP. Crohn's disease and pregnancy. Gut 1984;25:52-6.

61   Katz JA, Pore G. Inflammatory bowel disease and pregnancy. *Inflamm Bowel Dis*2001;7:146-57.

62   Jess T, Loftus E V, Velayos FS, Harmsen WS, Zinsmeister AR, Smyrk TC, et al. Risk of intestinal cancer in inflammatory bowel disease: a population-based study from olmsted county, Minnesota. *Gastroenterology*2006;130:1039-46.

63   Leighton JA, Shen B, Baron TH, Adler DG, Davila R, Egan J V, et al. ASGE guideline: endoscopy in the diagnosis and treatment of inflammatory bowel disease. *Gastrointest Endosc*2006;63:558-65.

64   Peyrin-Biroulet L, Khosrotehrani K, Carrat F, Bouvier A-M, Chevaux J-B, Simon T, et al. Increased risk for nonmelanoma skin cancers in patients who receive thiopurines for inflammatory bowel disease. *Gastroenterology*2011;141:1621-8.e1-5.

65   Beaugerie L, Brousse N, Bouvier AM, Colombel JF, Lémann M, Cosnes J, et al. Lymphoproliferative disorders in patients receiving thiopurines for inflammatory bowel disease: a prospective observational cohort study. *Lancet*2009;374:1617-25.

66   Kotlyar DS, Osterman MT, Diamond RH, Porter D, Blonski WC, Wasik M, et al. A systematic review of factors that contribute to hepatosplenic T-cell lymphoma in patients with inflammatory bowel disease. *Clin Gastroenterol Hepatol*2011;9:36-41.e1.

67   Bongartz T, Sutton AJ, Sweeting MJ, Buchan I, Matteson EL, Montori V. Anti-TNF antibody therapy in rheumatoid arthritis and the risk of serious infections and malignancies: systematic review and meta-analysis of rare harmful effects in randomized controlled trials. *JAMA*2006;295:2275-85.

68   Gong J, Zhu L, Guo Z, Li Y, Zhu W, Li N, et al. Use of thiopurines and risk of colorectal neoplasia in patients with inflammatory bowel diseases: a meta-analysis. *PLoS One*2013;8:e81487.

69   Scott EM, Gaywood I, Scott BB. Guidelines for osteoporosis in coeliac disease and inflammatory bowel disease. British Society of Gastroenterology. *Gut*2000;46 Suppl 1:i1-8.

70   Zhang CK, Hewett J, Hemming J, Grant T, Zhao H, Abraham C, et al. The influence of depression on quality of life in patients with inflammatory bowel disease. *Inflamm Bowel Dis*2013;19:1732-9.

71   Lix LM, Graff LA, Walker JR, Clara I, Rawsthorne P, Rogala L, et al. Longitudinal study of quality of life and psychological functioning for active, fluctuating, and inactive disease patterns in inflammatory bowel disease. *Inflamm Bowel Dis*2008;14:1575-84.

72   Persoons P, Vermeire S, Demyttenaere K, Fischler B, Vandenberghe J, Van Oudenhove L, et al. The impact of major depressive disorder on the short- and long-term outcome of Crohn's disease treatment with infliximab. *Aliment Pharmacol Ther*2005;22:101-10.

73   Walker JR, Ediger JP, Graff LA, Greenfeld JM, Clara I, Lix L, et al. The Manitoba IBD cohort study: a population-based study of the prevalence of lifetime and 12-month anxiety and mood disorders. *Am J Gastroenterol*2008;103:1989-97.

74   Kemp K, Griffiths J, Lovell K. Understanding the health and social care needs of people living with IBD: a meta-synthesis of the evidence. *World J Gastroenterol*2012;18:6240-9.

Related links

thebmj.com
- Earn CPE/CME credits

bmj.com/archive
Previous articles in this series
- Meniere's disease (BMJ 2014;349: g6544)
- Carpal Tunnel Syndrome (BMJ 2014;349:g6437)
- Management of arteriovenous fistulas (BMJ 2014;349:g6262)
- The diagnosis and management of hiatus hernia (BMJ 2014;349:g6154)
- The management of teenage pregnancy (BMJ 2014;349:g5887)

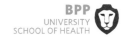

Ulcerative colitis

Alexander C Ford, senior lecturer and honorary consultant gastroenterologist[12],
Paul Moayyedi, director of division of gastroenterology[3],
Steven B Hanauer, Joseph B Kirsner professor of medicine and clinical pharmacology and chief of gastroenterology, hepatology, and nutrition[4]

[1]Leeds Gastroenterology Institute, St James's University Hospital, Leeds LS9 7TF, UK

[2]Leeds Institute of Molecular Medicine, Leeds University, Leeds, UK

[3]McMaster University Medical Centre, Hamilton, ON, Canada

[4]University of Chicago, 5481 S Maryland Ave, Chicago, IL, USA

Correspondence to: A C Ford
alexf12399@yahoo.com

Cite this as: BMJ 2013;346:f432

DOI: 10.1136/bmj.f432

http://www.bmj.com/content/346/bmj.f432

Ulcerative colitis is an inflammatory disorder of the gastrointestinal tract that affects the colorectum. It often presents in young adulthood and is more common in developed nations. The diagnosis is reached after lower gastrointestinal investigation confirms diffuse, continuous, and superficial inflammation in the large bowel and biopsies show changes in keeping with the disorder. There is no single known unifying cause, and the pathogenesis probably relates to a change in colonic environment in a genetically susceptible person. It is a chronic lifelong condition that, untreated, has a relapsing and remitting course. Medical treatment aims to induce remission and prevent relapse of disease activity once this has been achieved, thereby minimising the impact on quality of life and preventing long term sequelae. We summarise recent guidelines, systematic reviews, meta-analyses, and randomised controlled trials (RCTs) to provide the general reader with an update on how this disorder can be effectively identified and managed.

What is ulcerative colitis and who gets it?

Ulcerative colitis is an idiopathic inflammatory bowel disease (IBD), which affects the colon in a diffuse, continuous, and superficial pattern. Inflammation, which can be detected at lower gastrointestinal endoscopy, extends from the anorectal verge to a variable proximal extent. The epidemiology of ulcerative colitis varies considerably worldwide. The highest incidence and prevalence rates are in the developed world, but incidence is increasing in developing countries. It has been proposed that this is the result of improved hygiene and sanitation, which have led to reduced exposure to enteric infections and immaturity of the immune system.

In a recent systematic review of population based studies, incidence varied from 0.6 to more than 20 people per 100 000 person years in Europe and North America, compared with 0.1 to 6.3 per 100 000 person years in Asia and the Middle East.[1] Overall, incidence appeared to be on the rise worldwide. Peak incidence occurred in the second to fourth decade of life, although a modest rise was also seen in later life. Prevalence was estimated at 5-500 people per 100 000 worldwide. No consistent difference was seen between the sexes. Smoking protects against developing ulcerative colitis. Risk is eight times higher in first degree

SOURCES AND SELECTION CRITERIA

We searched Medline, Embase, the Cochrane Database of Systematic Reviews, and Clinical Evidence online using the term "ulcerative colitis". We limited studies to those conducted in adults and focused on systematic reviews, meta-analyses, and high quality randomised controlled trials published within the past five years.

relatives of people with the disorder compared with first degree relatives of healthy controls,[2] although this is not completely explained by known genetic risk factors.

What are the clinical features and associated conditions?

Because the rectum is inevitably affected, the presenting symptoms are usually rectal bleeding, urgency, and tenesmus, with diarrhoea depending on the proximal extent and severity of inflammation. The current Montreal classification system for ulcerative colitis is based on the severity of symptoms and the extent of inflammation of the colorectum (table).[3] However, the extent of disease may change in 50% of patients during follow-up.[4]

About 30% of patients exhibit immune mediated inflammatory disorders of other organs.[5] The liver is affected in 5% of patients (primary sclerosing cholangitis and autoimmune liver disease), joints in 20% (seronegative arthritis of the large joints, sacroiliitis, and ankylosing spondylitis), eye in around 5% (scleritis, episcleritis, and anterior uveitis), and skin in 5% (erythema nodosum and pyoderma gangrenosum).

What is the underlying pathophysiology of ulcerative colitis?

The exact pathophysiology is unknown, but the condition is probably caused by an inappropriate immune response to an unknown environmental stimulus within the colon.[6] Genome-wide association studies have shown that defects in genes integral to the preservation of the colonic epithelial barrier are implicated in the pathogenesis.[7] Mucin depletion and dysregulated tight junctions are thought to contribute to a disrupted epithelial architecture, which allows normal commensal bacteria to be sampled by dendritic cells. These then act as antigen presenting cells and induce inappropriate activation of the host immune system, leading to an aberrant T cell driven inflammatory response. It is unclear what triggers this inflammatory cascade, although imbalances in intestinal flora have been implicated.

How is ulcerative colitis diagnosed?

The condition is usually diagnosed when a patient with typical symptoms undergoes endoscopic examination of the lower gastrointestinal tract, after infectious causes of the symptoms have been excluded by stool examination. The diagnosis is secured if inflammation of the colorectum is confirmed and colorectal epithelial biopsies show chronic changes, including crypt distortion, along with acute

SUMMARY POINTS

- Ulcerative colitis affects one in 200 people in developed nations
- The condition commonly presents in young adults
- Most people with ulcerative colitis will have a normal life expectancy
- 5-aminosalicylates and thiopurines are effective at preventing relapse of disease activity
- Patients are at increased risk of colorectal cancer and should undergo regular surveillance colonoscopy
- Bone densitometry is recommended in patients who need repeated courses of glucocorticosteroids and those at high risk of osteoporosis
- Most drugs used to treat ulcerative colitis are safe during pregnancy

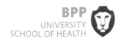

inflammatory changes of cryptitis, crypt abscesses, and a plasma-lymphocytoid cell infiltrate in the lamina propria. However, an exact diagnosis at initial presentation may prove elusive, and more than 40% of those thought to have IBD unclassified (indeterminate colitis) may later be found to have ulcerative colitis.[8] Conversely, a small proportion (probably <5%) of patients initially thought to have ulcerative colitis may later be reclassified as having Crohn's disease.[8] Correct diagnosis at presentation is important because disease course, complications, and treatments differ.

What is the prognosis?

Recent data suggest that less than 10% of patients will need colectomy within the first 10 years of diagnosis[9]; more extensive disease, raised inflammatory markers, and age less than 50 years at diagnosis are associated with colectomy. Modifiable risk factors associated with relapse of disease activity are uncertain but may include diet, cessation of smoking, stressful life events, and poor adherence to drugs. The disease may be associated with a modest increase in mortality in the community, although this effect seems to be attenuating in more contemporary cohorts of patients,[10] perhaps because of earlier diagnosis and improved treatment.

What are the treatment options?

Ulcerative colitis is a chronic lifelong disorder. One in five patients will require sickness related absence from work or school, which impacts adversely on quality of life.[11] About 50% of affected people are in remission at any one time, but 90% will experience a relapsing and remitting course.[12] As a result, no one treatment modality will entirely control symptoms throughout a lifetime of disease (box). It may therefore be useful to categorise treatments according to severity of disease activity (table) and tailor therapy accordingly. Although cessation of symptoms has traditionally been the aim of treatment, in the past 10 years endoscopic mucosal healing has increasingly been used as an endpoint in RCTs because of accumulating evidence that it is associated with a lower likelihood of disease relapse or colectomy.[13]

Induction of remission in mildly to moderately active disease

Mild to moderate flares of disease activity (table) are often treated with oral or topical 5-aminosalicylates or oral glucocorticosteroids. These drugs inhibit production of cytokines and other inflammatory mediators, although the exact mechanisms underlying their beneficial effects in ulcerative colitis are unknown. Glucocorticosteroids usually act within days, whereas 5-aminosalicylates may take up to four weeks to have any benefit. If there is no response to 5-aminosalicylates within two weeks, consider switching to oral glucocorticosteroids.

Glucocorticosteroids

A recent meta-analysis on the efficacy of glucocorticosteroids in active disease identified five RCTs comparing the efficacy of glucocorticosteroids with placebo.[14] Remission rates with active treatment in individual trials varied from 13% to 80%. The likelihood of not achieving remission was significantly lower with glucocorticosteroids (relative risk 0.65, 95% confidence interval 0.45 to 0.93), with a number needed to treat (NNT) of 3. Potential side effects of glucocorticosteroids include infections, weight gain, hyperglycaemia, acne,

hirsutism, and hypertension, although these were no more common in patients assigned to active treatment in trials that reported these data. Bone loss occurs within the first six months of treatment and warrants supplementation with calcium and vitamin D.

Oral 5-aminosalicylates

Two systematic reviews and meta-analyses of RCTs show that 5-aminosalicylates can induce remission in mildly to moderately active disease. A recently updated Cochrane review reported that these drugs were more effective than placebo for inducing clinical remission in eight trials (relative risk of not achieving remission 0.86, 0.81 to 0.91).[15] A second meta-analysis of data from 11 RCTs found a similar relative risk, with remission rates with active treatment varying from 11% to 70%. The NNT to prevent one patient not achieving remission was 6.[16] Overall, the best evidence was for the use of mesalazine, which was studied in seven trials. It is unclear which preparations of oral mesalazine are most effective because of a paucity of trials comparing equivalent doses of the available preparations.

The most common side effects of 5-aminosalicylates are headache, abdominal pain, nausea, vomiting, skin rash, and diarrhoea. However, overall, 5-aminosalicylates were safe and well tolerated, with no significant difference in adverse events compared with placebo. The second meta-analysis also studied the effect of total dose used on rates of remission.[16] Overall, failure to achieve remission was significantly reduced with total daily doses of 2 g or more mesalazine, compared with doses under 2 g, with an NNT of 11, and no significant difference in adverse events.

Topical 5-aminosalicylates

Topical 5-aminosalicylates are prescribed in the form of suppositories or retention suspensions (enemas). This route of administration is useful for patients whose disease is confined to the rectum or distal colon. A Cochrane review studied their efficacy in inducing remission of mildly to moderately active ulcerative colitis.[17] The authors concluded that topical 5-aminosalicylates were more effective than placebo. They were superior for clinical, endoscopic, and histological remission, and safety and tolerability were excellent. The pooled odds ratio for remission was 8.3 (4.3 to 16.1); remission rates with active treatment in individual trials varied from 40% to 80%.

A more recent meta-analysis compared the efficacy of topical and oral 5-aminosalicylates for induction of remission in mildly to moderately active disease.[18] No significant difference in remission rates was detected (relative risk 0.82, 0.52 to 1.28). Despite these findings, and the fact that European guidelines recommend topical treatment as first line in patients with mildly to moderately active ulcerative proctitis,[19] patient preference and its impact on adherence to treatment dictate how 5-aminosalicylates are administered. There is limited evidence to suggest that patients prefer oral 5-aminosalicylates,[20] although more studies are needed.

Combined oral and topical 5-aminosalicylates

Some patients with difficult to control disease may benefit from combined oral and topical 5-aminosalicylates. National and international guidelines recommend such an approach for mild to moderate flares of disease activity in left sided colitis.[19][21][22] A meta-analysis published in 2012 identified four RCTs comparing combined treatment with oral 5-aminosalicylates alone in active disease.[18] Combined

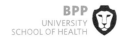

treatment seemed to be better, with a relative risk of not achieving remission of 0.65 (0.47 to 0.91) and an NNT of 5. However, no trials have looked at adherence to combination treatment, particularly in the long term.

Induction of remission in severely active disease

Severe exacerbations (table), characterised by the passage of at least six bloody stools a day (often with nocturnal symptoms), with systemic signs, anaemia, or raised inflammatory markers usually require admission to hospital for intravenous glucocorticosteroids. If these drugs do not work, infliximab or ciclosporin are used as rescue therapy, in an attempt to avoid surgery. In this setting, response to intravenous glucocorticosteroids should be judged at three to five days, and a decision made on whether rescue therapy is needed. Success of treatment with ciclosporin or infliximab should be judged within five to seven days of treatment.

Glucocorticosteroids

The only study in the meta-analysis to recruit patients with a severe flare of activity showed a significant benefit of glucocorticosteroids.[14] Despite considerable evidence from routine clinical practice that intravenous glucocorticosteroids are effective in acute severe ulcerative colitis, evidence from RCTs to support this is sparse.

Anti-tumour necrosis factor α biological agents

Infliximab and adalimumab are monoclonal antibodies that are directed against tumour necrosis factor α (TNF-α). Five placebo controlled trials have studied the efficacy of infliximab in moderately to severely active ulcerative colitis[23] [24] [25] [26]; three recruited inpatients[23] [24] [26] and two recruited ambulatory outpatients.[24] Trials conducted in inpatients found no significant improvement in outcomes with infliximab,[23] [24] [26] whereas both trials of outpatients found a benefit.[w11] A meta-analysis of all five RCTs found a significant effect of infliximab over placebo in moderately to severely active disease,[27] with a relative risk of remission not being achieved of 0.72 (0.57 to 0.91) and an NNT of 4. Remission rates with active treatment in individual trials varied from 25% to 60%. In the United Kingdom, the use of infliximab is restricted to three dose induction therapy for acute severe exacerbations.[28] More recent RCTs, that enrolled similarly refractory outpatient populations, have shown that adalimumab is significantly superior to placebo,[29] [30] although absolute differences in remission rates were modest (7-9%). The meta-analysis of RCTs of infliximab found no significant difference in adverse event rates.[27] Common side effects of anti-TNF-α agents include infusion or injection site reactions, headache, nausea, vomiting, arthralgia, and myalgia. More serious adverse events are rare but include increased risk of certain infections,[31] such as reactivation of latent tuberculosis, and increased risk of lymphoma, particularly if combined with other immunosuppressants.[32]

Ciclosporin

Ciclosporin is a fungally derived calcineurin inhibitor that reduces T cell activation. In a small but pivotal trial, which recruited 20 patients with severely active glucocorticosteroid refractory disease,[33] none of the nine patients randomised to placebo showed a clinical response at seven days, compared with nine of 11 given ciclosporin. The results of this study led to the widespread use of ciclosporin in this setting. More recently, an open label RCT that compared infliximab and ciclosporin head to head for the treatment of acute severe glucocorticosteroid refractory ulcerative colitis found that both treatments were similarly effective, with no response to treatment occurring in 54% and 60% respectively.[34]

Preventing relapse of quiescent disease

Once remission has been achieved, oral or topical 5-aminosalicylates form the mainstay of medical treatment. Patients who experience repeated flares of disease activity, despite optimising this treatment, may need an immunosuppressant drug, such as a thiopurine. Because of their side effects, glucocorticosteroids should not be used long term to maintain remission.

Oral 5-aminosalicylates

A recently updated Cochrane review and another meta-analysis examined maintenance treatment with 5-aminosalicylates.[16] [35] The Cochrane review identified seven placebo controlled trials and reported that the risk of relapse was significantly lower with 5-aminosalicylates (relative risk 0.69, 0.62 to 0.77).[35] The second meta-analysis identified 11 RCTs, and reported a similar effect in favour of 5-aminosalicylates after six to 12 months of treatment, with an NNT to prevent one relapse of only 4, and relapse rates with active treatment in individual trials of 0% to 63%.[16] Adverse events were no higher with 5-aminosalicylates. This meta-analysis also examined the effect of total daily dose of 5-aminosalicylate on likelihood of relapse. Doses of 2 g/day or more were more effective than doses of less than 2 g/day (NNT 10), with no increase in adverse events.[16]

Despite oral 5-aminosalicylates being highly efficacious in preventing disease relapse, evidence suggests that less than 50% of patients adhere to treatment.[36] This may be due to the inconvenience of divided dosing schedules,[37] which stem from a desire to minimise the side effects of sulfasalazine. Non-sulfa containing mesalazine formulations are better tolerated, so adherence may be improved if once daily, rather than two or three times daily, dosing schedules are used. A meta-analysis identified seven RCTs (>2700 patients) that compared once daily schedules with conventional ones.[38] It found that relapse rates were no higher with once daily dosing (relative risk of relapse 0.94, 0.82 to 1.08) and adverse events were no more common. However, adherence rates were not significantly different (relative risk of non-adherence 0.87, 0.46 to 1.66).

Topical 5-aminosalicylates

In terms of preventing relapse of disease activity, a recent meta-analysis identified seven trials of topical 5-aminosalicylates (555 patients).[39] All trials compared topical mesalazine with placebo, and in three treatment was intermittent (two or three times a week). The duration of treatment ranged from six to 24 months, and the relative risk of relapse was 0.60 (0.49 to 0.73), with relapse rates with active treatment in individual trials varying from 20% to 55%. The NNT to prevent one patient relapsing was 3, and no significant difference in adverse events was detected.

Thiopurines

Azathioprine, and its metabolite mercaptopurine, are the most commonly used immunosuppressants in ulcerative colitis. They are usually used in an attempt to maintain glucocorticosteroid induced remission, where 5-aminosalicylates have failed. Despite their widespread

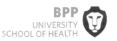
Montreal classification of extent and severity of ulcerative colitis[3]			
Extent	**Anatomy**	**Severity**	**Definition**
E1: Ulcerative proctitis	Limited to the rectum	S0: Clinical remission	Asymptomatic
E2: Left sided (distal) ulcerative colitis	Limited to a proportion of the colorectum distal to the splenic flexure	S1: Mild	≤4 stools/day (with or without blood), absence of systemic illness, and normal inflammatory markers
E3: Extensive (pancolitis) ulcerative colitis	Extends proximally to the splenic flexure	S2: Moderate	>4 stools/day but minimal signs of systemic toxicity
		S3: Severe	≥6 bloody stools/day, pulse ≥90 beats/min, temperature ≥37.5°C, haemoglobin <105 g/L, and erythrocyte sedimentation rate ≥30 mm in the first hour

use, the evidence base to support their efficacy is not strong. A recent systematic review and meta-analysis identified only three RCTs of 127 patients.[40] When data were pooled, the relative risk of relapse was significantly reduced with azathioprine compared with placebo (0.60, 0.37 to 0.95), and the NNT to prevent one relapse was 4. Relapse rates with active treatment in individual trials varied from 45% to 80%. Adverse event rates were incompletely reported by all trials. However, potentially serious adverse events include myelosuppression and associated opportunistic infections, acute and chronic effects on liver function, and hypersensitivity reactions, including pancreatitis. Long term use may be associated with an increased risk of lymphoproliferative disorders and non-melanoma skin cancer.

Treatment of refractory disease

Patients who have frequent relapses despite optimal conventional medical treatments have few options other than surgery. However, some investigators have reported success with other immunosuppressant drugs such as tacrolimus, a macrolide derived from soil bacteria. Other emerging treatments include golimumab, another anti-TNF-α agent; vedolizumab, a monoclonal antibody directed against integrin $\alpha_4\beta_7$; and phosphatidylcholine, a class of phospholipid thought to be deficient in the colonic mucus in ulcerative colitis.

When should surgery be considered?

Colectomy is an option for patients who do not respond to, or are intolerant of, medical treatment, or in those with complications such as colorectal neoplasia. Because ulcerative colitis is confined to the colorectum, colectomy is curative, and the usual approach is a restorative proctocolectomy with ileal pouch-anal anastomosis. A systematic review of 33 case series suggested that the quality of life of patients 12 months after the procedure was similar to that seen in the general population.[41]

The main complication related to this procedure is pouchitis, which can occur in 30% of cases, and presents with increased stool frequency, urgency, incontinence, and nocturnal seepage. This can be treated medically, most often using antibiotics, including metronidazole and ciprofloxacin, or probiotics, such as VSL#3, but it can become chronic in

5% of cases, which leads to pouch failure.[42] In this situation the only option is pouch excision with a permanent ileostomy. Other concerns with surgery are reduced fertility in women, with a systematic review suggesting a 3.9 (2.1 to 7.4) relative risk of infertility after pouch surgery,[43] and pre-operative misdiagnosis of Crohn's disease as ulcerative colitis, which can lead to Crohn's of the pouch and loss of the pouch in some patients.

Overall management of ulcerative colitis

There are a wealth of RCT data on individual treatments for inducing and maintaining remission in ulcerative colitis, but a paucity of data on overall disease management.[44] Patients who remain well for long periods on 5-aminosalicylates may be referred back to the community and told to continue maintenance treatment but to contact a specialist if they develop a flare of disease activity.[45] Those with frequent relapses (more than once a year) can benefit from specialist supervision and potential escalation to immunosuppressive or biological therapy.[21 22] Aggressive medical management of those with frequent relapses may explain why the rate of surgery in ulcerative colitis patients is falling.[46]

Monitoring of drug therapy in ulcerative colitis

Interstitial nephritis is a serious complication of 5-aminosalicylate treatment that is estimated to occur in less than one in 500 people treated. Patients should therefore have their renal function monitored three months after starting the drug, and yearly thereafter (BNF). Vaccinate patients against preventable communicable diseases, including varicella zoster, hepatitis B, influenza, pneumococcus, and human papillomavirus, before starting immunosuppressants (glucocorticosteroids, thiopurines, biologicals, or ciclosporin). Exclude exposure to tuberculosis using skin tests or interferon based assays.

Patients receiving glucocorticosteroids require monitoring of blood pressure, blood glucose, and bone mineral density. Thiopurines can cause bone marrow suppression. Before starting these drugs, check the patient's thiopurine methyltransferase (TPMT) activity. This enzyme metabolises mercaptopurine to its active metabolite thioguanine. Patients with low TPMT activity have an increased risk of myelosuppression, and thiopurines should be avoided, or used with extreme caution. Even in patients with normal TPMT activity, thiopurines need to be monitored closely. Monitor patients' full blood count weekly for the first month of treatment, then monthly for the next six months or so, and three monthly thereafter. Observe patients on immunosuppressive treatments for evidence of opportunistic infection, and routinely check those on long term treatment for non-melanoma skin cancers.

DISCUSSING ULCERATIVE COLITIS AND ITS TREATMENT WITH PATIENTS

- Explain that ulcerative colitis is a lifelong disorder but that the symptoms come and go
- Explain that the cause is incompletely understood
- Explain that 5-aminosalicylates are effective for inducing remission of mild to moderate exacerbations and for preventing relapse of disease activity
- Stress to pregnant women that 5-aminosalicylates and thiopurines are not detrimental to the fetus and that the priority is to maintain remission

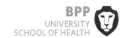
Colorectal cancer screening in ulcerative colitis

A meta-analysis of population based studies found that patients with ulcerative colitis have about double the incidence of colorectal cancer than people without the disorder.[47] However, recent population based data suggest that the overall risk of colorectal cancer may be comparable to the general population, although patients with disease diagnosed in childhood and adolescence, a longer disease duration, or coexistent primary sclerosing cholangitis seem to be at higher risk.[48] In the UK, colonoscopic surveillance is recommended for all patients, starting about 10 years after the onset of symptoms, except for those with ulcerative proctitis that is documented on two consecutive endoscopic examinations, who do not require surveillance.[49] The surveillance interval depends on the extent of disease (figure).

Osteoporosis in ulcerative colitis

Doctors should aim to minimise the use of glucocorticosteroids by optimising 5-aminosalicylate treatment and introducing thiopurines early in the disease course if 5-aminosalicylates do not control disease activity. In the UK, guidelines recommend bisphosphonate prophylaxis in patients over 65 years who need glucocorticosteroids.[50] In patients under 65 years who need more than three months of glucocorticosteroids, bone densitometry measurement is recommended, and a bisphosphonate started if the T score is 1.5 or less.

Pregnancy and breast feeding

Patients with ulcerative colitis are often young and the disease has serious implications for pregnancy. Patients with active disease at the time of conception may have an increased risk of spontaneous abortion. Rates of preterm delivery, low birth weight, and congenital anomalies, such as limb deficiencies and urinary obstruction, may be increased.[51] One in five pregnancies in patients with ulcerative colitis ends with caesarean section.[52] Relapse of disease activity during pregnancy may increase rates of low birth weight and preterm birth.[53]

A recent meta-analysis of seven studies (2200 pregnant women) found no significant association between 5-aminosalicylate use and rates of spontaneous abortion, preterm delivery, low birth weight, congenital abnormalities, or stillbirth.[54] Thiopurines pose a hypothetical risk to the fetus. A study that recruited more than 470 women who

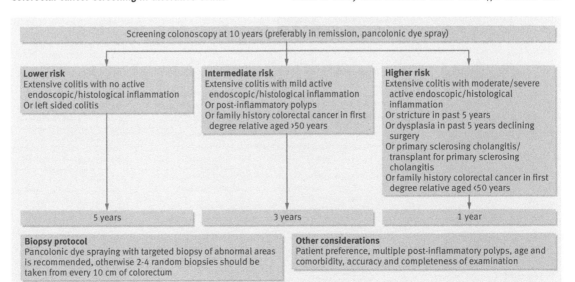

Surveillance recommendations from the British Society of Gastroenterology for detection of colorectal cancer in ulcerative colitis[49]

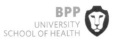

used azathioprine early in pregnancy, most of whom had IBD, found a higher rate of congenital malformations in these women compared with women with IBD not taking azathioprine (odds ratio 1.42, 0.93 to 2.18), although the increase was not significant.[55] Despite these theoretical risks, most experts recommend continuing these drugs throughout pregnancy because of the risks posed to the mother and fetus from an exacerbation of ulcerative colitis. Biologicals cross the placenta in the third trimester of pregnancy and should therefore be discontinued at this stage.

5-aminosalicylates are considered safe to take when breast feeding. Although small amounts of thiopurine may be secreted in breast milk,[56] long term follow-up of a small number of children exposed to the drug during breast feeding found no impairments in mental or physical development.[57] Secretion of biologicals in breast milk is limited, and these drugs are probably safe in this setting.

Contributors: ACF, PM, and SBH conceived and designed the article. ACF drafted the manuscript. All authors approved the final version of the manuscript. ACF is guarantor.

Competing interests: All authors have completed the Unified Competing Interest form at www.icmje.org/coi_disclosure.pdf (available on request from the corresponding author) and declare: no support from any organisation for the submitted work; ACF has received speaker's fees from Shire Pharmaceuticals and MSD; PM has received speaker's fees from Shire Pharmaceuticals; SBH has consulted for Shire, Ferring, Abbott, Warner-Chilcott, and Janssen and has received speaker's fees from Ferring, Abbott, Warner-Chilcott, and Janssen.

Provenance and peer review: Commissioned; externally peer reviewed.

1   Molodecky NA, Soon IS, Rabi DM, Ghali WA, Ferris M, Chernoff G, et al. Increasing incidence and prevalence of the inflammatory bowel diseases with time, based on systematic review. Gastroenterology2012;142:46-54.

2   Orholm M, Munkholm P, Langholz E, Nielsen OH, Sorensen TI, Binder V. Familial occurrence of inflammatory bowel disease. N Engl J Med1991;324:84-8.

3   Silverberg MS, Satsangi J, Ahmad T, Arnott ID, Bernstein CN, Brant SR, et al. Toward an integrated clinical, molecular and serological classification of inflammatory bowel disease: report of a working party of the 2005 Montreal World Congress of Gastroenterology. Can J Gastroenterol2005;19(suppl A):5-36.

4   Langholz E, Munkholm P, Davidsen M, Nielsen OH, Binder V. Changes in extent of ulcerative colitis: a study on the course and prognostic factors. Scand J Gastroenterol1996;31:260-6.

5   Vavricka SR, Brun L, Ballabeni P, Pittet V, Prinz Vavricka BM, Zeitz J, et al. Frequency and risk factors for extraintestinal manifestations in the Swiss inflammatory bowel disease cohort. Am J Gastroenterol2011;106:110-9.

6   Danese S, Fiocchi C. Ulcerative colitis. N Engl J Med2011;365:1713-25.

7   Anderson CA, Boucher G, Lees CW, Franke A, D'Amato M, Taylor KD, et al. Meta-analysis identifies 29 additional ulcerative colitis risk loci, increasing the number of confirmed associations to 47. Nat Genet2011;43:246-52.

8   Henriksen M, Jahnsen J, Lygren I, Sauar J, Schulz T, Stray N, et al. Change of diagnosis during the first five years after onset of inflammatory bowel disease: results of a prospective follow-up study (the IBSEN Study). Scand J Gastroenterol2006;41:1037-43.

9   Solberg IC, Lygren I, Jahnsen J, Aadland E, Hoie O, Cvancarova M, et al. Clinical course during the first 10 years of ulcerative colitis: results from a population-based inception cohort (IBSEN Study). Scand J Gastroenterol2009;44:431-40.

10 Jess T, Frisch M, Simonsen J. Trends in overall and cause-specific mortality among patients with inflammatory bowel disease from 1982-2010. Clin Gastroenterol Hepatol2013;11:43-8.

11 Bernklev T, Jahnsen J, Henriksen M, Lygren I, Aadland E, Sauar J, et al. Relationship between sick leave, unemployment, disability, and health-related quality of life in patients with inflammatory bowel disease. Inflamm Bowel Dis2006;12:402-12.

12 Langholz E, Munkholm P, Davidsen M, Binder V. Course of ulcerative colitis: analysis of changes in disease activity over years. Gastroenterology1994;107:3-11.

13 Neurath MF, Travis SP. Mucosal healing in inflammatory bowel diseases: a systematic review. Gut2012;61:1619-35.

14 Ford AC, Bernstein CN, Khan KJ, Abreu MT, Marshall JK, Talley NJ, et al. Glucocorticosteroid therapy in inflammatory bowel disease: systematic review and meta-analysis. Am J Gastroenterol2011;106:590-9.

15 Feagan BG, MacDonald JK. Oral 5-aminosalicylic acid for induction of remission in ulcerative colitis. Cochrane Database Syst Rev2012;10:CD000543.

16 Ford AC, Achkar J-P, Khan KJ, Kane SV, Talley NJ, Marshall JK, et al. Efficacy of 5-aminosalicylates in ulcerative colitis: systematic review and meta-analysis. Am J Gastroenterol2011;106:601-16.

17 Marshall JK, Thabane M, Steinhart AH, Newman JR, Anand A, Irvine EJ. Rectal 5-aminosalicylic acid for induction of remission in ulcerative colitis. Cochrane Database Syst Rev2010;1:CD004115.

18 Ford AC, Khan KJ, Achkar J-P, Moayyedi P. Efficacy of oral versus topical, or combined oral and topical 5-aminosalicylates, in ulcerative colitis: systematic review and meta-analysis. Am J Gastroenterol2012;107:167-76.

19 Travis SPL, Stange EF, Lemann M, Oresland T, Bemelman WA, Chowers Y, et al. European evidence-based consensus on the management of ulcerative colitis: current management. J Crohns Colitis2008;2:24-62.

20 Moody GA, Eaden JA, Helyes Z, Mayberry JF. Oral or rectal administration of drugs in IBD? Aliment Pharmacol Ther1997;11:999-1000.

21 Mowat C, Cole A, Windsor A, Ahmad T, Arnott I, Driscoll R, et al. Guidelines for the management of inflammatory bowel disease in adults. Gut2011;60:571-607.

22 Kornbluth A, Sachar DB; and the Practice Parameters Committee of the American College of Gastroenterology. Ulcerative colitis practice guidelines in adults: American College of Gastroenterology, Practice Parameters Committee. Am J Gastroenterol2010;105:501-23.

23 Jarnerot G, Hertervig E, Friis-Liby I, Blomquist L, Karlen P, Granno C, et al. Infliximab as rescue therapy in severe to moderately severe ulcerative colitis: a randomized, placebo-controlled study. Gastroenterology2005;128:1805-11.

24 Probert CJ, Hearing SD, Schreiber S, Kuhbacher T, Ghosh S, Arnott IDR, et al. Infliximab in moderately severe glucocorticoid resistant ulcerative colitis: a randomised controlled trial. Gut2003;52:998-1002.

25 Rutgeerts P, Sandborn WJ, Feagan BG, Reinisch W, Olson A, Johanns J, et al. Infliximab for induction and maintenance therapy for ulcerative colitis. N Engl J Med2005;353:2462-76.

26 Sands BE, Tremaine WJ, Sandborn WJ, Rutgeerts PJ, Hanauer SB, Mayer L, et al. Infliximab in the treatment of severe, steroid-refractory ulcerative colitis: a pilot study. Inflamm Bowel Dis2001;7:83-8.

27 Ford AC, Sandborn WJ, Khan KJ, Hanauer SB, Talley NJ, Moayyedi P. Efficacy of biological therapies in inflammatory bowel disease: systematic review and meta-analysis. Am J Gastroenterol2011;106:644-59.

28 National Institute for Health and Clinical Excellence. Infliximab for acute exacerbations of ulcerative colitis. 2008. www.nice.org.uk/ta163.

29 Sandborn WJ, van Assche G, Reinisch W, Colombel J-F, D'Haens G, Wolf DC, et al. Adalimumab induces and maintains clinical remission in patients with moderate-to-severe ulcerative colitis. Gastroenterology2012;142:257-65.

30 Reinisch W, Sandborn WJ, Hommes DW, D'Haens G, Hanauer S, Schreiber S, et al. Adalimumab for induction of clinical remission in moderately to severely active ulcerative colitis: results of a randomised controlled trial. Gut2011;60:780-7.

31 Lichtenstein GR, Feagan BG, Cohen RD, Salzberg BA, Diamond RH, Price S, et al. Serious infection and mortality in patients with Crohn's disease: more than 5 years of follow-up in the TREAT registry. Am J Gastroenterol2012;107:1409-22.

32 Deepak P, Sifuentes H, Sherid M, Stobaugh D, Sadozai Y, Ehrenpreis ED. T-cell non-Hodgkin's lymphomas reported to the FDA AERS with tumor necrosis factor-alpha (TNF-a) inhibitors: results of the REFURBISH study. Am J Gastroenterol2013;108:99-105.

33 Lichtiger S, Present DH, Kornbluth A, Gelernt I, Bauer J, Galler G, et al. Cyclosporine in severe ulcerative colitis refractory to steroid therapy. N Engl J Med1994;330:1841-5.

34 Laharie D, Bourreille A, Branche J, Allez M, Bouhnik Y, Filippi J, et al. Ciclosporin versus infliximab in patients with severe ulcerative colitis refractory to intravenous steroids: a parallel, open-label randomised controlled trial. Lancet2012;380:1909-15.

35 Feagan BG, MacDonald JK. Oral 5-aminosalicylic acid for maintenance of remission in ulcerative colitis. Cochrane Database Syst Rev2012;10:CD000544.

36 Kane SV, Cohen RD, Aikens JE, Hanauer SB. Prevalence of nonadherence with maintenance mesalamine in quiescent ulcerative colitis. Am J Gastroenterol2001;96:2929-33.

37 Kane SV. Systematic review: adherence issues in the treatment of ulcerative colitis. Aliment Pharmacol Ther2006;23:577-85.

38 Ford AC, Khan KJ, Sandborn WJ, Kane SV, Moayyedi P. Once-daily dosing vs. conventional dosing schedule of mesalamine and relapse of quiescent ulcerative colitis: systematic review and meta-analysis. Am J Gastroenterol2011;106:2070-7.

39 Ford AC, Khan KJ, Sandborn WJ, Hanauer SB, Moayyedi P. Efficacy of topical 5-aminosalicylates in preventing relapse of quiescent ulcerative colitis: a meta-analysis. Clin Gastroenterol Hepatol2012;10:513-9.

40 Khan KJ, Dubinsky MC, Ford AC, Ullman TA, Talley NJ, Moayyedi P. Efficacy of immunosuppressive therapy for inflammatory bowel disease: systematic review and meta-analysis. Am J Gastroenterol2011;106:630-42.

41 Heikens JT, de Vries J, van Laarhoven CJ. Quality of life, health-related quality of life and health status in patients having restorative proctocolectomy with ileal pouch-anal anastomosis for ulcerative colitis: a systematic review. Colorectal Dis2012;14:536-44.

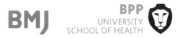

42 Holubar SD, Cima RR, Sandborn WJ, Pardi DS. Treatment and prevention of pouchitis after ileal pouch-anal anastomosis for chronic ulcerative colitis. *Cochrane Database Syst Rev*2010;6:CD001176.

43 Rajaratnam SG, Eglington TW, Hider P, Fearnhead NS. Impact of ileal pouch-anal anastomosis on female fertility: meta-analysis and systematic review. *Int J Colorectal Dis*2011;26:1365-74.

44 Talley NJ, Abreu MT, Achkar J-P, Bernstein CN, Dubinsky MC, Hanauer SB, et al. An evidence-based systematic review on medical therapies for inflammatory bowel disease. *Am J Gastroenterol*2011;106(suppl 1s):S2-25.

45 Kennedy AP, Nelson E, Reeves D, Richardson G, Roberts C, Robinson A, et al. A randomised controlled trial to assess the effectiveness and cost of a patient orientated self management approach to chronic inflammatory bowel disease. *Gut*2004;53:1639-45.

46 Targownik LE, Singh H, Nugent Z, Bernstein CN. The epidemiology of colectomy in ulcerative colitis: results from a population-based cohort. *Am J Gastroenterol*2012;107:1228-35.

47 Jess T, Rungoe C, Peyrin-Biroulet L. Risk of colorectal cancer in patients with ulcerative colitis: a meta-analysis of population-based cohort studies. *Clin Gastroenterol Hepatol*2012;10:639-45.

48 Jess T, Simonsen J, Jorgensen KT, Pedersen BV, Nielsen NM, Frisch M. Decreasing risk of colorectal cancer in patients with inflammatory bowel disease over 30 years. *Gastroenterology*2012;143:375-81.

49 Cairns SR, Scholefield JH, Steele RG, Dunlop MG, Thomas HJ, Evans GD, et al. Guidelines for colorectal cancer screening and surveillance in moderate and high risk groups (update from 2002). *Gut*2010;59:666-89.

50 Lewis NR, Scott BB. Guidelines for osteoporosis management in inflammatory bowel disease and coeliac disease. British Society of Gastroenterology, 2007. www.bsg.org.uk/pdf_word_docs/ost_coe_ibd.pdf.

51 Cornish J, Tan E, Teare J, Teoh TG, Rai R, Clark SK, et al. A meta-analysis on the influence of inflammatory bowel disease on pregnancy. *Gut*2007;56:830-7.

52 Ilnyckyji A, Blanchard JF, Rawsthorne P, Bernstein CN. Perianal Crohn's disease and pregnancy: role of the mode of delivery. *Am J Gastroenterol*1999;94:3274-8.

53 Reddy D, Murphy SJ, Kane SV, Present DH, Kornbluth A. Relapses of inflammatory bowel disease during pregnancy: in-hospital management and birth outcomes. *Am J Gastroenterol*2008;103:1203-9.

54 Rahimi R, Nikfar S, Rezaie A, Abdollahi M. Pregnancy outcome in women with inflammatory bowel disease following exposure to 5-aminosalicylic acid drugs: a meta-analysis. *Reprod Toxicol*2008;25:271-5.

55 Cleary BJ, Kallen B. Early pregnancy azathioprine use and pregnancy outcomes. *Birth Defects Res A Clin Mol Teratol*2009;85:647-54.

56 Christensen LA, Dahlerup JF, Nielsen MJ, Fallingborg JF, Schmiegelow K. Azathioprine treatment during lactation. *Aliment Pharmacol Ther*2008;28:1209-13.

57 Angelberger S, Reinisch W, Messerschmidt A, Miehsler W, Novacek G, Vogelsang H, et al. Long-term follow-up of babies exposed to azathioprine in utero and via breastfeeding. *J Crohns Colitis*2011;5:95-100.

Related links

bmj.com/archive
Previous articles in this series

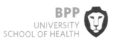

Laparoscopic colorectal surgery

Oliver M Jones, consultant colorectal surgeon,
Ian Lindsey, consultant colorectal surgeon,
Chris Cunningham, consultant colorectal surgeon

[1]Department of Colorectal Surgery, Surgery and Diagnostics, Churchill Hospital, Oxford OX3 7LJ, UK

Correspondence to: O M Jones
oliver.jones@ouh.nhs.uk

Cite this as: *BMJ* 2011;343:d8029

DOI: 10.1136/bmj.d8029

http://www.bmj.com/content/343/
bmj.d8029

The uptake of laparoscopic colorectal surgery is increasing annually. Colon resection using this approach was first reported in 1991, but hospital episode statistics (HES) data show that 22% of colon resections in the United Kingdom in were performed in this manner by 2008-9.[1][2] The laparoscopic approach minimises surgical trauma and allows faster recovery from surgery, and it has been evaluated for other operations, such as cholecystectomy. Early reports of the outcomes of laparoscopic colorectal surgery comprised mostly non-malignant cases, but more recently laparoscopic surgery has become widely used for colorectal cancer. Updated guidance (2010) from the UK National Institute for Health and Clinical Excellence recommends that all patients deemed suitable must be offered laparoscopic surgery even if this means onward referral to a suitably qualified surgeon.[3] We review the effectiveness of laparoscopic colorectal surgery compared with open surgery and the potential adverse effects.

What are the benefits of laparoscopic colorectal surgery?

The rationale for using laparoscopic surgery is that it can help minimise the trauma of access, reduce pain, and accelerate postoperative return of bowel function and general mobility. All these factors may shorten hospital stay. Other potential benefits include reduced formation of adhesions and lower rates of incisional hernia.

A trocar, which acts as a conduit for the camera and operating instruments, is introduced through small incisions (usually 5-12 mm in length) (fig 1). The operation within the abdominal cavity is similar to that performed during open surgery. Occasionally, a decision is made during surgery that the operation cannot be safely completed laparoscopically (commonly because of adhesions, bleeding, poor views of the anatomy, or an unexpectedly advanced tumour) and a conventional abdominal incision is made. Such patients are said to have undergone "conversion" to an open operation.

We review the evidence for benefit of laparoscopic surgery over open surgery according to specific colorectal pathology.

Colorectal cancer

The earliest large randomised trial that compared laparoscopic and open surgery for colon resection was the multicentre CLASICC trial in which patients with both colonic cancer and rectal cancer were randomised on a 2:1 basis to laparoscopic surgery or open surgery. The trial was

SOURCES AND SELECTION CRITERIA

We searched the Cochrane databases using the terms laparoscopic, colorectal surgery, colorectal cancer, diverticular disease, Crohn's disease, and ulcerative colitis to identify observational studies, case series, and randomised trials.

conducted early in the global experience of laparoscopic colorectal surgery, and this was reflected in 29% of patients in the laparoscopic surgery arm undergoing conversion to open surgery.[4] Involvement of the circumferential resection margin was significantly higher for upper rectal cancers in the laparoscopic arm; this may have been because relatively inexperienced surgeons (with as few as 20 previous resections) could participate in the trial. Despite this, short term outcomes and longer term oncological outcomes were similar between the groups.[5] Furthermore, rates of incisional hernia and admissions with adhesional intestinal obstruction were non-significantly lower in patients randomised to laparoscopic surgery, although they were higher in the subgroup converted to an open operation.[6]

Many more trials followed. A Cochrane review of short term outcomes among 3526 patients from 25 randomised trials, published in 2005, showed that quality of life was improved in patients undergoing laparoscopic surgery and hospital stay was reduced by 1.4 days.[7] A similar systematic review of longer term outcomes has also shown equivalence between approaches and, importantly, no difference between tumour recurrence rates.[8]

Ulcerative colitis

Subtotal colectomy is the most commonly performed operation for colitis (fig 2). At index operation or some months later, the rectum and anus may be removed, or the rectum only—with preservation of the anal canal—in patients keen to avoid a long term stoma. A pouch or reservoir is formed from terminal ileum and anastomosed onto the anal canal to restore continuity, with the aim of avoiding a lifelong stoma.

A meta-analysis of laparoscopic surgery for ulcerative colitis was published in 2006. It comprised six studies that compared open and laparoscopic surgery for ulcerative colitis within the same institution and four case matched studies.[9] The results indicated that, overall, patients undergoing laparoscopic surgery had a weighted mean difference (reduction) in hospital stay of 2.6 days. After colectomy, morbidity was significantly lower in the laparoscopic group (40% v 68%), although morbidity after laparoscopic pouch surgery was similar. Mortality was rare and did not differ significantly between approaches. A retrospective questionnaire review of a case series of patients who had undergone pouch surgery (100 laparoscopic; 189 open) found that overall sexual function scores for men and women were similar regardless of which approach was used, although male orgasmic function was significantly inferior in the laparoscopic group.[10]

SUMMARY POINTS

- Laparoscopic surgery has been established as safe in colorectal surgery
- Surgeons and hospitals need appropriate training and mentoring before adopting this approach
- Offer patients a laparoscopic alternative to open surgery
- Laparoscopic surgery remains technically challenging in conditions such as rectal cancer and will be inappropriate for some patients
- The role of advanced technologies—including single port surgery, natural orifice surgery, and robotics—remains unclear

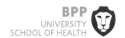

Crohn's disease

There are many possible anatomical resections for Crohn's disease, but because of the distribution of disease, the most common is ileocolic resection. A recent Cochrane review of two randomised trials (120 patients) comparing laparoscopic and open ileocolic resection for Crohn's disease found that—although there was a trend towards fewer wound infections and reoperations with laparoscopic surgery—the two approaches were equivalent. The authors concluded that laparoscopic surgery was as safe as the open approach.[11]

Diverticulitis

Two trials have evaluated laparoscopic surgery for elective resection of diverticulitis. In a single blinded randomised controlled trial of 113 patients, the laparoscopic approach took longer but was associated with a marginal reduction in postoperative pain and a reduction in length of hospital stay from seven to five days.[12] A double blind randomised controlled trial of 104 patients reported a reduction in length of hospital stay (from 10 to eight days) and in major morbidity for patients randomised to laparoscopic surgery, along with less pain and better reported quality of life indicators.[13] With more experience, morbidity, mortality, and length of stay might be reduced further, and it might be possible to use laparoscopic surgery in patients with complicated disease (such as fistulas and abscesses).[14]

The role of laparoscopy in patients with acute diverticulitis is less certain. A recent report enrolled 100 consecutive patients with perforated diverticulitis that had been confirmed by computed tomography.[15] All underwent laparoscopy, and the eight patients with fecalent peritonitis had an open resection. The remaining 92 patients with purulent peritonitis were managed with laparoscopic lavage, drain placement, but no resection. Morbidity and mortality in this series were 4% and 3%, respectively. At median follow-up of three years, only two patients had returned with recurrent diverticulitis. Randomised trials are awaited, but this study may herald an important shift in the operative management of acute diverticulitis.

Pelvic floor dysfunction

From the colorectal perspective, pelvic floor dysfunction focuses on the posterior compartment. We summarised the role of laparoscopic surgery in the treatment of this problem in our recent clinical review.[16]

Possible disadvantages and contraindications

A recent meta-analysis of 10 randomised trials comparing laparoscopic surgery and open surgery suggested that the laparoscopic approach is associated with a higher rate of intraoperative complications,[17] particularly bowel injury (odds ratio 1.88, 95% confidence interval 1.10 to 3.21; P=0.02). Such adverse events (if recognised immediately) may result in conversion to open surgery. Outcomes are often worse in this "converted" group than in the "successfully completed laparoscopic" and open groups.[4]

What is fast track surgery and does it benefit patients?

Fast track surgery protocols or enhanced recovery protocols aim to reduce the physiological insult of surgery and expedite patient recovery, discharge, and return to normal function. The protocols include preoperative measures such as patient education, avoidance of routine bowel preparation, reduction in preoperative starvation, and the use of preoperative carbohydrate and protein loading.

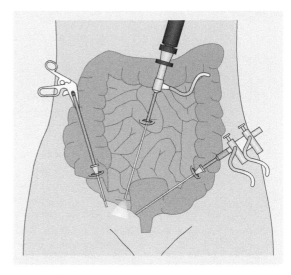

Fig 1 Conventional laparoscopy. A camera is inserted, usually at the umbilicus, and operating ports are inserted at remote sites to provide "triangulation" for the surgeon

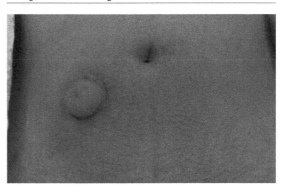

Fig 2 Single port approach to subtotal colectomy in a patient with medically refractory ulcerative colitis. The operation was performed through a single access port at the site of the eventual ileostomy in the right iliac fossa. Before stoma formation, the colectomy specimen was removed through this site

Tailored anaesthesia, avoidance of perioperative fluid overload, and early postoperative mobilisation are also important components.

Such protocols have been widely adopted by laparoscopic surgeons, although the early reports related to open surgery.[18] A recent meta-analysis comparing enhanced recovery programmes with "standard" management identified six randomised controlled trials with 452 patients (undergoing both open and laparoscopic colorectal surgery) and found a reduction in hospital stay of 2.5 days.[19]

Most large studies that have compared laparoscopic and open colorectal surgery have not used an enhanced recovery approach. Enhanced recovery may be more important than the surgical approach itself. Indeed, a randomised blinded study of laparoscopic colonic resection versus open resection in the context of enhanced recovery (60 patients) reported similar hospital stay in both groups (two days), with equivalent return of functional activities and no significant differences in morbidity.[20] The recently reported LAFA study randomised patients to laparoscopic or open surgery for colon cancer and to enhanced recovery or standard care, resulting in four treatment groups.[21] The shortest postoperative length of stay was in the laparoscopic and enhanced recovery group (median stay five days; P<0.001); however, regression analysis suggested that laparoscopy was the only factor that predicted reduced hospital stay and reduced morbidity.

Enhanced recovery protocols will probably be modified as further evidence becomes available. As an example, avoidance of routine mechanical bowel preparation was included in the protocols on the basis of large meta-analyses attesting to the safety of this approach.[22] However, more recent evidence has shown that in specific subgroups, such as patients undergoing surgery for rectal cancer, this practice may be associated with higher rates of morbidity.[23]

Reducing the postoperative stay in hospital and its potential sequelae

Some patients are now staying in hospital for less than 24 hours after colorectal resection. One study reported 10 patients who underwent laparoscopic colectomy and were discharged within 23 hours of surgery with no morbidity and no readmissions.[24] Indeed, enhanced recovery protocols do not seem to increase hospital readmission rates,[19] and neither does laparoscopic colorectal surgery compared with open surgery according to HES data.[25]

As discussed, laparoscopic surgery has been shown to reduce morbidity without increasing readmission. Broadly, the type of postoperative morbidity after colorectal surgery is similar for both laparoscopic and open approaches (table). Although many studies have shown a reduction in morbidity with laparoscopic surgery, earlier discharge may partially offset this benefit in terms of the amount of morbidity seen in primary care.

What advances in laparoscopic surgery may improve outcomes further?

Single port surgery

Attempts to minimise the trauma of access from laparoscopic surgery have led to the development of single port surgery (fig 3). This approach uses a single incision (often in the umbilicus or at a future stoma site) through which all laparoscopic instruments are passed. The obvious advantage of this approach is improved cosmesis—for example, a subtotal colectomy can be performed via a single 2 cm incision at the future ileostomy site, so the operation is essentially scar free apart from the ileostomy itself.[26] It is unclear whether the benefits over conventional laparoscopy are substantial enough to justify the technical difficulties experienced by the surgeon from lack of triangulation and instrument clash.

Natural orifice surgery

This approach uses internal transvisceral incisions rather than incisions in the abdominal wall (fig 4). The technique has the potential to reduce pain, wound complications, and the physiological stress of surgery while also having cosmetic benefits. The transvaginal and transgastric routes have been the most commonly used access points to date. Technical challenges remain, such as defining the optimal method of gaining access transviscerally and the safest way to close these orifices.

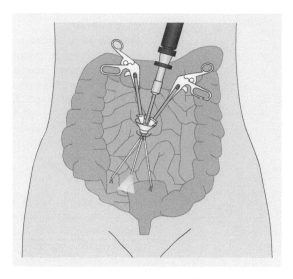

Fig 3 Single port laparoscopy. The camera and all instruments are introduced through a single device, often at the umbilicus or a future stoma site. The surgeon lacks triangulation, which may be partially overcome by using articulated instruments, and instrument and camera clash is common

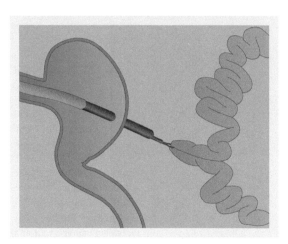

Fig 4 Natural orifice or transvisceral surgery. Access to the abdominal cavity is not through the abdominal wall but through another organ, most commonly the vagina or stomach

Combined laparoscopy and endoscopy

Laparoscopy is useful in the colonoscopic treatment of large polyps and early cancers. Laparoscopy can improve colonoscopic access to the polyp, and it has been used in endoscopic assisted transluminal resection, endoscopic guided laparoscopic local or wedge excision, and to help assess the integrity of the bowel after endoscopic excision of the polyp. Several reports have attested to the safety and applicability of this approach.[27]

Potential complications from laparoscopic and open colorectal surgery*

Type of complication	Examples
Technical	Anastomotic leak; intra-abdominal abscess; ureteric injury
Infective	Wound infection; chest infection; urinary tract infection
Thromboembolic	Deep vein thrombosis; pulmonary embolus
Abdominal wall	Extraction site hernia; port site hernia; abdominal wall haematoma
Cardiovascular	Myocardial infarction; unstable angina; atrial fibrillation
Gastrointestinal	Bowel obstruction; ileus
Stoma related	Patient unable to manage stoma; prolapse; ischaemia

*Many of these complications manifest a few days after surgery and with the trend to early discharge may become increasingly relevant to primary care doctors.

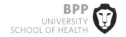

Robotic surgery

Robotic surgery can be used as an adjunct to all laparoscopic colorectal procedures. Its limitations include set up time and expense, as well as limited flexibility when surgery takes place in more than one quadrant of the abdomen, and in the future its main role will probably be in the pelvis. The early results of a prospective comparative study comparing conventional and robotic laparoscopic total mesorectal excision for low rectal cancer have shown that the robotic approach is safe.[28] A recent systematic review and meta-analysis of the efficacy of the robotic approach in abdominal surgery concluded that although it took longer to perform and was more expensive, it was associated with a lower risk of conversion to open surgery.[29]

Conclusion

The laparoscopic approach to colorectal surgery is now well established in the UK and throughout the world. Since the early large trials that established the safety of this approach, technology has improved and further advances have been made in surgical experience and formal training. It is not yet known whether this will translate into improved functional or oncological outcomes compared with conventional surgery. In the interim, patients should be offered a laparoscopic alternative to open surgery and referred to hospitals where the appropriate expertise exists if necessary.

OMJ performed the literature search and wrote the initial draft. All three authors revised the initial draft, prepared the illustrations, and wrote the final draft. OMJ is guarantor.

Competing interests: All authors have completed the ICMJE uniform disclosure form at www.icmje.org/coi_disclosure.pdf (available on request from the corresponding author) and declare: no support from any organisation for the submitted work; no financial relationships with any organisations that might have an interest in the submitted work in the previous three years; no other relationships or activities that could appear to have influenced the submitted work.

Provenance and peer review: Commissioned; externally peer reviewed.

Patient consent obtained.

1   National Institute for Health and Clinical Excellence. NICE implementation uptake report: Laparoscopic surgery for colorectal cancer: laparoscopic surgery for colorectal cancer. 2010. www.nice.org.uk/media/B4D/4A/UptakeReportColorectalCancer.pdf.
2   Jacobs M, Verdeja JC, Goldstein HS. Minimally invasive colon resection (laparoscopic colectomy). Surg Laparosc Endosc 1991;1:144-50.
3   National Institute for Health and Clinical Excellence. Laparoscopic surgery for colorectal cancer. 2006. www.nice.org.uk/nicemedia/pdf/TA105guidance.pdf.
4   Guillou PJ, Quirke P, Thorpe H, Walker J, Jayne DG, Smith AM, et al; MRC CLASICC trial group. Short-term endpoints of conventional versus laparoscopic-assisted surgery in patients with colorectal cancer (MRC CLASICC trial): multicentre, randomised controlled trial. Lancet 2005;365:1718-26.
5   Jayne DG, Thorpe HC, Copeland J, Quirke P, Brown JM, Guillou PJ. Five-year follow-up of the Medical Research Council CLASICC trial of laparoscopically assisted versus open surgery for colorectal cancer. Br J Surg 2010;97:1638-45.
6   Taylor GW, Jayne DG, Brown SR, Thorpe H, Brown JM, Dewberry SC, et al. Adhesions and incisional hernias following laparoscopic versus open surgery for colorectal cancer in the CLASICC trial. Br J Surg 2010;97:70-8.
7   Schwenk W, Haase O, Neudecker JJ, Muller JM. Short term benefits for laparoscopic colorectal resection. Cochrane Database Syst Rev 2005;2:CD003145.
8   Kuhry E, Schwenk W, Gaupset R, Romild U, Bonjer HJ. Long-term results of laparoscopic colorectal cancer resection. Cochrane Database Syst Rev 2008;2:CD003432.
9   Tan JJ, Tjandra JJ. Laparoscopic surgery for ulcerative colitis- a meta-analysis. Colorectal Dis 2006;8:626-36.
10   Larson DW, Davies MM, Dozois EJ, Cima RR, Piotrowicz K, Andersen K, et al. Sexual function, body image, and quality of life after laparoscopic and open ileal pouch-anal anastomosis. Dis Colon Rectum 2008;51:392-6.
11   Dasari BV, McKay D, Gardiner K. Laparoscopic versus open surgery for small bowel Crohn's disease. Cochrane Database Syst Rev 2011;1:CD006956.
12   Gervz P, Inan I, Perneger T, Schiffer E, Morel P. A prospective, randomized, single-blind trial of laparoscopic versus open sigmoid colectomy for diverticulitis. Ann Surg 2010;252:3-8.
13   Klarenbeek BR, Veenhof AA, Bergamaschi R, van der Peet DL, van der Broek WT, de Lange ES, et al. Laparoscopic sigmoid resection for diverticulitis decreases major morbidity rates: a randomized control trial: short-term results of the Sigma Trial. Ann Surg 2009;249:39-44.
14   Jones OM, Stevenson AR, Clark D, Stitz RW, Lumley JW. Laparoscopic resection for diverticular disease: follow-up of 500 consecutive patients. Ann Surg 2008;248:1092-7.
15   Myers E, Hurley M, O'Sullivan GC, Kavanagh D, Wilson I, Winter DC. Laparoscopic peritoneal lavage for generalized peritonitis due to perforated diverticulitis. Br J Surg 2008;95:97-101.
16   Jones OM, Cunningham C, Lindsey I. The assessment and management of rectal prolapse, rectal intussusception, rectocoele and enterocoele in adults. BMJ 2011;342:c7099.
17   Sammour T, Kahokehr A, Srinivasa S, Bissett IP, Hill AG. Laparoscopic colorectal surgery is associated with a higher intraoperative complication rate than open surgery. Ann Surg 2011;253:35-43.
18   Kehlet H, Mogensen T. Hospital stay of 2 days after open sigmoidectomy with a multimodal rehabilitation programme. Br J Surg 1999;86:227-30.
19   Adamina M, Kehlet H, Tomlinson GA, Senagore AJ, Delaney CP. Enhanced recovery pathways optimize health outcomes and resource utilization: a meta-analysis of randomized controlled trials in colorectal surgery. Surgery 2011;149:830-40.
20   Basse L, Jakobsen DH, Bardram L, Billesbolle P, Lund C, Mogensen T, et al. Functional recovery after open versus laparoscopic colonic resection: a randomized, blinded study. Ann Surg 2005;241:416-23.
21   Vlug, MS, Wind J, Hollman MW, Ubbink DT, Cense HA, Engel AF, et al; LAFA study group. Laparoscopy in combination with fast track multimodal management is the best peri-operative strategy in patients undergoing colonic surgery: a randomized clinical trial (LAFA study). Ann Surg 2011;254:868-75.
22   Guenaga KF, Matos, D, Wille-Jorgensen P. Mechanical bowel preparation for elective colorectal surgery. Cochrane Database Syst Rev 2011;9:CD001544.
23   Bretagnol F, Panis Y, Rullier E, Rouanet P, Berdah S, Dousset B, et al; French Research Group of Rectal Cancer Surgery (GRECCAR). Rectal cancer surgery with or without bowel preparation: the French GRECCAR III multicenter single-blinded randomized trial. Ann Surg 2010;252:863-8.
24   Levy BF, Scott MJ, Fawcett WJ, Rockall TA. 23-hour-stay laparoscopic colectomy. Dis Colon Rectum 2009;52:1239-43.
25   Faiz O, Haji A, Burns E, Bottle A, Kennedy R, Aylin P. Hospital stay amongst patients undergoing major elective colorectal surgery: predicting prolonged stay and readmissions in NHS hospitals. Colorectal Dis 2011;13:816-22.
26   Cahill RA, Lindsey I, Jones O, Guy R, Mortensen N, Cunningham C. Single-port laparoscopic total colectomy for medically uncontrolled colitis. Dis Colon Rectum 2010;53:1143-7.
27   Wilhelm D, von Delius S, Weber L, Meining A, Schneider A, Friess H, et al. Combined laparoscopic-endoscopic resections of colorectal polyps: 10-year experience and follow-up. Surg Endosc 2009;23:688-93.
28   Baik SH, Kwon HY, Kim JS, Hur H, Sohn SK, Cho CH, et al. Robotic versus laparoscopic low anterior resection of rectal cancer: short term outcome of a prospective comparative study. Ann Surg Oncol 2009;16:1480-7.
29   Maeso S, Reza M, Mayol JA, Blasco JA, Guerra M, Andradas E, et al. Efficacy of the Da Vinci surgical system in abdominal surgery compared with that of laparoscopy: a systematic review and meta-analysis. Ann Surg 2010;252:254-62.

Related links

bmj.com/archive
- Managing infants who cry excessively in the first few months of life (2011;343:d7772)
- Managing motion sickness (2011;343:d7430)
- Osteoarthritis at the base of the thumb (2011;343:d7122)
- Inherited cardiomyopathies (2011;343:d6966)

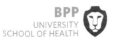

The modern management of incisional hernias

David L Sanders, speciality trainee in upper gastrointestinal surgery[1],
Andrew N Kingsnorth, consultant surgeon[2]

[1]Upper Gastrointestinal Surgery, Royal Cornwall Hospital, Truro TR1 3LJ, UK

[2]Peninsula College of Medicine and Dentistry, Plymouth, UK

Correspondence to: D L Sanders dsanders@doctors.org.uk

Cite this as: BMJ 2012;344:e2843

DOI: 10.1136/bmj.e2843

http://www.bmj.com/content/344/bmj.e2843

Before the introduction of general anaesthesia by Morton in 1846, incisional hernias were rare. As survival after abdominal surgery became more common so did the incidence of incisional hernias.[1] Since then, more than 4000 peer reviewed articles have been published on the topic, many of which have introduced a new or modified surgical technique for prevention and repair. Despite considerable improvements in prosthetics used for hernia surgery, the incidence of incisional hernias and the recurrence rates after repair remain high. Arguably, no other benign disease has seen so little improvement in terms of surgical outcome.

Unlike other abdominal wall hernias, which occur through anatomical points of weakness, incisional hernias occur through a weakness at the site of abdominal wall closure. Why, unlike primary abdominal wall hernias, are the results after repair so poor? Perhaps it is because in the repair of incisional hernias several problems need to be overcome: a multilayered wall structure of different tissue properties in constant motion has to be sutured; positive abdominal pressure has to be dealt with; and tissues with impaired healing properties, reduced perfusion, and connective tissue deficiencies have to be joined.

This review, which is targeted at the general medical audience, aims to update the reader on the definition, incidence, risk factors, diagnosis, and management of incisional hernias.

Unravelling the terminology

Despite the size of the problem, the terminology used to describe incisional hernias still varies greatly. An internationally acceptable and uniform definition is needed to improve the clarity of communication within the medical community and enable publication data and future studies to be interpreted properly. Table 1 lists the definitions of the commonly (mis)used terms.

How common are incisional hernias?

Incisional hernias are one of the most common complications after abdominal surgery. The true incidence is difficult to determine, as shown by the wide range of published figures in the literature. The reasons for this discrepancy are the lack of standardised definition, the inconsistency of data sources used (which include self reporting by patients, audits of routine clinical examination, and insurance company databases), short length of follow-up (often one year),

SOURCES AND SELECTION CRITERIA

We searched PubMed from 1970-2012 and Embase and the Cochrane Library from inception using the terms "hernia" and "incisional" (using the Boolean operator AND) and "ventral" (using the Boolean operator OR). The reference lists were also used to identify studies of interest. Both authors independently identified publications for inclusion and differences were resolved by discussion. We gave priority to research published in the past five years and highly regarded older publications.

and the subjectivity of clinical examination.[2] The reported incidence after a midline laparotomy ranges from 3% to 20% and is doubled if the index operation is complicated by wound infection.[3] About 50% of incisional hernias are detected within one year of surgery, but they can occur several years afterwards, with a subsequent risk of 2% a year.[3][4]

Millions of abdominal incisions are created each year worldwide, so incisional hernias are a major problem, both in terms of morbidity and socioeconomic cost. Although exact figures are unknown, it is estimated that each year 10 000 repairs are performed in the United Kingdom and 100 000 are performed in the United States.[5]

Who is at risk?

Until recently, incisional hernias were thought to result mainly from a technical failure in the surgical closure of the abdominal wall.[6] However, we now know that a complex array of patient related, surgical, and postoperative variables influence their development. These variables share a common denominator—they all influence normal wound healing (table 2). Most of the evidence on risk factors has been determined by retrospective studies, and the relative importance of many of the proposed risk factors is poorly understood.

Patient related factors

Associations between surgery for abdominal aortic aneurysm, the presence of other primary abdominal wall hernias, and the development of incisional hernias have repeatedly been documented.[7][8] Similarly patients with certain connective tissue diseases (Marfan's syndrome, osteogenesis imperfecta, and Ehlers-Danlos syndrome) have an increased incidence of incisional hernias.[9][10] A review article published in 2011, which drew on evidence from 52 publications, concluded that collagen metabolism in patients with a hernia is altered at three levels. The ratio between type I (strong) and type III (weak) collagen is decreased, the quality of collagen is poorer, and collagen breakdown is increased via increased matrix metalloproteinase (MMP) activity.[11] However, it has not been established whether these changes are localised to the site of hernia development or whether they affect all body tissues. The relative contribution of collagen deficiencies versus other patient related risk factors for hernia development is also not fully understood (table 2).

SUMMARY POINTS

- Incisional hernias are a common complication of abdominal surgery
- Incisional hernias can occur many years after the index operation
- Surgical site infection doubles the risk of incisional hernia
- In case of uncertainty, ultrasonography can help confirm the diagnosis before specialist referral
- Laparoscopic repair is generally reserved for small hernias (fascial defect <10 cm), although some surgeons report good results with larger defects

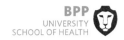

Table 1 Definitions of incisional hernia and the commonly (mis)used terminology

Term	Definition
Incisional hernia	Any gap in the abdominal wall, with or without a bulge in the area of the postoperative scar, that can be seen or palpated on clinical examination or imaging
Primary incisional hernia	An incisional hernia that has not previously been surgically repaired
Recurrent incisional hernia	An incisional hernia that has previously been surgically repaired
Trocar site hernia	An abdominal wall gap, with or without a bulge in the area of previous cannulation with a laparoscopic trocar, that can be seen or palpated on clinical examination or imaging
Acute wound failure (fascial dehiscence, evisceration, eventration)	The acute breakdown or separation of the fascial tissues, with resulting protrusion of the intra-abdominal contents through a fascial defect but without the presence of a peritoneal sac; this usually occurs in the first 2 weeks of wound healing and always results in formation of an incisional hernia
Primary abdominal wall hernia (epigastric hernia, umbilical hernia, paraumbilical hernia, spigellian hernia)	Hernia of the abdominal wall that is not related to an incision (usually refined by defining the site of the hernia)
Recurrent abdominal wall hernia (recurrent epigastric hernia, umbilical hernia, paraumbilical hernia, spigellian hernia)	Recurrence of a primary hernia of the abdominal wall that has been previously surgically repaired
Ventral hernia	This term should not be used owing to the historical confusion with the definition; In Europe the term ventral hernia has been used interchangeably with incisional hernia; in the United States the term has been used to describe any abdominal wall hernia other than in the groin

Table 2 Patient related risk factors for developing an incisional hernia

Risk factor	Proposed effects on wound healing
Age >65 years	Reduced tissue perfusion and reduced collagen formation
Sex	Some studies suggest that male sex is a risk factor, although others have found no difference between the sexes[4 7]
Atherosclerosis	Reduced perfusion to the wound
Diabetes	Reduced inflammatory response; alterations in microcirculation and granulation tissue
Obesity	Increased intra-abdominal pressure; obesity related comorbidities, such as diabetes and increased risk of surgical site infection
Renal failure	Metabolic factors, which prevent formation of normal granulation tissue
Protein deficiency	Important for collagen development
Vitamin C deficiency	An important cofactor in the biosynthesis of collagen
Immunosuppression	Alterations in normal tissue regeneration
Smoking	Alteration in the formation and degradation of collagen, vasoconstriction, and increased mechanical stress from coughing
Drugs and other treatments	Drugs and treatments that cause immunosuppression or reduced vascular perfusion, such as steroids, chemotherapy, and radiotherapy; warfarin, which reduces vitamin K dependent cell-cell adhesion and cell cycle regulation

Surgical factors

Incisional hernias can occur after any type of laparotomy incision but are most common after midline (especially upper midline) and transverse incisions.[4] An analysis of 11 publications assessing the incidence of incisional hernia after different abdominal incisions concluded that the risk was 10.5% for midline incisions and 7.5% for transverse incisions.[12] However, many of these publications included variable closure techniques and disease processes.

Several clinical trials and meta-analyses have shown that a continuous closure technique with a simple running suture is the best option for closure of laparotomy incisions.[13 14 15] The use of monofilament slowly resorbable suture material versus non-absorbable or braided material decreases the rate of incisional hernias and reduces the incidence of postoperative pain and wound infection.[13 14 15]

Experimental studies and randomised clinical trials have shown that a suture length to wound length ratio of at least 4:1, and not more than 5:1, minimises the risk of incisional hernia.[16 17 18] Traditional surgical teaching recommends that continuous sutures are placed 10 mm from the wound edge and 10 mm apart.[17] However, recently this technique has increasingly been challenged. The large tissue bites have been shown to be associated with an increase in the amount of necrotic tissue and slackening of the stitches, resulting in increased risk of wound infection and the development of an incisional hernia.[19 20] In a large randomised controlled trial, small stitches placed 4-6 mm from the wound edge and 4 mm apart (in the aponeurotic layer only) minimised the risk of incisional hernias from 18% to 5.6% (P<0.001) and reduced wound infection rates by 50% (from 10.2% to 5.2%; P<0.02).[21] This is currently being evaluated in a multicentre randomised controlled trial.[16] Most surgeons still use the large bite method and adoption of the small bite technique will be a major shift in surgical practice.

Postoperative factors

Surgical site infection is commonly documented as the most important independent risk factor for the development of an incisional hernia and is thought to double the risk.[4] A prospective cohort study showed that factors that increase intra-abdominal pressure in the immediate postoperative phase, such as postoperative ileus, the need for repeated urinary catheterisation, coughing, vomiting, and mechanical ventilation, also increase the risk of incisional hernias.[22]

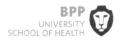

Predicting the risk

A scoring system for predicting the development of early (less than six months after surgery) incisional hernia was published in 2010.[23] The study used linear and multivariate regression models of 42 patient related, surgery related, and perioperative variables. Of these the most significant predictive factors, in order of importance, were fascial suture to incision ratio less than 4.2:1, surgical site infection, time to removal of skin sutures less than 16 days, and body mass index greater than 24. This may provide a useful future tool for preoperative risk assessment and the use of prophylactic mesh, but it still requires prospective and independent validation. Van Ramshorst and colleagues have also published a model for predicting wound abdominal dehiscence risk.[24] They identified the major independent risk factors as age, sex, chronic pulmonary disease, ascites, jaundice, anaemia, emergency surgery, type of surgery, postoperative coughing, and wound infection.

Can an incisional hernia be prevented?

Currently the risk of incisional hernia cannot be eliminated except by avoiding a laparotomy incision in the first place. However, the risk can be minimised by reducing systemic risk factors, especially smoking, obesity, and nutritional deficiencies, and by optimising diabetic management, even if surgery has to be delayed. The risk can be further minimised by careful attention to surgical technique when closing the abdominal wall. Surgeons should follow the 2008 National Institute for Health and Clinical Excellence guidelines for the prevention and treatment of surgical site infection.[25] The guidelines provide a detailed review of preoperative, intraoperative, and postoperative measures to minimise the risk of infection. A systematic review of randomised controlled trials found that preoperative antibiotic prophylaxis (less than two hours before surgery) is beneficial in clean surgery involving a prosthesis, clean contaminated surgery, and contaminated surgery. The most significant difference was seen in colorectal surgery (12.9% surgical site infection with antibiotics versus 40.2% without antibiotics).[w1]

The role of prophylactic mesh placement in high risk patient groups is unclear. Promising results have been reported in a randomised controlled trial and case series for elective open abdominal aortic aneurysm surgery (rate of incisional hernias: 9.3% v 2.7% at three year follow-up) and after gastric bypass for obesity (rate of incisional hernias 4.4% at two year follow-up v 30% in matched controls).[w2] [w3] However, other small series have reported unacceptably high complication rates.[w4] Two large multicentre trials assessing prophylactic mesh placement are currently being conducted.

Mention the postoperative risk of incisional hernia when obtaining informed consent from all patients undergoing laparotomy.

How should an incisional hernia be diagnosed?

Most incisional hernias can be diagnosed by a review of the patient's history and by clinical examination. Patients typically present with an abdominal bulge in the region of the surgical scar. On examination the edges of the fascial defect can often be palpated, although an accurate estimation of the size of the defect may be difficult to discern clinically. The size of the peritoneal sac and associated contents is often large, although the fascial defect may be fairly small, particularly in obese patients and after multiple abdominal operations, where there may be numerous small fascial defects. Many incisional hernias are asymptomatic, but 20-50% present with pain. Skin changes as a result of pressure related capillary thrombosis and atrophic muscle fibrosis may occur in large and in longstanding hernias.[w5]

What diagnostic imaging should be used?

Ultrasonography is commonly used to confirm the clinical diagnosis. The sonographic image of a hernia is a fascial gap with protruding hernia contents. The hernia sac should increase in size or change location when the patient coughs. Intestinal structures are characterised by peristaltic movements and air bubbles, whereas the omentum appears as a stationary, highly reflective, space occupying structure.

More detailed diagnostic imaging is indicated in four patient groups[w6]:

- Obese patients (body mass index >35)
- Patients with recurrent incisional hernias
- Patients with large hernias with loss of domain (abdominal viscera permanently residing outside the abdominal cavity in the hernia sac)
- Patients with pain within the abdominal wall but with no clinically detectable hernia.

In these patients computed tomography (with or without valsalva) and particularly multidetector computed tomography, which allows three dimensional reconstruction, is useful. Occult defects are accurately delineated, the contents of the sac defined, and an estimate can be made of the abdominal contents that have lost domain.[w7]

Does an incisional hernia have to be repaired?

Not every patient who presents with an incisional hernia is suitable for surgical repair, and the risk of surgery must be balanced against the risk of complications if the hernia is left untreated. Between 6% and 15% of incisional hernia repairs are performed because of strangulation or obstructive symptoms.[w5] However, little information is currently available on the risk of major complications from untreated incisional hernias. Small hernias invariably enlarge with time as a result of the continuous intra-abdominal pressure, diaphragmatic contractions, and increased pressure from coughing or straining.[w8]

A commonsense approach is advocated. If the patient can safely have general anaesthesia and the chance of successful repair is reasonable, then surgery is indicated. If the patient presents a high anaesthetic risk or surgical repair will be technically difficult, then the size of the fascial defect relative to the hernia, the symptom complex, the patient's age, and the patient's preferences must be carefully considered. In such cases, conservative management may be more appropriate. This decision making process is patient specific and therefore we recommend that all patients are referred for a specialist opinion.

What methods of surgical repair are available?

Despite recent advances in the management of incisional hernias, recurrence rates remain high. The recurrence rate after open suture repair can be as high as 54%, and as high as 36% for open mesh repair; however, in general, recurrence rates are slightly lower, with a mean of about 15%.[w9] Recurrence rates for laparoscopic repair seem to be comparable to open mesh procedures but laparoscopic repair requires a shorter hospital stay.[w10] The method of choice for repair of incisional hernias is still debatable. Figure 1 shows the anatomy of the different methods of repair.

Interestingly, in a comparative retrospective study of more than 400 incisional hernia operations over 25 years, the most important prognostic factor was found to be the surgeon's experience rather than the repair method used.[w11]

Mesh versus suture repair

A systematic review found that hernia repair without prosthetic mesh is associated with unsatisfactory recurrence rates of 12-54%, whereas hernia repair with mesh results in recurrence rates of 2-36%.[w9] It is now accepted that only the smallest (less than 3 cm) incisional hernia should be repaired by primary tissue approximation with sutures.[w12 w13] A population based study of 10 882 patients in the US found an increase in the frequency of synthetic mesh use from 35% in 1987 to 65% by 1999.[w14] A recent Cochrane review of open procedures for the repair of incisional hernia concluded that open mesh repair is superior to suture repair in terms of recurrence but inferior in terms of wound infection and seroma formation on the basis of evidence from three trials.[w15]

Laparoscopic mesh repair versus open mesh repair

Laparoscopic incisional hernia repair is an emerging technique with promising initial results. A composite or coated mesh (to reduce visceral adhesions) is placed in the intraperitoneal position and the hernia defect is usually not closed. This is referred to as an intraperitoneal onlay mesh (IPOM; fig 1). The advantages of the laparoscopic approach are that it allows the whole of the previous incision to be visualised and small fascial defects to be identified, but it has the disadvantage of relying fully on the strength of the mesh and its fixation.

A 2002 meta-analysis identified 83 studies comparing open and laparoscopic incisional hernia repair from a structured Medline search; it was able to compare 390 patients having open repair with 322 patients having laparoscopic repair.[w16] Perioperative complications and length of stay were reduced in the laparoscopic group. Another meta-analysis identified 53 studies with a total of 5227 laparoscopic incisional hernia repairs. The rate of hernia recurrence was 3.98%.[w17] Most of

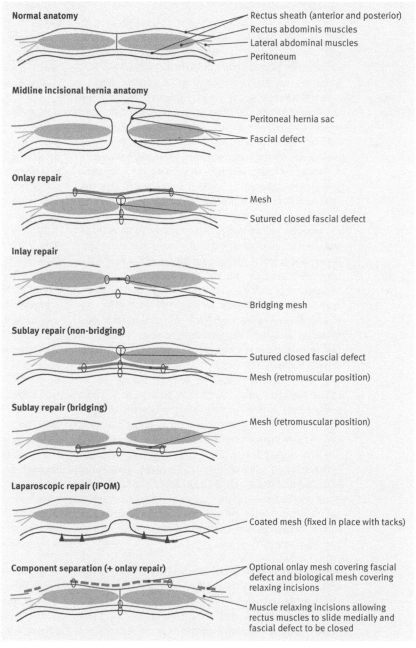

Fig 1 Simplified anatomy of a midline incisional hernia and options for surgical repair

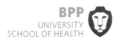

the studies were carried out in specialty centres that carried out large numbers of minimally invasive procedures, the authors concluded that the true recurrence rate is probably higher. Laparoscopic repair has been criticised for producing cosmetically worse results than the open repair because the hernia sac is not excised and the defect is not closed. Furthermore, laparoscopic repair is not always possible for large incisional hernias or when the hernia extends towards the costal margin or pelvis because adequate mesh overlap cannot easily be achieved.[w17] A 2011 Cochrane review of 10 randomised control trials (including 880 patients) concluded that laparoscopic repair is a safe technique that has a lower risk of wound infection, shorter hospital stay, and is associated with fewer (albeit more severe) complications than open repair.[w18] However, the data were heterogeneous and most trials had a short length of follow-up.

Techniques for open mesh repair

Three principal types of repair have been described for the open repair of incisional hernia with mesh—the inlay, onlay, and sublay techniques.

In the inlay technique the mesh is placed between the muscles in a bridging position. The mesh is in contact with the viscera (fig 1). Polypropylene mesh anchors to all adjacent tissues and can therefore induce extensive adhesions to viscera if placed in a position where it becomes adjacent to the bowel. Erosion of the mesh then can occur into the intestines—a well recognised drawback of this technique.[w12] A non-randomised prospective study reported good results with this technique, but these impressive results have not been repeated elsewhere.[w19] A smaller retrospective analysis compared the inlay, onlay, and sublay techniques. The recurrence rate for the inlay technique was 44%, and two of 23 patients developed enterocutaneous fistulas.[w20] Inlay techniques, therefore, are not generally recommended. Furthermore, the force needed to dislocate a bridged mesh is much lower than for a closed defect, and bridging should be a last resort only.[w21]

In the onlay technique (fig 1), the mesh is placed over the abdominal wall closure in the subcutaneous prefascial space.[w22] In a systematic review, recurrence rates after this technique varied from 5.5% to 14.8%, with a mean follow-up of one to 6.7 years.[w23] The main criticisms of this technique are the high rates of wound infections and seroma formation.[w12 w15]

In the sublay technique, the mesh is placed over the closed posterior rectus sheath and peritoneum (fig 1).[w24] If the hernia is large and the posterior sheath cannot be closed, the mesh is sometimes used to bridge the defect (fig 1). A systematic review found that the recurrence rate after sublay repair varied from 1% to 23% at a mean follow-up of 1.7 to 6.7 years.[w23] The European Hernia Society has adopted sublay mesh repair as the gold standard open repair; however, the procedure has been reported as technically more difficult than the onlay technique, with a steeper learning curve and a requirement for more operative time.[w12 w25]

Chronic pain after incisional hernia repair

Chronic pain (for more than three months postoperatively[w26]) after incisional hernia repair is poorly documented. A review reported that clinically important pain after open mesh repair of incisional hernia has an incidence of 10-20%.[w27] The causes of the pain are poorly understood but probably include a combination of mesh associated inflammation, nerve damage from mesh fixation, nerve entrapment or damage, visceral adhesions to the mesh and fixation points, and tension in the repair. Whether the pain relates to the preoperative symptom complex (as with inguinal hernia repair) is not yet established. The importance of chronic pain is difficult to gauge because of the lack of prospective high quality studies. Patients may think that mild postoperative discomfort is an acceptable consequence of surgery for an unsightly and uncomfortable abdominal swelling, whereas pain that limits daily activity after repair of a small asymptomatic incisional hernia may not be thought acceptable.

Patients who present with chronic pain should be referred back to the operating surgeon. A computed tomogram may be useful to assess whether the pain is related to a recurrence of the hernia or a port site hernia (after laparoscopic repair). If there is no evidence of recurrence, many surgeons adopt a watch and wait approach with referral to chronic pain services. Other surgeons have reported removing fixation tacks or sutures or replacing the mesh, with successful outcome.[w28 w29] However, no high quality evidence is available to recommend the best way to manage this problem.

Special circumstances

Giant incisional hernias

Patients with giant incisional hernias (fascial defect >10 cm in transverse diameter) and obese patients (body mass index >35) present a surgical and anaesthetic challenge. These patients often have poor quality abdominal wall musculature coupled with multiple comorbid medical problems. A further problem that has to be overcome is the risk of serious "loss of domain" once the hernia is repaired, which can result in abdominal compartment syndrome. Loss of domain implies that a proportion of the abdominal contents resides permanently (in a hernia sac) outside the natural abdominal cavity. Returning the contents requires considerable physiological adaption (predominantly respiratory) if the volume exceeds 20% of the size of the abdominal cavity.[w8]

Preoperative pneumoperitoneum has been used to overcome the problems of loss of domain by increasing the size of the abdominal cavity before surgery.[w30] Although this technique may be effective, it has not been widely adopted in the UK. Patients and the surgical technique must be carefully selected, and the team will usually include a hernia specialist, anaesthetist, and plastic surgeon. Patients often need postoperative care in the intensive treatment unit. Dumainian and Denham have updated an algorithm for the management of complex incisional hernias.[w31]

The component separation technique allows a flap of the rectus muscle, anterior rectus sheath, internal oblique, and transversus abdominus muscle to slide medially, enabling giant hernia defects (up to 20 cm) to be closed (figs 1 and 2).[w32] This can be reinforced with a prosthetic mesh to supplement the attenuated layers of the abdominal wall and is the technique of choice for giant midline incisional hernias.

Incisional hernia repair and pregnancy

Repair of large incisional hernias in premenopausal women presents special problems because elasticity and expansion of the abdominal wall will be required if the patient subsequent becomes pregnant. Few data are available on the required compliance of the abdominal wall during pregnancy or whether prosthetic mesh reduces the elasticity

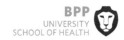

TIPS FOR NON-SPECIALISTS

- Refer all incisional hernias for a specialist opinion and urgently refer painful hernias and large hernias in which a small fascial defect is suspected
- Divarication of the rectus muscles (separation of the rectus muscle with an intact fascia, which usually does not need surgery) may resemble an epigastric hernia; if the diagnosis is uncertain, ultrasonography is useful before referral
- Optimise weight, smoking status, and diabetic control before surgery
- The positioning of the mesh depends on the type of repair; a small postoperative bulge after laparoscopic hernia repair is normal because the fascial defect is not closed

ONGOING RESEARCH

- Watchful Waiting Versus Repair of Oligosymptomatic Incisional Hernias (AWARE) http://clinicaltrials.gov/ct2/show/NCT01349400
- Prevention of Incisional Hernia by Mesh Augmentation After Midline Laparotomy for Aortic Aneurysm Treatment (PRIMAAT) http://clinicaltrials.gov/ct2/show/NCT00757133
- Prophylactic Mesh Implantation for the Prevention of Incisional Hernia (ProphMesh) http://clinicaltrials.gov/ct2/show/NCT01203553
- Laparoscopic Versus Open Incisional Hernia Repair (COLIBRI) http://clinicaltrials.gov/ct2/show/NCT01420757 (completed but not yet published)

ADDITIONAL EDUCATIONAL RESOURCES

Resources for patients

- Patient UK (www.patient.co.uk/health/Hernia.htm)—An overview of all types of hernia, risk factors, and management

For healthcare professionals

- Sauerland S, Walgenbach M, Habermalz B, Seiler CM, Miserez M. Laparoscopic versus open surgical techniques for ventral or incisional hernia repair. *Cochrane Database Syst Rev* 2011;3:CD007781
- Den Hartog D, Dur AHM, Tuinebreijer WE, Kreis RW. Open surgical procedures for incisional hernias. *Cochrane Database Syst Rev* 3008;3:CD006438
- Muysoms FE, Miserez M, Berrevoet F, Campanelli G, Champault GG, Chelala E, et al. Classification of primary and incisional abdominal wall hernias. *Hernia* 2009;13:407-14 (European Hernia Society classification for incisional hernias)
- Sanders DL, Kingsnorth AN. Prosthetic mesh materials used in hernia surgery. *Expert Rev Med Devices* 2012;9:159-79
- Medscape (http://emedicine.medscape.com/article/1297226-overview)—An overview of abdominal wall reconstruction and complex hernias

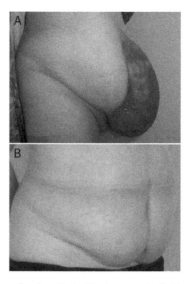

Fig 2 Photographs of a patient with a large complex incisional hernia before (A) and after (B) laparostomy

Contributors: Both authors contributed with the literature review. DLS wrote the article and ANK reviewed the article and made amendments. DLS is guarantor.

Funding: None received.

Competing interests: All authors have completed the ICMJE disclosure form at http://www.icmje.org/coi_disclosure.pdf (available on request from the corresponding author) and declare: no support from any organisation for the submitted work; no financial relationships with any organisations that might have an interest in the submitted work in the previous three years, no other relationships or activities that could appear to have influenced the submitted work.

Provenance and peer review: Not commissioned; externally peer reviewed.

Patient consent obtained.

1. Sanders DL, Kingsnorth AN. From ancient to contemporary times: a concise history of incisional hernia repair. *Hernia* 2012;16:1-7.
2. Fitzgibbons RJ, Richards AT, Quinn TH. Open repair of abdominal wall hernia. In: Ashley SW, ed. ACS surgery principles and practice. American College of Surgeons, 2007. www.acssurgery.com/acs/pdf/ACS0527.pdf.
3. Mudge M, Hughes LE. Incisional hernia: a 10 year prospective study of incidence and attitudes. *Br J Surg* 1985;72:70-1.
4. Bucknall TE, Cox PJ, Ellis H. Burst abdomen and incisional hernia: a prospective study of 1129 major laparotomies. *BMJ* 1982;284:931-3.
5. Rutkow IM. Demographic and socioeconomic aspects of hernia repair in the United States in 2003. *Surg Clin North Am* 2003;83:1045-51, v-vi.
6. Sanders RJ, DiClementi D. Principles of abdominal wound closure. II. Prevention of wound dehiscence. *Arch Surg* 1977;112:1188-91.
7. Stevick CA, Long JB, Jamasbi B, Nash M. Ventral hernia following abdominal aortic reconstruction. *Am Surg* 1988;54:287-9.
8. Hall KA, Peters B, Smyth SH, Warneke JA, Rappaport WD, Putnam CW, et al. Abdominal wall hernias in patients with abdominal aortic aneurysmal versus aortoiliac occlusive disease. *Am J Surg* 1995;170:572-5; discussion 75-6.
9. Girotto JA, Malaisrie SC, Bulkely G, Manson PN. Recurrent ventral herniation in Ehlers-Danlos syndrome. *Plast Reconstr Surg* 2000;106:1520-6.
10. Klinge U, Binnebosel M, Mertens PR. Are collagens the culprits in the development of incisional and inguinal hernia disease? *Hernia* 2006;10:472-7.
11. Henriksen NA, Yadete DH, Sorensen LT, Agren MS, Jorgensen LN. Connective tissue alteration in abdominal wall hernia. *Br J Surg* 2011;98:210-9.
12. Carlson MA, Ludwig KA, Condon RE. Ventral hernia and other complications of 1000 midline incisions. *South Med J* 1995;88:450-3.
13. van 't Riet M, Steyerberg EW, Nellensteyn J, Bonjer HJ, Jeekel J. Meta-analysis of techniques for closure of midline abdominal incisions. *Br J Surg* 2002;89:1350-6.
14. Hodgson NC, Malthaner RA, Ostbye T. The search for an ideal method of abdominal fascial closure: a meta-analysis. *Ann Surg* 2000;231:436-42.
15. Ceydeli A, Rucinski J, Wise L. Finding the best abdominal closure: an evidence-based review of the literature. *Curr Surg* 2005;62:220-5.
16. Harlaar JJ, Deerenberg EB, van Ramshorst GH, Lont HE, van der Borst EC, Schouten WR, et al. A multicenter randomized controlled trial evaluating the effect of small stitches on the incidence of incisional hernia in midline incisions. *BMC Surg* 2011;11:20.
17. Jenkins TP. The burst abdominal wound: a mechanical approach. *Br J Surg* 1976;63:873-6.

enough to cause complications during pregnancy.[w33] There have been a few case reports of successful pregnancies in which the uterus has been within (or part of) the hernia sac.[w34-w36] Small, asymptomatic incisional hernias can probably be safely left until the completion of a family. Large or symptomatic hernias should be fixed, and in these cases it may be better to avoid the use of mesh and to use a sutured repair such as the shoelace technique.[w33] Patients must be warned of the high risk of recurrence with subsequent pregnancy.

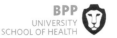

18 Cengiz Y, Blomquist P, Israelsson LA. Small tissue bites and wound strength: an experimental study. *Arch Surg* 2001;136:272-5.

19 Israelsson LA, Jonsson T. Suture length to wound length ratio and healing of midline laparotomy incisions. *Br J Surg* 1993;80:1284-6.

20 Harlaar JJ, van Ramshorst GH, Nieuwenhuizen J, Ten Brinke JG, Hop WC, Kleinrensink GJ, et al. Small stitches with small suture distances increase laparotomy closure strength. *Am J Surg* 2009;198:392-5.

21 Millbourn D, Cengiz Y, Israelsson LA. Effect of stitch length on wound complications after closure of midline incisions: a randomized controlled trial. *Arch Surg* 2009;144:1056-9.

22 Makela JT, Kiviniemi H, Juvonen T, Laitinen S. Factors influencing wound dehiscence after midline laparotomy. *Am J Surg* 1995;170:387-90.

23 Veljkovic R, Protic M, Gluhovic A, Potic Z, Milosevic Z, Stojadinovic A. Prospective clinical trial of factors predicting the early development of incisional hernia after midline laparotomy. *J Am Coll Surg* 2010;210:210-9.

24 Van Ramshorst GH, Nieuwenhuizen J, Hop WC, Arends P, Boom J, Jeekel J, et al. Abdominal wound dehiscence in adults: development and validation of a risk model. *World J Surg* 2010;34:20-7.

25 Welsh A. Surgical site infection: prevention and treatment of surgical site infection. RCOG Press, 2008.

Related links

bmj.com
- Get CME credits for this article

bmj.com/archive
Previous articles in this series
- Diagnosis and management of bone stress injuries of the lower limb in athletes (2012;344:e2511)
- The management of overactive bladder syndrome (2012;344:e2365)
- Cluster headache (2012;344:e2407)
- The management of ingrowing toenails (2012;344:e2089)

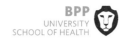

Modern management of splenic trauma

D R Hildebrand, specialty trainee in general surgery[1],

A Ben-sassi, consultant in colorectal surgery[2],

N P Ross, specialty trainee in general surgery[1],

R Macvicar, director of postgraduate general practice education[3],

F A Frizelle, professor of colorectal surgery[2],

A J M Watson, professor of colorectal surgery[1]

[1]Departments of Surgery, Raigmore Hospital, Inverness, IV2 3UJ, Scotland, UK

[2]Christchurch Public Hospital, Christchurch, New Zealand

[3]Postgraduate General Practice Education, NHS Education for Scotland, Inverness

Correspondence to: A J M Watson
angus.watson@nhs.net

Cite this as: BMJ 2014;348:g1864

DOI: 10.1136/bmj.g1864

http://www.bmj.com/content/348/bmj.g1864

Trauma is a major cause of morbidity and mortality; in the developed world, road traffic accidents are one of the leading causes. Up to 45% of patients with blunt abdominal trauma will have a splenic injury,[1] which may require urgent operative management, angioembolisation, or non-operative management in the form of active observation.

The management of splenic injuries has evolved over the past three decades with the realisation of the importance of the spleen in immunological defence against encapsulated organisms and a better understanding of the role of non-operative management of splenic injuries. Such management has been aided by better diagnostic and monitoring facilities and by advances in interventional radiology. This article aims to review the best available evidence for the management of patients with blunt splenic trauma.

Why is the spleen important?

The spleen removes old red blood cells and holds a reserve of blood. The white pulp synthesises antibodies, opsonins, properdin, and tuftsin. It removes antibody-coated bacteria and antibody-coated blood cells. The spleen contains half of the body's monocytes within the red pulp; these can specialise into dendritic cells and macrophages, which are crucial for antigen presentation to the immune system.

Post-splenectomy patients have modest increases in circulating white blood cells and platelets, a diminished responsiveness to some vaccines, and an increased susceptibility to infection by bacteria and protozoa. In particular, they have an increased risk of sepsis from polysaccharide encapsulated bacteria such as *Haemophilus influenzae* type b and *Streptococcus pneumoniae*.

Who gets splenic injuries?

Splenic trauma is caused by either non-penetrating (blunt) or penetrating injuries. Road traffic accidents, falls from height, assaults, and sporting injuries are the most common modalities of blunt trauma. However, splenic rupture can occur in patients with infection or malignancy and after medical procedures.[2] Splenic injury can therefore affect any age group.

When should I suspect a splenic injury?

The spleen is susceptible during trauma to the left lower thorax or left upper abdomen. Other injuries that may be associated with it include injuries to the rib cage, diaphragm, pancreas, and bowel. Haemodynamic instability, with a rising pulse rate and a decreasing blood pressure, is the most reliable sign of an injury.[3] However, clinical signs associated with splenic trauma are notoriously unreliable,[4] and a high index of suspicion based on the mechanism of injury is needed.

Patients can present with either left upper quadrant pain and left shoulder tip pain or diffuse abdominal pain. Some may have pleuritic left sided pain, and left lower chest injury has been shown to be present in 43% of patients with splenic injuries.[5] In the same American case series, left lower chest injury was found to be the single indicator of splenic injury in 6% of patients. Initial presentation, however, may be masked by other injuries. A contained rupture may have few symptoms on initial assessment.

How is the degree of severity of blunt splenic injuries assessed?

The initial assessment of a patient with suspected blunt injury to the spleen should be the same as for any trauma patient. Patients are assessed using the Advanced Trauma Life Support (ATLS) protocol, established by the American College of Surgeons Committee on Trauma but now adopted worldwide.[6] The diagnosis of blunt abdominal trauma cannot purely depend on clinical findings. These may include coma or haemodynamic instability, bruising over the abdomen, or negligible findings during abdominal examination. Several adjuncts have been recommended to facilitate the diagnosis.

What is the role of imaging in suspected splenic injury?
Abdominal ultrasound
Focused abdominal sonography for trauma (FAST) is a protocol driven abdominal ultrasound scan that can be performed by non-radiologists after specific training and is a core competency for all UK trainees in emergency medicine. Operators are trained to look for free intra-abdominal fluid. The ultrasound scan can be performed simultaneously with resuscitation and

SOURCES AND SELECTION CRITERIA

We did a literature review by searching the Medline database to locate English language articles, using the terms "blunt splenic injury," "spleen," "trauma," "investigation," "computed tomography," "splenic angioembolisation," and "non-operative management" and then by carrying out a hand search of reference lists of relevant included studies.

We identified no randomised controlled trials (evidence level I) in this area, although large retrospective and prospective series do exist. The evidence is generally level II and III.

SUMMARY POINTS

- Initial resuscitation, diagnostic evaluation, and management of the trauma patient is based on protocols from Advanced Trauma Life Support (ATLS)
- Further management of splenic injury depends on the haemodynamic stability of the patient
- Splenic injury is graded (I through V) depending on the extent and depth of splenic haematoma and/or laceration identified on computed tomography scan
- Low grade splenic injuries (I, II, and III) are suitable for non-operative management, although more recent evidence suggests that higher grades (IV and V) may also be suitable with the adjunct of angioembolisation
- Early use (<72 hours post-injury) of chemical venous thromboprophylaxis in the form of low molecular weight heparin does not increase the risk of failure of non-operative management in splenic trauma, although no consensus exists on time post-injury to start treatment

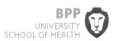

should take less than two minutes. FAST is particularly useful in haemodynamically unstable patients, as it is highly accessible, quick to perform, portable, and non-invasive. A survey of 96 North American regional trauma centres found that FAST is the preferred initial screening test after blunt abdominal trauma; 79% use this technique in preference to computed tomography scanning or diagnostic peritoneal lavage.[7] Diagnostic peritoneal lavage is done by infiltrating fluid into the peritoneal cavity through a cannula, salvaging it, and assessing it for the presence of blood or gut contents.

FAST is used to look for free abdominal fluid (sensitivity 98%[8]), which, when present, is presumed to be blood or gastrointestinal contents. The technique does, however, have limitations in obese patients, it is operator dependent, and intra-abdominal injuries may be missed as evidenced by a systematic review.[9] These include up to 25% of splenic and hepatic injuries, most renal injuries, and virtually all pancreatic, gut, and mesenteric injuries.[10] A negative ultrasound scan thus does not rule out injury, and computed tomography imaging is recommended in haemodynamically stable patients.[10] [11] Patients most likely to have false negative FAST scans are those with head injuries. This may be due to the distracting nature of the injury, which may affect both the patient and the examiner, or to the liberal use of computed tomography in these patients, which may detect small volumes of free intra-abdominal fluid. Small volumes of intra-peritoneal fluid, in the context of major trauma, probably have little clinical effect, and this may explain why false negative results, in these patients, do not predict an adverse outcome.[12]

Computed tomography
Over the past 20 years, in the developed world, computed tomography scanning has become the gold standard for imaging in blunt abdominal trauma,[13] and in the identification of splenic injuries,[14] especially now that computed tomography scanners are in close vicinity to resuscitation areas in accident and emergency departments. This has contributed to the development of non-operative management of blunt splenic trauma,[15] in some series increasing the frequency of non-operative management for equivalent injuries from 11% to 71%.[16]

A relatively simple protocol can be used for patients with blunt trauma, based on scanning the entire abdomen in the portal venous phase and a subsequent delayed excretory scan three to five minutes later if an injury is detected on the initial scan. No oral contrast is administered. The Royal College of Radiologists has issued guidelines on standardisation of computed tomography protocols, including splenic injuries protocols.[17]

Recently, however, a case series from Baltimore has shown that arterial phase imaging is superior to portal venous phase imaging for the identification of pseudoaneurysm but inferior for the identification of active bleeding and parenchymal injury. Dual phase imaging resulted in a sensitivity of 90% for the identification of pseudoaneurysm, 97% for active bleeding, and 99% for both non-vascular injury and perisplenic haematoma. The specificity of dual phase imaging was 100% across all injuries, and the accuracy was 97%, 99%, 99%, and 98%, respectively.[18]

Computed tomography scanning does, however, have its limitations. It has been shown to underestimate the degree of splenic trauma,[19] and it is not reliable as an outcome predictor in adults who have complications as a result of blunt splenic trauma, such as delayed splenic bleeding or subphrenic abscess.[20]

How are splenic injuries scaled?
Initially, the Abbreviated Injury Scale was introduced in 1971.[21] However, in the 1980s the American Association for the Surgery of Trauma appointed an Organ Injury Scaling (OIS) Committee with the goal of developing a comprehensive scaling of specific organ injuries. The individual organ injuries were graded I (minimal), II (mild), III (moderate), IV (severe), V (massive), and VI (lethal).[22] Since originally devised in 1987,[23] the scales for spleen and liver have been revised,[24] but no major alterations have been needed (table). Recently, however, the "Baltimore computed tomography grading system" has been proposed and validated, and has been shown to better predict the requirement for intervention for splenic trauma, as it takes into account computed tomography findings of splenic vascular injuries such as active bleeding, pseudoaneurysm, and arteriovenous fistula.[25] Current recommendations suggest that the Baltimore system should be the one utilised in modern practice.[26]

What happens when a splenic injury is diagnosed?
Once a diagnosis of splenic injury is established, the management depends on the haemodynamic status of the patient, the presence of associated injuries to other abdominal organs, and the availability of resources such as further radiological investigations or interventions. Haemodynamically unstable patients with positive FAST scans require urgent surgical exploration, with the potential to proceed to splenectomy. However, haemodynamically stable patients with low grade splenic injuries, as determined by computed tomography scanning, may be candidates for non-operative management.

What is the evidence supporting non-operative management of splenic injuries?
Non-operative management was first attempted in the paediatric population in the 1960s,[27] but it was not until the 1980s—when CT scans became more widely available—that non-operative management was adapted for adult trauma patients.[28] [29] A trend from splenectomy towards splenic conservation has been noted in many population based studies.[30] [31] [32] [33]

A recent systematic review of 21 non-randomised studies of non-operative management suggests that it now represents the gold standard treatment for minor splenic trauma and is associated with decreased mortality in severe splenic trauma (4.8% compared with 13.5% for operative management). The authors concluded, however, that for higher grades of splenic injury, the evidence is more difficult to interpret because of the substantial heterogeneity of expertise among different hospitals and potentially inappropriate comparison groups. On the basis of their interpretation of the evidence, they postulated that non-operative management can be the initial treatment in some cases of severe splenic trauma; however, the decision between operative and non-operative management depends on careful risk-benefit analysis for each patient, as well as on the expertise of the surgeon and of the multidisciplinary hospital team.[34]

What is the role of splenic angioembolisation in the management of splenic injuries?
Angioembolisation, a technique carried out in the main by interventional radiologists, uses wire-guided catheters under radiographic guidance within the vascular tree to both image and potentially occlude vessels, thus stopping

haemorrhage. Embolisation techniques include using mechanical (metal coils, embolisation particles) or chemical agents (gelfoam, sclerosant chemicals, thrombin) to achieve occlusion of a vessel either proximal or distal to the site of haemorrhage. This was first reported in the management of blunt splenic injuries in 1981.[35] Since then, large numbers of studies, none of which has been a randomised controlled trial, have been published, with varying results, outcomes, and recommendations. This paucity of high quality evidence makes forming guidelines challenging. However, American guidelines based on level II evidence suggest that patients with a grade >III injury, presence of contrast blush (intravenous contrast extravasation) on computed tomography, moderate haemoperitoneum, or evidence of ongoing splenic bleeding should be considered for splenic angioembolisation.[36]

A retrospective review in four US level 1 trauma units found that of 140 patients having splenic angioembolisation for grade IV and V injuries, 80% were successfully managed non-operatively,[37] and results have improved since then. A more recent retrospective review of 499 blunt splenic trauma patients, of whom 41 (8.2%) required splenic angioembolisation, found that this was associated with a decreased risk of splenectomy (P=0.003).[38] Similar findings were recently reported by a large multicentre series from four level 1 trauma centres in the United States, showing that centres using high volumes of angioembolisation for splenic injuries (defined as >10% of cases) have significantly higher rates of splenic salvage than those using the technique less frequently.[39]

Large case series have shown that major complications including splenic infarction, abscess formation, cyst formation, contrast induced renal impairment, and bleeding occur in 14-29% of cases and minor complications such as pyrexia, left pleural effusion, and coil migration in 34-62% of cases.[40] A recent meta-analysis of angioembolisation in 479 blunt splenic trauma patients compared the difference in outcomes between proximal and distal splenic artery embolisation.[41] Proximal embolisation was performed significantly more often than distal embolisation (60.3% v 33.2%; P<0.001), with a combination of techniques being applied in 6.5% of cases. Overall, the rate of failure of splenic angioembolisation was 10.2% (range 0-33%), and rates of failure due to re-bleeding, requiring splenectomy, ranged from 4.7% to 9.0%. This occurred more commonly, but not significantly so, after distal embolisation. The rate of major infarcts requiring splenectomy ranged from 0% to 0.5% in proximal embolisation and from 1.6% to 3.8% in distal embolisation, but again this was not statistically significant. Infectious complications requiring a splenectomy occurred in four patients, all after proximal embolisation. Minor complications occur more commonly after distal embolisation than after proximal embolisation. This is principally explained by higher rates of segmental infarctions following distal embolisation and is of little clinical relevance. The role of antibiotics after splenic angioembolisation to avoid abscess is uncertain.

Are there any intraoperative alternatives to splenectomy for management of haemodynamically stable patients?
Splenic salvage should be attempted only in haemodynamically stable patients undergoing trauma laparotomy for other injuries. In more than 97% of patients taken to theatre, splenectomy rather than splenic salvage is the outcome.[42] Salvage methods include the application of a topical haemostatic agent such as fibrin glue, which in an American case series resulted in haemostasis after one application in most patients, successful splenic salvage, and no returns to theatre.[43] This can be used in both splenic and hepatic trauma, but outcome data are lacking in the literature. The use of an absorbable polyglycolic acid mesh that is wrapped around the injured spleen to aid haemostasis and facilitate the insertion of sutures to complete haemostasis is another useful technique.[44 45] Recently, the use of a linear stapling device with the adjunct of a topical haemostatic agent to preserve part of the spleen has been described.[46] Patients who are unstable should proceed directly to laparotomy, with splenectomy if the haemorrhage is not controlled. Re-implantation of splenic tissue in an attempt to preserve immunological function is technically feasible,[47 48 49] although the true value of this in terms of immunological function and the prevention of overwhelming post-splenectomy sepsis is unproven.[50 51]

Does laparoscopy have a role in the management of splenic injuries?
The Society of American Gastrointestinal and Endoscopic Surgeons' guidelines on laparoscopy for trauma accept that diagnostic laparoscopy is technically feasible and safe when applied to selected trauma patients. This includes those with a suspected intra-abdominal injury that is not proven during imaging, who are haemodynamically stable, and without evidence of another injury requiring laparotomy. Diagnostic laparoscopy can potentially decrease the number of negative exploratory laparotomies performed.[52]

On review of the literature, only a handful of case reports and case series consider the use of laparoscopy in blunt splenic injuries. Splenic conservation with the appliance and use of haemostatic agents laparoscopically has been reported.[53 54] Several institutions have reported case series on the use of laparoscopic splenectomy in trauma.[55 56] One of the largest series from Italy included 10 consecutive patients with no mortality or morbidity related to the laparoscopic approach.[57] This is not routine practice at present.

What is the role of vaccination in patients with splenic injuries?
For patients in whom splenectomy is necessary, overwhelming post-splenectomy sepsis is a concern and has been recognised for around 40 years.[58] Current UK recommendations, based on level 2 and 3 evidence, are that vaccines should be administered either two weeks before or two weeks after splenectomy to increase the immunological benefit. Splenectomy patients or those with functional hyposplenism should receive pneumococcal vaccine, *Haemophilus influenzae* type b conjugate vaccine, and meningococcal conjugate vaccine, as well as annual influenza immunisation. Lifelong prophylactic antibiotics (oral penicillins or macrolides) should be offered to those at high risk of pneumococcal infection. The high risk group comprises patients aged under 16 years or over 50 years, those with an inadequate serological response to pneumococcal vaccination or a history of previous invasive pneumococcal disease, and those in whom a splenectomy was carried out for haematological malignancy. Counselling regarding the risks and benefits of lifelong antibiotics should be offered to patients not at high risk of infection, and a decision to discontinue may be appropriate. All splenectomy patients should carry an emergency supply of antibiotics as well as a medical alert card.[59]

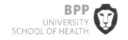
Organ injury scaling (spleen)[24]

Grade	Injury	Description
I	Haematoma	Subcapsular, <10% surface area
	Laceration	Capsular tear, <1 cm parenchymal depth
II	Haematoma	Subcapsular, 10-50% surface area; intraparenchymal, <5 cm diameter
	Laceration	1-3 cm parenchymal depth, not involving parenchymal vessel
III	Haematoma	Subcapsular, >50% surface area or expanding; ruptured subcapsular or parenchymal haematoma; intraparenchymal haematoma >5 cm
	Laceration	>3 cm parenchymal depth or involving trabecular vessels
IV	Laceration	Laceration of segmental or hilar vessels producing major devascularisation (>25% spleen)
V	Laceration	Completely shattered spleen
	Vascular	Hilar vascular injury which devascularised spleen

ADDITIONAL EDUCATIONAL RESOURCES

- The Eastern Association for the Surgery of Trauma (www.east.org/resources/treatment-guidelines/blunt-splenic-injury,-selective-nonoperative-management-of)—A review of management guidelines for healthcare professionals

- UpToDate (www.uptodate.com/contents/management-of-splenic-injury-in-the-adult-trauma-patient)—A review of splenic anatomy and physiology, and diagnostic and management strategies for splenic injuries for healthcare professionals

- National Trauma Data Bank (www.facs.org/trauma/ntdb/index.html)—American trauma database; information on trauma programmes, research, and education for healthcare professionals

- Trauma.org (www.trauma.org/archive/trauma.html)—Trauma and critical care educational resources for professionals

---

Routine immunisation for patients with splenic injuries managed conservatively is not recommended. Although concerns have been raised about splenic immune function after non-operative management with or without splenic angioembolisation, evidence seems to be emerging that immune function is reasonably well preserved. Phagocytic function of the spleen in patients who have undergone splenic angioembolisation has been measured by analysis of blood for the presence of Howell-Jolly bodies, and very few patients seem to show evidence of hyposplenism.[60][61][62]

How should patients who have had non-operative management of splenic injury be followed up?

No guidelines or follow-up protocols as to the outpatient management of patients who have had non-operative management of a splenic injury are available. In a prospective audit, no alteration in clinical management was made on the basis of repeat inpatient or outpatient imaging,[19] and a recent survey of American clinicians has shown no consensus regarding the duration of in-hospital monitoring and the timing of mobilisation and return to full activities including work and contact sports.[63] Similarly, no consensus exists on the time post-injury to start chemical venous thromboprophylaxis in the form of low molecular weight heparin; however, early use (<72 hours post-injury) does not increase the risk of failure of non-operative management.[64][65] An American case series reviewed 691 patients admitted with blunt abdominal trauma and concluded that late failure of non-operative management occurs infrequently, unpredictably, and almost always in patients who are still in hospital for associated injuries.[66]

What is the overall survival after splenic injury?

Mortality rates after splenic injury are difficult to quantify, as a proportion of trauma patients will die before admission to hospital, and many of those who die in hospital will die as a result of the overall severity of other injuries. A US cohort study of more than 33 000 trauma patients with splenic injuries found an in-hospital mortality rate of 6.1%. Mortality varied between states (2.1-9.2%).[67]

A large European cohort study of more than 13 000 trauma patients, of whom 1630 had splenic trauma, has been recently reported. Of these splenic injuries, 18.1% were grade II, 28% were grade III, 29.8% were grade IV, and 24.1% were grade V. Splenectomy was carried out in 46.5% of patients: 10.8% of grade II, 23.2% of grade III, 65.2% of grade IV, and 77.4% of grade V. In-hospital mortality after splenectomy was 24.8% compared with 22.2% in patients without splenectomy; however, the overall injury severity scores were very similar and are likely to account for the mortality rates.[68]

Contributors: DH and AB-s prepared the manuscript. NPR, RM, and FAF edited the manuscript. AJMW was responsible for the concept of the manuscript, was involved in the editing, and is the guarantor.

Competing interests: We have read and understood the BMJ Group policy on declaration of interests and declare the following interests: none.

Provenance and peer review: Not commissioned; externally peer reviewed.

1 Costa G, Tierno SM, Tomassini F, Venturini L, Frezza B, Cancrini G, et al. The epidemiology and clinical evaluation of abdominal trauma: an analysis of a multidisciplinary trauma registry. Ann Ital Chir2010;81:95-102.
2 Aubrey-Bassler FK, Sowers N. 613 cases of splenic rupture without risk factors or previously diagnosed disease: a systematic review. BMC Emerg Med2012;12:11.
3 Gutierrez G, Reines HD, Wulf-Gutierrez ME. Clinical review: hemorrhagic shock. Crit Care2004;8:373-81.
4 Schurink GW, Bode PJ, van Luijt PA, van Vugt AB. The value of physical examination in the diagnosis of patients with blunt abdominal trauma: a retrospective study. Injury1997;28:261-5.
5 Schneir A, Holmes JF. Clinical findings in patients with splenic injuries: are injuries to the left lower chest important? Cal J Emerg Med2001;2:33-6.
6 Kortbeek JB, Al Turki SA, Ali J, Antoine JA, Bouillon B, Brasel K, et al. Advanced trauma life support, 8th edition, the evidence for change. J Trauma2008;64:1638-50.
7 Boulanger BR, Kearney PA, Brenneman FD, Tsuei B, Ochoa J. Utilization of FAST (focused assessment with sonography for trauma) in 1999: results of a survey of North American trauma centers. Am Surg2000;66:1049-55.
8 Rothlin MA, Naf R, Amgwerd M, Candinas D, Frick T, Trentz O. Ultrasound in blunt abdominal and thoracic trauma. J Trauma1993;34:488-95.
9 Stengel D, Bauwens K, Sehouli J, Porzsolt F, Rademacher G, Mutze S, et al. Systematic review and meta-analysis of emergency ultrasonography for blunt abdominal trauma. Br J Surg2001;88:901-12.
10 Shuman WP, Ralls PW, Balfe DM, Bree RL, DiSantis DJ, Glick SN, et al. Imaging of blunt abdominal trauma. American College of Radiology: ACR appropriateness criteria. Radiology2000;215(suppl):143-51.
11 Smith J. Focused assessment with sonography in trauma (FAST): should its role be reconsidered? Postgrad Med J2010;86:285-91.
12 Laselle BT, Byyny RL, Haukoos JS, Krzyzaniak SM, Brooks J, Dalton TR, et al. False-negative FAST examination: associations with injury characteristics and patient outcomes. Ann Emerg Med2012;60:326-34.e3.
13 Barquist ES, Pizano LR, Feuer W, Pappas PA, McKenney KA, LeBlang SD, et al. Inter- and intrarater reliability in computed axial tomographic grading of splenic injury: why so many grading scales? J Trauma2004;56:334-8.
14 Federle MP, Griffiths B, Minagi H, Jeffrey RB Jr. Splenic trauma: evaluation with CT. Radiology1987;162:69-71.
15 Scatamacchia SA, Raptopoulos V, Fink MP, Silva WE. Splenic trauma in adults: impact of CT grading on management. Radiology1989;171:725-9.
16 Brasel KJ, DeLisle CM, Olson CJ, Borgstrom DC. Splenic injury: trends in evaluation and management. J Trauma1998;44:283-6.
17 Royal College of Radiologists. Standards of practice and guidance for trauma radiology in severely injured patients. Royal College of Radiologists, 2011.
18 Boscak AR, Shanmuganathan K, Mirvis SE, Fleiter TR, Miller LA, Sliker CW, et al. Optimizing trauma multidetector CT protocol for blunt splenic injury: need for arterial and portal venous phase scans. Radiology2013;268:79-88.
19 Shapiro MJ, Krausz C, Durham RM, Mazuski JE. Overuse of splenic scoring and computed tomographic scans. J Trauma1999;47:651-8.
20 Mirvis SE, Whitley NO, Gens DR. Blunt splenic trauma in adults: CT-based classification and correlation with prognosis and treatment. Radiology1989;171:33-9.
21 Rating the severity of tissue damage: I. The abbreviated scale. JAMA1971;215:277-80.
22 Moore EE, Moore FA. American Association for the Surgery of Trauma Organ Injury Scaling: 50th anniversary review article of the Journal of Trauma. J Trauma2010;69:1600-1.

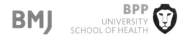

23 Moore EE, Shackford SR, Pachter HL, McAninch JW, Browner BD, Champion HR, et al. Organ injury scaling: spleen, liver, and kidney. *J Trauma*1989;29:1664-6.

24 Moore EE, Cogbill TH, Jurkovich GJ, Shackford SR, Malangoni MA, Champion HR. Organ injury scaling: spleen and liver (1994 revision). *J Trauma*1995;38:323-4.

25 Marmery H, Shanmuganathan K, Alexander MT, Mirvis SE. Optimization of selection for nonoperative management of blunt splenic injury: comparison of MDCT grading systems. *AJR Am J Roentgenol*2007;189:1421-7.

26 Olthof DC, van der Vlies CH, Scheerder MJ, de Haan RJ, Beenen LF, Goslings JC, et al. Reliability of injury grading systems for patients with blunt splenic trauma. *Injury*2014;45:146-50.

27 Upadhyaya P, Simpson JS. Splenic trauma in children. *Surg Gynecol Obstet*1968;126:781-90.

28 Mucha P Jr, Daly RC, Farnell MB. Selective management of blunt splenic trauma. *J Trauma*1986;26:970-9.

29 Longo WE, Baker CC, McMillen MA, Modlin IM, Degutis LC, Zucker KA. Nonoperative management of adult blunt splenic trauma: criteria for successful outcome. *Ann Surg*1989;210:626-9.

30 Peitzman AB, Heil B, Rivera L, Federle MB, Harbrecht BG, Clancy KD, et al. Blunt splenic injury in adults: multi-institutional study of the Eastern Association for the Surgery of Trauma. *J Trauma*2000;49:177-87, discussion 187-9.

31 Garber BG, Mmath BP, Fairfull-Smith RJ, Yelle JD. Management of adult splenic injuries in Ontario: a population-based study. *Can J Surg*2000;43:283-8.

32 Bee TK, Croce MA, Miller PR, Pritchard FE, Fabian TC. Failures of splenic nonoperative management: is the glass half empty or half full? *J Trauma*2001;50:230-6.

33 Velmahos GC, Zacharias N, Emhoff TA, Feeney JM, Hurst JM, Crookes BA, et al. Management of the most severely injured spleen: a multicenter study of the Research Consortium of New England Centers for Trauma (ReCONECT). *Arch Surg*2010;145:456-60.

34 Cirocchi R, Boselli C, Corsi A, Farinella E, Listorti C, Trastulli S, et al. Is non-operative management safe and effective for all splenic blunt trauma? A systematic review. *Crit Care*2013;17:R185.

35 Sclafani SJ. The role of angiographic hemostasis in salvage of the injured spleen. *Radiology*1981;141:645-50.

36 Stassen NA, Bhullar I, Cheng JD, Crandall ML, Friese RS, Guillamondegui OD, et al. Selective nonoperative management of blunt splenic injury: an Eastern Association for the Surgery of Trauma practice management guideline. *J Trauma Acute Care Surg*2012;73(5 suppl 4):S294-300.

37 Haan JM, Biffl W, Knudson MM, Davis KA, Oka T, Majercik S, et al. Splenic embolization revisited: a multicenter review. *J Trauma*2004;56:542-7.

38 Jeremitsky E, Kao A, Carlton C, Rodriguez A, Ong A. Does splenic embolization and grade of splenic injury impact nonoperative management in patients sustaining blunt splenic trauma? *Am Surg*2011;77:215-20.

39 Banerjee A, Duane TM, Wilson SP, Haney S, O'Neill PJ, Evans HL, et al. Trauma center variation in splenic artery embolization and spleen salvage: a multicenter analysis. *J Trauma Acute Care Surg*2013;75:69-74, discussion 74-5.

40 Ekeh AP, Khalaf S, Ilyas S, Kauffman S, Walusimbi M, McCarthy MC. Complications arising from splenic artery embolization: a review of an 11-year experience. *Am J Surg*2013;205:250-4, discussion 254.

41 Schnuriger B, Inaba K, Konstantinidis A, Lustenberger T, Chan LS, Demetriades D. Outcomes of proximal versus distal splenic artery embolization after trauma: a systematic review and meta-analysis. *J Trauma*2011;70:252-60.

42 Renzulli P, Gross T, Schnuriger B, Schoepfer AM, Inderbitzin D, Exadaktylos AK, et al. Management of blunt injuries to the spleen. *Br J Surg*2010;97:1696-703.

43 Ochsner MG, Maniscalco-Theberge ME, Champion HR. Fibrin glue as a hemostatic agent in hepatic and splenic trauma. *J Trauma*1990;30:884-7.

44 Delany HM, Ivatury RR, Blau SA, Gleeson M, Simon R, Stahl WM. Use of biodegradable (PGA) fabric for repair of solid organ injury: a combined institution experience. *Injury*1993;24:585-9.

45 Louredo AM, Alonso A, de Llano JJA, Diez LM, Alvarez JL, del Riego FJ. Usefulness of absorbable meshes in the management of splenic trauma. *Cir Esp*2005;77:145-52.

46 Costamagna D, Rizzi S, Zampogna A, Alonzo A. Open partial splenectomy for trauma using GIA-Stapler and FloSeal matrix haemostatic agent. *BMJ Case Rep*2010;2010:10.1136/bcr.01.2010.2601.

47 Millikan JS, Moore EE, Moore GE, Stevens RE. Alternatives to splenectomy in adults after trauma: repair, partial resection, and reimplantation of splenic tissue. *Am J Surg*1982;144:711-6.

48 Weber T, Hanisch E, Baum RP, Seufert RM. Late results of heterotopic autotransplantation of splenic tissue into the greater omentum. *World J Surg*1998;22:883-9.

49 Leemans R, Manson W, Snijder JA, Smit JW, Klasen HJ, The TH, et al. Immune response capacity after human splenic autotransplantation: restoration of response to individual pneumococcal vaccine subtypes. *Ann Surg*1999;229:279-85.

50 Ludtke FE, Mack SC, Schuff-Werner P, Voth E. Splenic function after splenectomy for trauma: role of autotransplantation and splenosis. *Acta Chir Scand*1989;155:533-9.

51 Pisters PW, Pachter HL. Autologous splenic transplantation for splenic trauma. *Ann Surg*1994;219:225-35.

52 Hori Y, SAGES Guidelines Committee. Diagnostic laparoscopy guidelines: this guideline was prepared by the SAGES Guidelines Committee and reviewed and approved by the Board of Governors of the Society of American Gastrointestinal and Endoscopic Surgeons (SAGES), November 2007. *Surg Endosc*2008;22:1353-83.

53 Shen HB, Lu XM, Zheng QC, Cai XT, Zhou H, Fei KL. Clinical application of laparoscopic spleen-preserving operation in traumatic spleen rupture. *Chin J Traumatol*2005;8:293-6.

54 Orcalli F, Elio A, Veronese E, Frigo F, Salvato S, Residori C. Conservative laparoscopy in the treatment of posttraumatic splenic laceration using microfiber hemostatic collagen: three case histories. *Surg Laparosc Endosc*1998;8:445-8.

55 Nasr WI, Collins CL, Kelly JJ. Feasibility of laparoscopic splenectomy in stable blunt trauma: a case series. *J Trauma*2004;57:887-9.

56 Huscher CG, Mingoli A, Sgarzini G, Brachini G, Ponzano C, Di Paola M, et al. Laparoscopic treatment of blunt splenic injuries: initial experience with 11 patients. *Surg Endosc*2006;20:1423-6.

57 Carobbi A, Romagnani F, Antonelli G, Bianchini M. Laparoscopic splenectomy for severe blunt trauma: initial experience of ten consecutive cases with a fast hemostatic technique. *Surg Endosc*2010;24:1325-30.

58 Singer DB. Postsplenectomy sepsis. *Perspect Pediatr Pathol*1973;1:285-311.

59 Davies JM, Lewis MP, Wimperis J, Rafi I, Ladhani S, Bolton-Maggs PH, et al. Review of guidelines for the prevention and treatment of infection in patients with an absent or dysfunctional spleen: prepared on behalf of the British Committee for Standards in Haematology by a working party of the Haemato-Oncology task force. *Br J Haematol*2011;155:308-17.

60 Bessoud B, Duchosal MA, Siegrist CA, Schlegel S, Doenz F, Calmes JM, et al. Proximal splenic artery embolization for blunt splenic injury: clinical, immunologic, and ultrasound-Doppler follow-up. *J Trauma*2007;62:1481-6.

61 Pirasteh A, Snyder LL, Lin R, Rosenblum D, Reed S, Sattar A, et al. Temporal assessment of splenic function in patients who have undergone percutaneous image-guided splenic artery embolization in the setting of trauma. *J Vasc Interv Radiol*2012;23:80-2.

62 Skattum J, Naess PA, Gaarder C. Non-operative management and immune function after splenic injury. *Br J Surg*2012;99(suppl 1):59-65.

63 Fata P, Robinson L, Fakhry SM. A survey of EAST member practices in blunt splenic injury: a description of current trends and opportunities for improvement. *J Trauma*2005;59:836-41, discussion 841-2.

64 Eberle BM, Schnuriger B, Inaba K, Cestero R, Kobayashi L, Barmparas G, et al. Thromboembolic prophylaxis with low-molecular-weight heparin in patients with blunt solid abdominal organ injuries undergoing nonoperative management: current practice and outcomes. *J Trauma*2011;70:141-6, discussion 147.

65 Alejandro KV, Acosta JA, Rodriguez PA. Bleeding manifestations after early use of low-molecular-weight heparins in blunt splenic injuries. *Am Surg*2003;69:1006-9.

66 Crawford RS, Tabbara M, Sheridan R, Spaniolas K, Velmahos GC. Early discharge after nonoperative management for splenic injuries: increased patient risk caused by late failure? *Surgery*2007;142:337-42.

67 Hamlat CA, Arbabi S, Koepsell TD, Maier RV, Jurkovich GJ, Rivara FP. National variation in outcomes and costs for splenic injury and the impact of trauma systems: a population-based cohort study. *Ann Surg*2012;255:165-70.

68 Heuer M, Taeger G, Kaiser GM, Nast-Kolb D, Kuhne CA, Ruchholtz S, et al. No further incidence of sepsis after splenectomy for severe trauma: a multi-institutional experience of the trauma registry of the DGU with 1,630 patients. *Eur J Med Res*2010;15:258-65.

Related links

bmj.com
- Get Cleveland Clinic CME credits for this article

bmj.com/archive
Previous articles in this series
- Fungal nail infection: diagnosis and management (BMJ 2014;348:g1800)
- Endometriosis (BMJ 2014;348:g1752)
- Management of sickle cell disease in the community (BMJ 2014;348:g1765)
- Coeliac disease (BMJ 2014;348:g1561)
- Fibromyalgia (BMJ 2014;348:g1224)

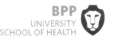

Islet transplantation in type 1 diabetes

Hanneke de Kort, research fellow[1],

Eelco J de Koning, associate professor, head of clinical islet transplantation programme[234],

Ton J Rabelink, professor of medicine, chair of department of nephrology[2],

Jan A Bruijn, professor immunopathology[1],

Ingeborg M Bajema, renal and transplantation pathologist[1]

[1]Department of Pathology, Leiden University Medical Centre, 2300 RC Leiden, Netherlands

[2]Department of Nephrology, Leiden University Medical Centre

[3]Department of Endocrinology, Leiden University Medical Centre

[4]Hubrecht Institute, Uppsalalaan 8, 3584 CT Utrecht, Netherlands

Correspondence to: E J P de Koning
e.dekoning@lumc.nl

Cite this as: BMJ 2011;342:d217

DOI: 10.1136/bmj.d217

http://www.bmj.com/content/342/bmj.d217

A clinical review in the BMJ in 2001 anticipated that by 2010 transplantation of islets of Langerhans would be the treatment of choice for most patients with type 1 diabetes.[1] Currently, islet transplantation is an option for a specific group of patients with type 1 diabetes only—those with severe glycaemic lability, recurrent hypoglycaemia, and hypoglycaemia unawareness. Patients with type 1 diabetes—who must deal with daily subcutaneous insulin injections, regular finger pricks for glucose measurements, and worries about hypoglycaemic episodes and long term complications of diabetes, hope for a cure for their disease and may ask their doctors about islet transplantation. Therefore, doctors who treat such patients should understand the potential benefits of islet transplantation as well as the hurdles that need to be overcome before it is widely used (box 1).

Why islet transplantation?

Type 1 diabetes is caused by the autoimmune destruction of insulin producing β cells in the pancreatic islets of Langerhans. A well defined worldwide population based survey showed that the incidence of childhood onset type 1 diabetes is rising rapidly, with an overall annual increase of 3.4% between 1995 and 1999.[2] A multicentre prospective registration study from Europe predicted that the number of prevalent cases of type 1 diabetes in children below the age of 15 will increase by 81% from 18 500 in 2005 to 33 500 in 2020 in the United Kingdom.[w1] For patients with type 1 diabetes, exogenous insulin administration to control blood glucose is a lifesaving treatment, but it also has a negative impact on personal and social functioning, not least because of the daily risk of hypoglycaemic episodes. In addition, normoglycaemia cannot be achieved by exogenous insulin and secondary complications such as retinopathy, neuropathy, nephropathy, and cardiovascular disease occur despite good glycaemic control.[3] [4] Consequently, patients with type 1 diabetes face living with the long term debilitating consequences of their disease.

Pancreatic islets constitute only 1-2% of the pancreas. They consist of clusters of mainly hormone producing cells (fig 1), with insulin producing β cells being the most abundant cell type.[5] Replacement of β cells is the only

SOURCES AND SELECTION CRITERIA

We searched PubMed, Embase, Web of Science, Cochrane, CINAHL, Academic Search Premier, and ScienceDirect using the keyword "islet transplantation". We limited our search to the English language and to human studies. We found no randomised controlled trials, and most publications lacked an appropriate control group that was intensively managed by insulin using modern treatment regimens. Data were mainly derived from case series, follow-up studies, crossover studies, and small trials. We also consulted published reviews and expert knowledge if considered necessary.

treatment capable of normalising glycaemia without the risk of hypoglycaemia because β cells respond to changes in glucose concentrations by subtly adjusting insulin secretion to maintain glucose homoeostasis.

Whole pancreas transplantation, a form of β cell replacement that has been performed since 1966, is a major surgical procedure with considerable peri-transplant complications and post-transplant morbidity related to the transplantation of superfluous exocrine pancreatic tissue. Islet transplantation, however, is minimally invasive and has low morbidity because the islets are infused percutaneously via a catheter into the hepatic portal vein. Figures 2 and 3 illustrate the complex processes of islet isolation and transplantation.

Who is eligible?

Islet transplantation has not become a mainstream treatment for type 1 diabetes largely because of a shortage of (high quality) donor organs for islet isolation, the high costs of isolation procedures and maintenance of a specialised human islet isolation laboratory, and the need for lifelong use of immunosuppressive agents. Islet transplantation is therefore usually reserved for a highly selective group of patients with severe glycaemic lability, recurrent hypoglycaemia, and a reduced ability to sense hypoglycaemic symptoms (reduced hypoglycaemia awareness). A cross sectional Danish-British multicentre survey found that patients with type 1 diabetes have an average of 1.3 severe hypoglycaemic episodes per patient year.[w2] However, the distribution was highly distorted, with about 5% of patients accounting for 54% of all reported episodes. Because islet transplantation improves recipients' hypoglycaemia awareness and reduces the frequency of hypoglycaemic episodes in the long term, this subgroup of patients would probably benefit most from the procedure. Islet transplantation is not a treatment option for type 2 diabetes, which is caused mainly by insulin resistance, with patients usually having considerable remaining islet function.

Most patients who undergo islet transplantation participate in clinical research studies with varying inclusion criteria. Inadequate glycaemic control with recurrent hypoglycaemia is the entry criterion most often used. However, because microvascular and perhaps macrovascular complications have

SUMMARY POINTS

- Islet of Langerhans transplantation is used in a select group of patients with type 1 diabetes with severe glycaemic lability, recurrent hypoglycaemia, and hypoglycaemia unawareness

- The procedure is minimally invasive, with few procedure related complications

- Two to three islet infusions are usually needed to achieve insulin independence

- Most patients need insulin by five years post-transplantation owing to declining graft function; beneficial effects on the frequency of hypoglycaemic episodes and hypoglycaemia awareness remain

- Most long term complications are related to systemic immunosuppression

- The risk-benefit ratio of islet transplantation should be carefully weighed by the treating physician and the potential recipient, who should be given adequate information

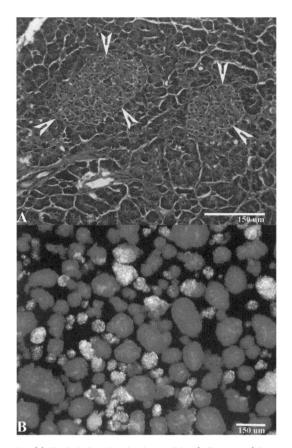

Fig 1 (A) Histological section showing two islets (yellow arrows) in the pancreas. (B) Isolated islets stain red with dithizone; non-islet (exocrine) tissue is yellow. Image B courtesy of Marten Engelse, Human Islet Isolation Facility, Leiden University Medical Centre, Netherlands

stabilised in some recipients of islet transplantation, studies that focus on microvascular complications and inadequate glycaemic control rather than hypoglycaemia related problems have begun. A retrospective cohort study found that islet transplantation may also prolong the survival of a previous kidney graft.[8] For these patients, who already receive immunosuppressive agents, the clinical decision to perform islet transplantation is influenced by a different risk-benefit ratio. In the UK, islet transplantation is now funded by the

> **BOX 1 WHAT GENERAL PRACTITIONERS NEED TO KNOW**
>
> - Most patients with type 1 diabetes do not fit the criteria for islet transplantation
> - It is not a treatment option for patients with type 2 diabetes, who usually have insulin resistance and considerable remaining islet function
> - Patients who have undergone successful islet transplantation usually have greatly improved hypoglycaemia awareness and experience fewer hypoglycaemic episodes
> - Although insulin independence can be achieved, most patients will ultimately have to resume insulin treatment, but the frequency of hypoglycaemic episodes remains reduced
> - Islet transplantation can improve glycaemic control and reduce risk of progression of vascular complications
> - The clinical problems related to long term use of immunosuppressive agents include drug interactions, infections, and an increased risk of certain cancers

NHS and is particularly indicated for patients with reduced hypoglycaemia awareness or those taking immunosuppressive drugs because of a previous kidney transplant.

How do we define success of islet transplantation?

Observations from long term studies triggered a debate about how to define the "success" of islet transplantation. Historically, the primary goal of islet transplantation has been the ability of donor islets to maintain normal glucose control and removal of the need for exogenous insulin. "Insulin independence" is a comprehensible clinical outcome parameter for success, but success can also be measured in terms of frequency of hypoglycaemic episodes and positive effects on vascular complications or quality of life.[9] Researchers found that islet transplantation often could not achieve long term insulin independence. Patients with this "partial graft function" have persistent insulin secretion from β cells but require additional oral or subcutaneous antihyperglycaemic agents, such as insulin. A retrospective cohort study found that the hypoglycaemia score (measure of severity of hypoglycaemia) of 31 islet transplant recipients was significantly reduced from 5.29 (standard deviation 1.51) before transplantation to 1.35 (1.92) at an average 47

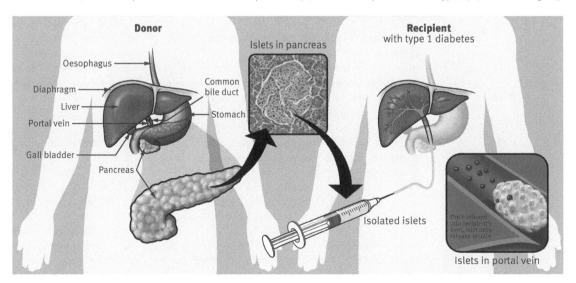

Fig 2 Process of clinical islet transplantation for the treatment of type 1 diabetes (adapted from Naftanel and Harlan[6])

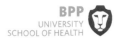

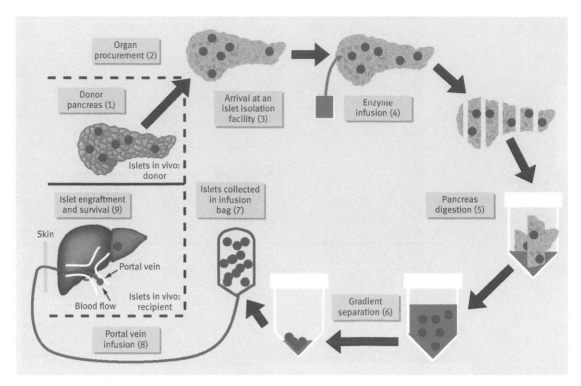

Fig 3 The islet isolation and transplantation procedure. Islet isolation from a donor pancreas is laborious, time consuming, and costly. A donor pancreas (1) is allocated to a potential recipient on the waiting list, procured (2), and transported to an islet isolation facility (3), which adheres to good manufacturing practice guidelines (box 2). At the facility, enzyme is infused into the pancreatic duct (4) and the islets are separated from the exocrine pancreatic tissue by combined enzymatic and mechanic digestion (5), then purified by density gradient centrifugation (6). Reported numbers of isolated islets vary greatly; an estimated 300 000 to 600 000 islet equivalents (mathematical conversion of varying islet sizes to equal a standardised islet of 150 µm in diameter) can be isolated from one pancreas.[7] The actual number depends on the number of islets in the donor pancreas and the islet yield after isolation. Most centres culture the islets in incubators for several hours to several days to perform safety and viability tests and prepare the recipients. Shortly before transplantation the islets are collected in an infusion bag (7). Transplantation involves the infusion of pancreatic islets into the hepatic portal vein (8). Access to the portal vein is usually achieved by ultrasound guided percutaneous catheterisation under local anaesthesia. The islets are infused over 10-30 minutes and embolise the small branches of the portal vein. Patients usually stay in hospital for several days. The islets will engraft in the recipient liver (9) and begin to function.

months after transplantation, indicating a substantial benefit even with partial graft failure and subsequent loss of insulin independence.[w3] Partial graft function has been shown to be associated with reduced frequency and severity of hypoglycaemic episodes and increased quality of life.[9] Today, most clinicians regard an absence of severe hypoglycaemic episodes and return of hypoglycaemia awareness as indicators of successful islet transplantation.

What results have clinical islet transplantation studies shown?

There are currently about 1000 recipients of islet transplantations worldwide. No randomised controlled trials have evaluated the effectiveness of the intervention. Small observational studies have been heterogeneous in their design. We review the best evidence from relatively large studies performed in established centres. Most studies report on patients with type 1 diabetes who had glycaemic lability, recurrent hypoglycaemia, and hypoglycaemia unawareness despite optimal self management. We focus on outcome parameters in terms of insulin independence and effects on vascular complications, quality of life, and patient survival.

Insulin independence

In 2000 a landmark case series reported on seven patients one year after islet transplantation. The seven recipients had remained insulin independent for an average of 11 months. The results of this small study were enthusiastically received.[1]

[10] It also became clear, however, that most patients needed two to three donor islet infusions to achieve insulin independence and that insulin independence was rarely sustained. Follow-up of a larger cohort of 65 patients reported in 2005 showed that insulin independence was present in about 69% at one year, 37% at two years, and 7.5% at five years. However, C peptide—a measure of insulin secretion (for every molecule of insulin, one molecule of C peptide is released from β cells)—was detected in 82% of subjects, indicating persistent but insufficient islet graft function at the end of this study.[11] More recently, in a cohort of 14 patients, about 64% were insulin independent and 83% had detectable C peptide at two years of follow-up.[12] The multicentre voluntary Collaborative Islet Transplant Registry (CITR) reported on 412 allograft recipients recruited from 1999 to 2008 with three year follow-up data for 257 islet transplant recipients.[w4] At three years, about 27% of recipients were insulin independent, C peptide was detected in about 57%, and 16% of the patient data were missing.[w4] Thus, long term partial graft function seems to continue and be expressed clinically by more stable glucose control and lower insulin requirements. Indicators of declining islet graft function in patients who have resumed insulin administration are worsening of glycaemic control, higher insulin demand, and a reduction in C peptide concentrations. Recent trials using a single islet infusion and new immunosuppressive protocols showed promising results at one year.[w5 w6] After one islet infusion all five patients treated with a belatacept based immunosuppressive regimen were insulin independent at one year.[w5]

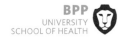

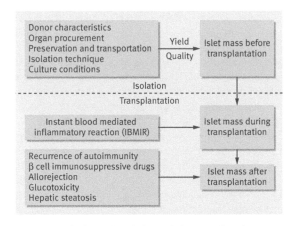

Fig 4 Islet loss before, during, and after transplantation

Vascular complications

Islet transplantation is associated with improvement or stabilisation in microvascular complications (neuropathy, retinopathy, and nephropathy) and cardiovascular outcome parameters.[8][13][14] An important clinical question, however, is whether it reduces microvascular complications more effectively than optimal glycaemic control achieved by subcutaneous insulin administration. Because no randomised controlled trials have been performed, we report the findings of one study of 42 patients that compared the effect of islet transplantation versus intensive medical treatment on microvascular complications using a one way crossover design.[14] This study found that islet transplantation improved glycated haemoglobin (6.6 (0.7) v 7.5 (0.9)), halted progression of retinopathy (0/51 v 10/82 eyes), and stabilised glomerular filtration rate compared with intensive medical treatment. In a prospective study of 44 patients with type 1 diabetes and previous kidney transplantation, islet transplantation performed in 24 patients improved kidney graft survival at six years compared with kidney transplantation alone (86% v 42% kidney graft survival, respectively).[8] Improved cardiovascular function after islet transplantation was shown in the same patient group.[13]

Quality of life

Several groups have studied the effect of islet transplantation on health related quality of life.[w7][w8] Recipients of islet transplants have indicated that stable glucose control and absence of hypoglycaemic episodes are the most beneficial outcomes of the procedure, providing a feeling of reliability and improved independence.[w9]

Patient survival

Whole pancreas transplantation has been shown to improve patient survival.[w10] Because of the small number (about 1000) of patients who have undergone islet transplantation worldwide, the short length of follow-up, and the small size of individual studies, it is not yet known whether islet transplantation improves survival.

What affects outcomes?

Box 3 and fig 4 list some of the factors that can lead to the loss of islets of Langerhans before, during, and after transplantation.

Pretransplantation and peritransplantation factors

Although glucose concentrations immediately normalise after successful whole pancreas transplantation, glucose lowering after islet transplantation is delayed. This is probably because an insufficient number of functional β cells are transplanted. A single islet infusion—the islets of one donor—is often insufficient to establish normoglycaemia. Donor characteristics, the procurement of the donor pancreas, pancreas preservation during transportation, the islet isolation procedure used, and culture conditions have important effects on the number and quality of transplantable islets.[w11] A substantial loss of islets is also thought to occur during transplantation,[w12] mainly because direct contact of islets with blood components in the hepatic portal system triggers an immediate blood mediated inflammatory reaction.[w13] Thus, often an inadequate or marginally adequate islet mass reaches the liver tissue. Several measures can help avoid this loss of functional islet mass, such as administration of heparin during and after transplantation[w14] and perioperative delivery of anti-inflammatory agents.[w15] Still, many experts believe that the best way to improve the outcome of islet transplantation would be to prevent inflammatory reactions during and immediately after islet transplantation.

Post-transplantation factors

After infusion into the portal vein, the islets travel to the liver. Here they need to adjust to their new environment and also face adverse conditions. The islets are immediately exposed to drugs and nutrients, such as glucose, which are present in higher concentrations in the portal system than in the peripheral circulation, and which can negatively affect islet function. One of the obvious potential problems is acute rejection, for which immunosuppressive drugs

---

BOX 2 GOOD MANUFACTURING PRACTICE

Good manufacturing practice is part of a quality system for the manufacturing and testing of foods, diagnostics, active drug ingredients, drug products, and medical devices. Islets of Langerhans, as a drug and biological product, are included in this quality system. In Europe, fewer than 15 islet isolation facilities currently generate islets for transplantation. Good manufacturing practice guidelines and enforcement are subject to country or continent specific legislation (see websites below).

- World Health Organization (www.who.int/medicines/areas/quality_safety/quality_assurance/production/en/)
- European Union (http://ec.europa.eu/enterprise/sectors/pharmaceuticals/documents/eudralex/index_en.htm)
- United States (www.fda.gov/Food/GuidanceComplianceRegulatoryInformation/CurrentGoodManufacturingPracticesCGMPs/default.htm)
- Canada (www.hc-sc.gc.ca/dhp-mps/compli-conform/gmp-bpf/index-eng.php)
- Australia (www.tga.gov.au/docs/html/gmpcodau.htm)

BOX 3 FACTORS THAT CONTRIBUTE TO ISLET LOSS BEFORE, DURING, AND AFTER TRANSPLANTATION

Factors affecting islet yield and quality

- Donor characteristics
- Organ procurement
- Preservation and transportation
- Isolation technique
- Culture conditions

Factors contributing to loss of transplanted cell mass during and after transplantation

- Immediate blood mediated inflammatory reaction
- Recurrence of autoimmunity
- Toxicity of immunosuppressive drugs
- Allorejection
- Glucotoxicity
- Hepatic steatosis

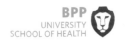

are given. Unfortunately, some immunosuppressive drugs, such as calcineurin inhibitors and steroids, interfere with β cell function.[w16] Measures that can help to give the islets a favourable start include using immunosuppressive drugs that have little effect on glucose metabolism and strict glycaemic control to avoid glucotoxicity.[w14] In addition, alternative implantation sites are being sought to avoid triggering the immediate blood mediated inflammatory reaction and the toxic drug levels found in the liver, and at the same time optimise vascularisation of the transplanted tissue.[15] Recently, islets have also been transplanted in human forearm muscle.[w17] The omental pouch, bone marrow, and implants consisting of islets within a biomaterial structure (scaffolds). are other potential transplantation sites.[15] Islet revascularisation occurs within several weeks, but the intra-islet vascular network is less developed in islets transplanted into the liver than in eutopic pancreatic islets.[w18] Thus, if not rejected early, the islet graft may not reach maximal efficacy with respect to glucose metabolism until one to three months after transplantation.

After one to three months islet efficacy becomes apparent, but on average only half of patients remain insulin independent at 15 months.[9] Chronic allograft rejection is a potential cause of long term graft failure.[16] Autoimmunity may also recur because islet recipients with positive T cell responses to autoantigens are more likely to lose full graft function.[w19] Furthermore, the long term toxic effects of immunosuppressive drugs on β cells are probably of considerable importance.[w16]

In patients who remain insulin independent after islet transplantation, a substantial portion of β cell mass may already have been destroyed before glucose concentrations start to rise. The absence of methods to monitor β cell mass, or alloimmune and autoimmune reactivity against β cells, render the intrahepatic grafted islets a "black box." Whereas in whole organ transplantation, biopsies provide information on potential problems such as rejection, ischaemia, and immunosuppressive toxicity, it is difficult to biopsy the islets dispersed throughout the liver. Liver biopsies have been performed to evaluate transplanted islets by light microscopy.[w18] However, this is an invasive procedure with low islet sampling rates and lack of reference values, which has limited value in clinical practice. Consequently, when islet function decreases and glucose concentrations rise over time there is little basis for intervention strategies other than re-evaluating the need for immunosuppressive drugs that negatively affect glucose metabolism and the use of glucose lowering agents. Therefore, current research is focused on increasing the functional β cell mass before, during, and after transplantation and on improving the functional assessment of grafted islets.[w20]

What are the potential complications of islet transplantation?

Complications can occur early (procedure related) or late (usually related to the use of immunosuppressives). Reports of early procedure related complications have come from different centres with a variety of expertise that have performed varying numbers of transplants. We try to give an indication of how often complications arise, how to monitor them, and how to try to prevent them.

Short term procedure related complications
Islet transplantation is a minimally invasive procedure compared with whole pancreas transplantation. Few detrimental procedure related complications exist. Hepatic

bleeding during transhepatic portal vein catheterisation occurs in about 12% of infusions,[11] but this has become less common with the use of fibrin sealant, Gelfoam pledgets, or coils to seal the catheter tract on withdrawal of the catheter.[17] Hepatic bleeding into the peritoneal cavity usually resolves spontaneously. Only rarely is surgery needed and no detrimental effect on graft survival has been reported. The infusion of foreign cell material into the portal system inevitably poses a risk for portal vein thrombosis. In an experienced centre this complication occurred in less than 4% of islet infusions.[11] Low dose heparin, given prophylactically during and after transplantation, limits the risk of portal vein thrombosis and carries an acceptable increased risk of bleeding. The liver parenchyma surrounding the new islets is temporarily damaged, but this is entirely reversible probably because of the excellent regenerative capacity of the liver. Resolution of the damage can be monitored by measuring liver enzyme concentrations after transplantation.

Long term complications
Similar to other transplants, long term complications are mostly related to the side effects of systemic immunosuppressive agents. Systemic immunosuppression increases the risk of infections and cancers, particularly virus related skin cancers and certain lymphoproliferative disorders. The most widely used agents in organ transplantation are calcineurin inhibitors. Unfortunately, these agents also have a nephrotoxic effect, which increases the risk of worsening renal function, especially in patients with diabetic nephropathy. The risk of complications can be reduced and their early management ensured by monitoring drug concentrations to prevent overdosing, using measures to prevent and recognise the development of infections, having a low threshold for starting antibiotics and antivirals in transplant recipients, and regularly checking for dermatological complications.

Organ transplantation can lead to the formation of anti-HLA antibodies. Recipients of islet transplants are usually exposed to a wide range of HLA antigens from multiple donors because over time they usually receive several islet infusions matched for ABO blood group only.[18] Although antibodies to donor derived HLA antigens are detected in only a minority of islet transplant recipients taking immunosuppressive drugs, patients taken off these drugs, either because of transplant failure or immunosuppressive related toxicity, show an increase in these antibodies.[18] This is important in patients who develop end stage diabetic nephropathy and require kidney transplantation because the presence of anti-HLA antibodies limits the chance of finding an acceptable donor kidney. Currently, we have no way to prevent the development of such antibodies.

What should I tell my patient who asks about this procedure?
Islet transplantation has been shown to be beneficial for a specific group of patients with type 1 diabetes who have severe glycaemic lability, recurrent hypoglycaemia, and hypoglycaemic unawareness, although lifelong use of immunosuppressive drugs is necessary. The lack of randomised control trials prevents a thorough comparison between this procedure and best medical practice (intensive insulin treatment) or pancreas transplantation. This lack of evidence has led to scepticism about the clinical value of this procedure among some diabetologists.[19] Currently the initial goal of long term insulin independence is achieved by only a small proportion of patients—an important message

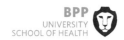

ADDITIONAL EDUCATIONAL RESOURCES

Additional resources for healthcare professionals

- Fiorina P, Shapiro AM, Ricordi C, Secchi A. The clinical impact of islet transplantation. *Am J Transplant* 2008;8:1990-7
- Bretzel R, Jahr H, Eckhard M, Martin I, Winter D, Brendel M. Islet cell transplantation today. *Langenbecks Arch Surg* 2007;392:239-53
- Low G, Hussein N, Owen RJT, Toso C, Patel VH, Bhargava R, et al. Role of imaging in clinical islet transplantation. *Radiographics* 2010;30:353-66
- Collaborative Islet Transplant Registry (www.citregistry.org/)—Map of affiliated transplant centres and regular updates on all recipients registered
- Lecture by L Fernandez of the University of Wisconsin on islet of Langerhans transplantation. http://videos.med.wisc.edu/videoInfo.php?videoid=1112
- Animation on islet cell isolation. www.youtube.com/watch?v=aMNKu-ZVUls
- European Association for the Study of Diabetes. Stem cells to cure diabetes: where do we stand? http://webcast.easd.org/Halban/index.htm

Additional resources for patients

- Diabetes UK (www.diabetes.org.uk/Research/Islet_cell_transplantation/)—Comprehensive information on the islet transplantation procedure and eligibility criteria
- National Institutes of Health (http://diabetes.niddk.nih.gov/dm/pubs/pancreaticislet/)—More detailed information with links to USA based clinical trials
- Juvenile Diabetes Research Foundation (www.jdrf.org.au/living-with-type-1-diabetes/what-is-type-1-diabetes)—Website on what type 1 diabetes is and how you can help further research in this area

ONGOING RESEARCH AND UNANSWERED QUESTIONS

- How can the islet yield be improved to decrease the number of donors needed for one successful transplant?[20]
- Identifying the best islet implantation site and technique that will result in an optimally functioning graft[15]
- How can biomaterials be used to create alternative transplantation sites?
- Which in vitro tests can best predict in vivo functioning of transplanted islets?[21]
- What alternative cell sources (such as embryonic stem cells or tissue specific progenitor cells) can be used to overcome the shortage of donor organs?[22]
- What immunosuppressive strategies are less toxic to β cells?
- Can tolerance be induced by cellular immunotherapy, thereby making immunosuppressants obsolete?[23]
- What are the key factors in long term islet allograft failure?
- How can islet mass be visualised and monitored?[24]
- How can long term islet function be improved?

to communicate to potential recipients. However, the select group of patients treated with islet transplantation has shown improved glycaemic control, reduced frequency of hypoglycaemic episodes, and reduced rate of progression of vascular complications. Researchers now need to identify factors that will lead to better graft survival and function.

Conclusion

Although progression in the islet transplantation field is not as rapid as was envisaged,[1] the pitfalls and difficulties of this procedure are now clearly identified, and advances in islet isolation, transplantation, and patient management are likely to improve the clinical outcome of islet transplantation in years to come.

Contributors: Jan W Schoones, a trained librarian, helped compose our search strategy. We thank Bart L Hogewind, Bob A van Es, and Danielle Cohen for critical reading of the manuscript. IMB had the idea for the paper. HdK, EJdK, and IMB planned the content and wrote the first draft. JAB and TJR redrafted the manuscript. HdK, EJdK, and IMB produced the final manuscript. All authors are guarantors.

Funding: None received.

Competing interests: All authors have completed the Unified Competing Interest form at www.icmje.org/coi_disclosure.pdf (available on request from the corresponding author) and declare: no support from any organisation for the submitted work; no financial relationships with any organisations that might have an interest in the submitted work in the previous three years; no other relationships or activities that could appear to have influenced the submitted work.

Provenance and peer review: Not commissioned; externally peer reviewed.

1. Serup P, Madsen OD, Mandrup-Poulsen T. Science, medicine, and the future: islet and stem cell transplantation for treating diabetes. *BMJ* 2001;322:29-32.
2. DIAMOND Project Group. Incidence and trends of childhood type 1 diabetes worldwide 1990-1999. *Diabet Med* 2006;23:857-66.
3. The Diabetes Control and Complications Trial Research Group. The effect of intensive treatment of diabetes on the development and progression of long-term complications in insulin-dependent diabetes mellitus. *N Engl J Med* 1993;329:977-86.
4. Nathan DM, Cleary PA, Backlund JY, Genuth SM, Lachin JM, Orchard TJ, et al; Diabetes Control and Complications Trial/Epidemiology of Diabetes Interventions and Complications (DCCT/EDIC) Study Research Group. Intensive diabetes treatment and cardiovascular disease in patients with type 1 diabetes. *N Engl J Med* 2005;353:2643-53.
5. Leibiger IB, Leibiger B, Berggren PO. Insulin signaling in the pancreatic beta-cell. *Annu Rev Nutr* 2008;28:233-51.
6. Naftanel MA, Harlan DM. Pancreatic islet transplantation. *PLoS Med* 2004;1:e58.
7. Korsgren O, Nilsson B, Berne C, Felldin M, Foss A, Kallen R, et al. Current status of clinical islet transplantation. *Transplantation* 2005;79:1289-93.
8. Fiorina P, Venturini M, Folli F, Losio C, Maffi P, Placidi C, et al. Natural history of kidney graft survival, hypertrophy, and vascular function in end-stage renal disease type 1 diabetic kidney-transplanted patients: beneficial impact of pancreas and successful islet cotransplantation. *Diabetes Care* 2005;28:1303-10.
9. Robertson RP. Islet transplantation a decade later and strategies for filling a half-full glass. *Diabetes* 2010;59:1285-91.
10. Shapiro AMJ, Lakey JRT, Ryan EA, Korbutt GS, Toth E, Warnock GL, et al. Islet transplantation in seven patients with type 1 diabetes mellitus using a glucocorticoid-free immunosuppressive regimen. *N Engl J Med* 2000;343:230-8.
11. Ryan EA, Paty BW, Senior PA, Bigam D, Alfadhli E, Kneteman NM, et al. Five-year follow-up after clinical islet transplantation. *Diabetes* 2005;54:2060-9.
12. Vantyghem MC, Kerr-Conte J, Arnalsteen L, Sergent G, Defrance F, Gmyr V, et al. Primary graft function, metabolic control, and graft survival after islet transplantation. *Diabetes Care* 2009;32:1473-8.
13. Fiorina P, Gremizzi C, Maffi P, Caldara R, Tavano D, Monti L, et al. Islet transplantation is associated with an improvement of cardiovascular function in type 1 diabetic kidney transplant patients. *Diabetes Care* 2005;28:1358-65.
14. Warnock GL, Thompson DM, Meloche RM, Shapiro RJ, Ao Z, Keown P, et al. A multi-year analysis of islet transplantation compared with intensive medical therapy on progression of complications in type 1 diabetes. *Transplantation* 2008;86:1762-6.
15. Merani S, Toso C, Emamaullee J, Shapiro AM. Optimal implantation site for pancreatic islet transplantation. *Br J Surg* 2008;95:1449-61.
16. Harlan DM, Kenyon NS, Korsgren O, Roep BO. Current advances and travails in islet transplantation. *Diabetes* 2009;58:2175-84.
17. Daly B, O'Kelly K, Klassen D. Interventional procedures in whole organ and islet cell pancreas transplantation. *Semin Intervent Radiol* 2004;21:335-43.
18. Campbell P, Senior P, Salam A, LaBranche K, Bigam D, Kneteman N, et al. High risk of sensitization after failed islet transplantation. *Am J Transplant* 2007;7:2311-7.
19. Khan MH, Harlan DM. Counterpoint: clinical islet transplantation: not ready for prime time. *Diabetes Care* 2009;32:1570-4.
20. Brandhorst H, Asif S, Andersson K, Theisinger B, Andersson HH, Felldin M, et al. A new oxygen carrier for improved long-term storage of human pancreata before islet isolation. *Transplantation* 2010;89:155-60.
21. Papas KK, Suszynski TM, Colton CK. Islet assessment for transplantation. *Curr Opin Organ Transplant* 2009;14:674-82.
22. Hansson M, Madsen OD. Pluripotent stem cells, a potential source of beta-cells for diabetes therapy. *Curr Opin Investig Drugs* 2010;11:417-25.
23. Chatenoud L. Chemical immunosuppression in islet transplantation—friend or foe? *N Engl J Med* 2008;358:1192-3.
24. Medarova Z, Moore A. Non-invasive detection of transplanted pancreatic islets. *Diabetes Obes Metab* 2008;10:88-97.

Related links

bmj.com/archive

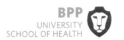

Renal transplantation

Paul T R Thiruchelvam, specialist registrar general surgery[1],
Michelle Willicombe, specialist registrar nephrology[2],
Nadey Hakim, surgical director department of transplant surgery[2],
David Taube, professor of transplant medicine[2],
Vassilios Papalois, consultant transplant and general surgeon, chief of service[2]

[1]North West Thames, Department of Transplant Surgery, Imperial College Renal and Transplant Centre, Hammersmith Hospital, London W12 0NN, UK

[2]Imperial College Renal and Transplant Centre, Hammersmith Hospital, London

Correspondence to: P T R Thiruchelvam paul.thiruchelvam@imperial.ac.uk

Cite this as: BMJ 2011;343:d7300

DOI: 10.1136/bmj.d7300

http://www.bmj.com/content/343/bmj.d7300

Epidemiological data from the past decade suggest that the global burden of patients with renal failure who receive renal replacement therapy exceeds 1.4 million and that this figure is growing by about 8% a year.[1] [2] The UK renal registry from 2009 estimated that over 47 000 people received renal replacement therapy in the UK.[3] Renal transplantation increases survival and improves the quality of life for patients with end stage renal failure.[4] [5] A recent UK estimate found that transplantation conferred a cost saving of £25 000 (€29 000; $40 000) a year per patient with end stage renal failure.[6] In the UK rates of renal transplantation are increasing (fig 1), and since 2006 the number of patients waiting more than five years for a transplant has halved, but there are still a large number (about 7000) of patients on the transplant waiting list (fig 1).[7] [8]

We review the process of selecting patients eligible for renal transplantation and the care of patients after renal transplantation for the primary care physician. This article is based on evidence from large registries, case series, clinical trials where available, and national guidelines.

Who is eligible for a kidney transplant?

Guidelines recommend that all patients with chronic kidney disease at stage 5 or stage 4 (glomerular filtration rates <15 mL/min and 15-30 mL/min respectively) with progressive disease likely to require renal replacement therapy within six months should be considered for transplantation.[9] [10] The mean estimated glomerular filtration rate of patients starting renal replacement therapy is 8.6 mL/min/1.73 m².[11] A minority of patients with end stage renal failure are deemed unsuitable for transplantation. Absolute contraindications to transplantation are few, but include untreated malignancy, active infection, untreated HIV infection or AIDS, or any condition where life expectancy is under two years.[9] [10] Relative contraindications and special considerations for transplantation are listed in box 1 and discussed in detail in the web extra appendix on bmj.com. Patients should have access to transplantation if they are medically fit for surgery. Ineligible patients will remain on long term dialysis. Patients who are awaiting a kidney transplant will be regularly reassessed. About 5% of patients are removed from the transplant list each year, typically because they are deemed too unwell for transplant.[7]

Pre-emptive kidney transplantation is transplantation before the need for maintenance dialysis arises. It is the treatment of choice in patients nearing renal replacement therapy in both national and international guidelines because pre-emptive kidney transplantation is associated with improved allograft and patient survival,[9] [12] [13] [14] [15] [16] reduced dialysis related cardiovascular morbidity and sensitisation events, cost savings on dialysis, and better quality of life.[17] In the UK in 2008 only 5.3% of the 6639 patients who met guideline criteria for kidney transplantation received a pre-emptive transplant.[3] Most pre-emptive transplants are living donations. If no suitable living donor can be found patients are placed on the deceased donor waiting list when their glomerular filtration rate falls below the cut-off value. Patients with type 1 diabetes should also be listed for a simultaneous kidney-pancreas transplant.

How are donor kidneys sourced?

Brain or cardiac death donors
Most transplanted kidneys in the past four decades have come from "donation after brain death" donors. However the number of kidneys derived from "donation after cardiac death" donors has increased in recent years in the UK and comprised 34% (n=567) of all deceased donor kidney transplants in 2010-1 compared with 66% (n=1100) from "donation after brain death" donors.[7] Kidneys transplanted from "donation after cardiac death" donors have a longer warm ischaemia time and higher rates of both delayed graft function and primary non-function but similar long term patient outcomes and graft survival.[18]

Living donors
Living donor transplantation has also increased over the past decade, with one in three transplants in the UK now from a living donor.[7] Living donor kidney transplantation has reduced the gap between demand and supply of kidneys. Donors include those who are genetically related to the recipient or emotionally related (such as spouse, partner, or close friend). A long term series from the US found that living transplants are associated with reduced rates of delayed graft function and better allograft and patient survival.[19] The United Network for Organ Sharing (UNOS) reports five year allograft survival of 79.9% for living donor kidneys compared with 66.5% for deceased donor kidneys. With improvements in surgical nephrectomy techniques (laparoscopic and mini-open donor), reduced postoperative pain, shorter hospital stay, and faster return to work, living donation has become more acceptable.[20] More complex

---

SOURCES AND SELECTION CRITERIA
We searched PubMed, the Cochrane Database, and ScienceDirect using the key words "kidney transplantation." The search was limited to those journals published in the English language. The data were mainly derived from large registry descriptions, multiple case series, and clinical trials. We have combined our knowledge with that of recently published guidelines and reviews identified by the previously mentioned PubMed searches on kidney transplantation.

SUMMARY POINTS

- The global burden of end stage renal disease is increasing
- Renal transplantation increases patient survival and quality of life and reduces costs of care for patients with end stage renal disease
- Most donor kidneys come from "brain death" or "cardiac death" donors, but donations from living donors are increasing
- Pre-emptive transplantation from a living donor is the best treatment choice for patients with end stage renal disease and has been associated with improved allograft and patient survival
- Long term outcomes in kidney transplantation are improving

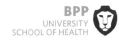

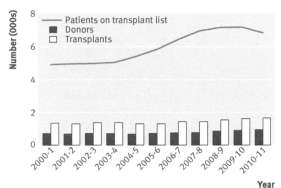

Fig 1 Deceased donor kidney programme in the UK, 1 April 2000-31 March 2010. Number of donors, transplants and patients on the active transplant list at 31 March.

procedures with living donors are now being considered in certain centres, such as transplantation from obese donors with a body mass index >35 and from older donors and transplants with multiple vessels.

A "matched pair donation" scheme exists whereby a relative, friend, or partner of a potential recipient can donate an incompatible organ by being matched with another incompatible donor-recipient pair, enabling both people in need of a transplant to receive a compatible organ. Pooled donation is a form of matched pair donation involving more than two living donor pairs. Altruistic non-directed donation occurs when a kidney is donated by a healthy person who does not have a relationship with the recipient and is not informed who the recipient will be.

What are the consequences of live kidney donation for the donor?

A large follow-up study of live kidney donors from one centre found that donors showed a 25% reduction in glomerular filtration rate, glomerular hyperfiltration, and proteinuria, which were not clinically important.[21] An increase in protein excretion by the remaining kidney, particularly in male donors, is well described, but in the absence of a correlation between protein excretion and blood pressure or renal function, the clinical importance of this finding is unclear.[22] Long term outcomes of uninephrectomy have found no major adverse consequences.[23] The lifespan of a kidney donor seems to be similar to that for the general population of similar age, and there is no increased risk of developing end stage renal disease.[24] [25]

How is a patient with renal disease prepared for transplant surgery?

Patients are counselled about the risks of surgery and the risks, complications, and side effects of immunosuppressive therapy. Patients must be clearly informed about their mortality risk, rates of graft survival, and the potential impact of transplantation on their employment activities. Explaining the potential risk of recurrent kidney disease in an allograft is also important. Individual risks may change with the length of time that a person waits for a procedure, and patients may need repeated re-evaluation and counselling.

It is important to remember that the mean age of patients starting renal replacement therapy is 64 years. Patients require a full cardiac and respiratory assessment, including an assessment for the presence of peripheral vascular disease. A formal urological assessment is done (ultrasound, voiding cystourethrogram, cystoscopy) to exclude pre-existing disease that may compromise the function of the

graft, such as bladder outflow obstruction, ureteric reflux, or congenital abnormality. Avoid blood transfusions in patients awaiting transplant surgery. Antibodies are measured regularly while patients are waiting for a procedure.

The renal transplant operation

Techniques for performing a donor nephrectomy are not discussed here as this article is aimed at generalist physicians, but Gibbons and Nicol provide details.[26] Living donors may be referred to the British Kidney Patient Association (BKPA)[27] and to Morgan and Ibrahim[23] for information on the long term effects of donating a kidney.

The procedure for a renal transplant has not changed much since the original operation described by Kuss et al in 1951.[28] The most common approach is a pelvic operation with extraperitoneal placement of the kidney. The right side is usually chosen, as the iliac vessels on the right are more superficial than on the left. The transplant involves three important anastomoses: the donor renal artery is anastomosed to the recipient external iliac artery (end-to-side); the donor renal vein is anastomosed to the external iliac vein (end-to-side); and the donor ureter is reimplanted to the recipient's bladder forming a ureterneocystostomy with a J-J ureteric stent left in situ. The J-J stent is removed 8–12 weeks postoperatively under local anaesthetic via flexible cystoscopy.[29]

What are the potential short and medium term complications of renal transplantation?

Early and late complications of renal transplant are presented in box 2.

Surgical complications

Surgical complications after a renal transplant have reduced over time as techniques have been refined. Reported rates of surgical complications are low (5–10%) compared with liver and pancreas transplantation.[30]

Bleeding is uncommon and is usually from vessels not ligated at the hilum or from small retroperitoneal vessels of the recipient. Vascular complications can involve the donor vessels (renal artery thrombosis (<1%), renal artery stenosis (1–10%), renal vein thrombosis) or the recipient vessels (iliac artery thrombosis, pseudoaneurysm, deep vein thrombosis (5%)).[30] Urological complications present as a leak or obstruction (2–10%), often as a result of ischaemia of the transplant ureter. The incidence of lymphoceles (fluid filled collections from cut lymphatics) is 0.6–18%, which can be reduced by careful ligation of all lymphatics. Wound complications are the most common surgical complication after a renal transplant; these include wound infections (5%) and fascial dehiscence or incisional hernias (3–5%).[30]

Medical complications

The main complications in the first few weeks after transplantation are rejection and infection. Risk of rejection can be determined to some extent before transplantation. High

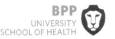

BOX 2: COMPLICATIONS AFTER RENAL TRANSPLANTATION

Surgical complications

Early

- Haemorrhage
- Renal artery thrombosis
- Renal vein thrombosis
- Recipient vasculature injury
- Urine leak
- Lymphocele
- Wound complications

Late

- Ureteral obstruction
- Transplant renal artery stenosis

Medical complications

Early

- Acute rejection—acute cellular, antibody mediated
- Infection—bacterial, viral (cytomegalovirus), fungal (pneumocystis)

Late

- Immunosuppression related— specific side effect profile, malignancy, chronic alloimmune injury
- Allograft related—recurrent disease
- Renal disease— anaemia, bone disease
- Cardiovascular disease
- Infections—polyoma virus

risk patients include those who are blood group incompatible or who are transplanted against a positive cross match and who have antibodies against the donor kidney before transplantation. Such patients require antibody removal before the operation. For other patients, risk is determined by whether the patient is sensitised or how well matched the donor kidney is to the recipient. To prevent rejection, the recipients receive induction at the time of transplant with either depleting or non-depleting monoclonal or polyclonal antibodies directed against T cells. Such agents include anti-CD3 (antithymocyte globulin), anti-CD25 (basiliximab), or anti-CD52 (alemtuzumab). Maintenance immunosuppression is then required in the long term to prevent rejection. Transplant centres use different induction and maintenance regimens. The table provides a summary of commonly used immunosuppressant agents.

Infectious complications are highest in the early postoperative period. Two particularly important infections that require special mention are cytomegalovirus and pneumocystis pneumonia. Cytomegalovirus has a broad clinical spectrum (presenting with symptoms of fever and malaise sometimes associated with leucopenia, thrombocytopenia, gastroenteritis, pneumonitis, and hepatitis) after transplantation and can prove fatal.[31] Transplant units either give patients cytomegalovirus prophylaxis with valganciclovir for three to six months after transplantation or adopt a strict surveillance protocol and treat only when cytomegalovirus DNA is detected. Pneumocystis pneumonia is also most likely to occur in the first six months after transplantation, and most patients receive co-trimoxazole prophylaxis.

In the longer term the most common cause of graft failure is chronic alloimmune injury, and, with failure, other complications of renal disease emerge such as anaemia, bone disease, and fluid imbalance. Transplant patients are also at risk of malignancy and cardiac disease—the former as a result of long term immunosuppression, and the latter being multifactorial in nature.

Patients increasingly present with renal disease in the allograft now that modern immunosuppression means fewer acute rejections, and this accounts for about 5% of allograft loss.[32] Primary focal segmental glomerulosclerosis, IgA nephropathy, mesangiocapillary glomerulonephritis type II, and diabetic nephropathy are the commonest causes of recurrent disease in an allograft. The impact of recurrent renal disease on allograft survival depends on the underlying cause.

What are the long term outcomes for renal transplantation?

The average lifespan of a renal transplant is now 8–15 years, depending on the type of graft.[3] Data from the NHS Blood and Transplant registry show that one year and 10 year graft survival rates are 89% and 67% for adult kidneys from "brain death donors," and 96% and 78% for kidneys from live donors (fig 2).[7] Survival of the transplant recipient at 10 years for cadaveric and live donor transplants is 71% and 89% respectively.

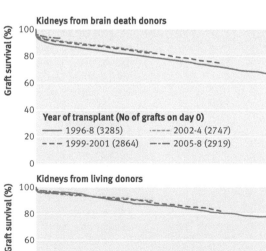

Fig 2 Long term graft survival after first kidney only transplantation from "brain death donors" and live donors

TIPS FOR NON-SPECIALISTS

Do's

- Strictly manage cardiovascular risk factors
- Encourage self examination and attendance at national screening programmes (such as cervical smear tests)
- Encourage avoidance of sun exposure
- Vaccinate against influenza and pneumococcus
- Refer to transplant unit for preconception management
- Promptly refer to transplant unit in context of febrile episode

Don'ts

- Administer live vaccines
- Prescribe drugs that induce or inhibit cytochrome P450 activity if patient is taking sirolimus, tacrolimus, or ciclosporin
- Prescribe nephrotoxic agents (such as non-steroidal anti-inflammatory drugs)

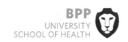

Immunosuppressant agents and adverse effects

Agent	Mechanism of action	Adverse effects
Corticosteroids	Inhibit cytokine production	Diabetes, osteoporosis, weight gain, hypertension
Ciclosporin	Calcineurin inhibitor	Hirsuitism, gum hypertrophy, hypertension, diabetes, nephrotoxicity
Tacrolimus	Calcineurin inhibitor	Diabetes, nephrotoxicity, neurotoxicity (tremor)
Mycophenolate mofetil	Inosine monophosphate dehydrogenase inhibitor	Gastrointestinal disturbance (diarrhoea), haematological (anaemia, leucopenia), mouth ulcers
Azathioprine	Purine synthesis inhibitor	Myelosuppression, hepatitis
Sirolimus	Mammalian target of rapamycin (mTOR) inhibitor	Peripheral oedema, poor wound healing, hypertriglyceridaemia, anaemia, proteinuria

---

PATIENTS' PERSPECTIVES (LIVING DONOR TRANSPLANT)

The donor

When I first offered to be a kidney donor for my friend Paul it was a decision that just felt right. I had a little understanding of what might be involved, and a knowledgeable partner who—while naturally a little apprehensive—did appreciate that the risks to me were very small. So I volunteered for the donor programme at the Hammersmith Hospital without very much thought as to what was actually involved.

Not having attended any donor seminars, I had not expected the very thorough work-up by the transplant team. During the several visits that spring, every part of my body was checked out. It felt odd, but reassuring, visiting the hospital when I didn't feel ill. A slight alarm when the cardiac test picked up an anomaly, but a subsequent angiogram showed it to be treatable with drugs and not something that would prevent the transplant. I was very happy that a potentially significant condition had been picked up early—an unexpected bonus that I am still grateful for to this day. The day arrived, and as I was wheeled into surgery I was strangely calm. I was about to go under the knife, but the knowledge that I was going to change Paul's and Barbara's lives forever was with me as I slipped into unconsciousness. The operation was totally successful for both Paul and myself, and the recovery period in hospital and at home was made so much easier by the wonderful care provided by the medical and nursing teams.

Three years on, I have little left to show for the experience other than a tiny scar and a great sense of pride that I did something that made a real difference.

The recipient

Since 18 years old, I had known that I would need either to be put on dialysis or have a kidney transplant—just like my father in the early 1980s. I had been observed on an annual basis until my creatinine level reached 500 (when I was aged 50), and I was then transferred to the renal team at the hospital.

My clinical issue is hereditary polycystic kidney disease, and I was informed of what might happen, but I soon realised that things had changed from the 1980s. The transplantation team at the hospital were so supportive; they have become almost like family. My operation (a live, blood group incompatible transplant) went well, and, while in the care of the high dependency unit, I progressed well to being discharged after only seven days.

Since then, my health has returned to normal. I see the team every eight weeks and take great comfort from knowing that I am being kept under the watchful eye of a great group of people. My experience shows what miracles can be performed and, with a team including family and friends in support, life can return to normal really quickly.

THE ROLE OF THE LIVE DONOR COORDINATOR

The live donor work-up process is a team effort, involving a range of healthcare professionals working together with donors and recipients to ensure the best outcome. We are responsible for the coordination of the management and care of the donors; from their first contact with us, through the assessment process, surgery, and follow-up. We are responsible for ensuring that our patients are fully informed about the work-up process and understand the realities and risks of live donor transplantation.

The initial assessment is essential to identify any problems for either the donor or recipient and address them at an early stage to enable us to proceed to transplantation. Each pair's experience is individual, depending on the complexity of the situation, and our role is to keep the process running smoothly and support donors and recipients through an experience which is full of highs and lows. Whether pairs can proceed to transplantation or are unable to proceed as planned, the coordinators are there to provide support and care to the patients and their families throughout the process. Seeing a recipient and donor after the operation looking fit and healthy and being able to enjoy life again is the most rewarding part of our role.

Jen McDermott, lead live donor coordinator, Imperial College NHS Trust

---

ONGOING CHALLENGES IN RENAL TRANSPLANTATION

Reducing transplant demand
- Early detection and prevention of progression of chronic kidney disease
- Patient education of risk factors
- Improve diabetic management

Improving organ utility
- Match donor and recipient age and organ quality
- Increase live donor transplantation as an alternative to transplant waiting list
- Machine organ perfusion—optimising cadaveric organs
- Improve organ retrieval—reducing organ damage
- Increase use of non-heart beating donor kidneys

Increasing organ availability
- Better training for donor coordinators
- Greater number of donor coordinators managing the donation process
- Increase number of donor card carriers
- Greater use of "extended criteria donors"
- Increase numbers of paired exchange and altruistic donors
- Encourage organ donation from ethnic minority groups
- Change legislation—"opt out" or mandated choice organ donation

Optimising immunosuppression
- Development of more specific monoclonal antibodies
- Corticosteroid sparing regimens

ABO or HLA incompatible kidney transplantation
- Long term outcomes for ABO incompatible kidneys similar to those for antibody compatible kidneys

---

ADDITIONAL EDUCATIONAL RESOURCES

For healthcare professionals
- Renal Association (www.renal.org/home.aspx)
- British Transplantation Society (www.bts.org.uk)
- Transplantation Society (www.tts.org/)
- UK Renal Registry (www.renalreg.com/)
- American Society of Nephrology (www.asn-online.org/)
- European Society of Organ Transplantation (www.esot.org)

For patients
- British Kidney Patient Association (www.britishkidney-pa.co.uk)
- Kidney Patient Guide (www.kidneypatientguide.org.uk)
- UK National Kidney Federation (www.kidney.org.uk)
- Transplant Support Network (www.transplantsupportnetwork.org.uk)
- American Association of Kidney Patients (www.aakp.org)
- American Kidney Fund (www.akfinc.org)

What are the considerations for long term follow-up?

Regular follow-up of the transplant recipient by the transplant clinic for the life of the allograft is routine, and the specialist unit will offer advice regarding any patient who becomes acutely unwell. Patients' general practitioners plays an important role in monitoring risk factors for cardiovascular disease and maintaining a high level of suspicion for incident malignancy. In one national cohort of adult kidney transplant patients, new onset diabetes occurred in 16% within three years of transplantation.[33] The potential for hazardous drug interactions in patients undergoing long term immunosuppression means that

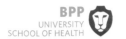

particular care is needed with prescribing. We include a list of tips for non-specialists, but advice from the patient's specialist transplant unit should be sought if in doubt.

Fertility is impaired in patients with end stage renal failure, but gonadal function improves and ovulation resumes within a few months of renal transplantation.[34] Current recommendations advise that, after a year of stable graft function, pregnancy is likely to be safe.[35] In women with normal graft function, pregnancy usually has no adverse effects on graft function and survival. Women require preconception counselling, particularly regarding optimisation of immunotherapy and other drugs that may be teratogenic, and any patient wanting to conceive should be referred early to the transplant unit. Pregnancy after transplantation is considered high risk and is managed accordingly. These pregnancies are more likely to be complicated by preterm labour (30–50%), pre-eclampsia (30–37%) and intrauterine growth restriction (20–33%).[36] The transplanted kidney does not usually obstruct labour, but caesarean section is required in half of women.

Contributors: All authors contributed equally in the writing of the article, Vassilios Papalois is the guarantor of the article.

Funding: No special funding received.

Competing interests: All authors have completed the ICMJE uniform disclosure form at www.icmje.org/coi_disclosure.pdf (available on request from the corresponding author) and declare: no support from any organisation for the submitted work; no financial relationships with any organisations that might have an interest in the submitted work in the previous three years; no other relationships or activities that could appear to have influenced the submitted work.

Provenance and peer review: Not commissioned; externally peer reviewed.

Patient consent obtained.

1 Moeller S, Gioberge S, Brown G. ESRD patients in 2001: global overview of patients, treatment modalities and development trends. Nephrol Dial Transplant 2002;17:2071-6.
2 Schieppati A, Remuzzi G. Chronic renal diseases as a public health problem: epidemiology, social, and economic implications. Kidney Int Suppl 2005:S7-S10.
3 UK Renal Registry. UK Renal Registry: the twelfth annual report, December 2009. 2009. www.renalreg.com/Reports/2009.html.
4 Wolfe RA, Ashby VB, Milford EL, Ojo AO, Ettenger RE, Agodoa LY, et al. Comparison of mortality in all patients on dialysis, patients on dialysis awaiting transplantation, and recipients of a first cadaveric transplant. N Engl J Med 1999;341:1725-30.
5 Ojo AO, Hanson JA, Meier-Kriesche H, Okechukwu CN, Wolfe RA, Leichtman AB, et al. Survival in recipients of marginal cadaveric donor kidneys compared with other recipients and wait-listed transplant candidates. J Am Soc Nephrol 2001;12:589-97.
6 NHS Blood and Transplant. Organ donation: cost-effectiveness of transplantation. 2011. www.uktransplant.org.uk/ukt/newsroom/fact_sheets/cost_effectiveness_of_transplantation.jsp
7 NHS Blood and Transplant. Organ donation: activity report 2010-2011. 2011. www.uktransplant.org.uk/ukt/statistics/transplant_activity_report/transplant_activity_report.jsp
8 Johnson RJ, Fuggle SV, Mumford L, Bradley JA, Forsythe JL, Rudge CJ. A new UK 2006 national kidney allocation scheme for deceased heart-beating donor kidneys. Transplantation 2010;89:387-94.
9 The Renal Association. Assessment of the potential kidney transplant recipient. 2011. www.renal.org/Clinical/GuidelinesSection/AssessmentforRenalTransplantation.aspx
10 British Transplantation Society. Active BTS standards and guidelines. 2011. www.bts.org.uk/transplantation/standards-and-guidelines/
11 Byrne C, Ford D, Gilg J, Ansell D, Feehally J. UK ESRD incident rates in 2008: national and centre-specific analyses. In: UK Renal Registry: the twelfth annual report, December 2009. www.renalreg.com/Report-Area/Report%202009/Chap03_Renal09_web.pdf
12 Innocenti GR, Wadei HM, Prieto M, Dean PG, Ramos EJ, Textor S, et al. Preemptive living donor kidney transplantation: do the benefits extend to all recipients? Transplantation 2007;83:144-9.
13 Kasiske BL, Snyder JJ, Matas AJ, Ellison MD, Gill JS, Kausz AT. Preemptive kidney transplantation: the advantage and the advantaged. J Am Soc Nephrol 2002;13:1358-64.
14 Mange KC, Joffe MM, Feldman HI. Dialysis prior to living donor kidney transplantation and rates of acute rejection. Nephrol Dial Transplant 2003;18:172-7.
15 Gill JS, Tonelli M, Johnson N, Pereira BJ. Why do preemptive kidney transplant recipients have an allograft survival advantage? Transplantation 2004;78:873-9.
16 Becker BN, Rush SH, Dykstra DM, Becker YT, Port FK. Preemptive transplantation for patients with diabetes-related kidney disease. Arch Intern Med 2006;166:44-8.
17 Abou Ayache R, Bridoux F, Pessione F, Thierry A, Belmouaz M, Leroy F, et al. Preemptive renal transplantation in adults. Transplant Proc 2005;37:2817-8.
18 Kokkinos C, Antcliffe D, Nanidis T, Darzi AW, Tekkis P, Papalois V. Outcome of kidney transplantation from nonheart-beating versus heart-beating cadaveric donors. Transplantation 2007;83:1193-9.
19 Hariharan S, Johnson CP, Bresnahan BA, Taranto SE, McIntosh MJ, Stablein D. Improved graft survival after renal transplantation in the United States, 1988 to 1996. N Engl J Med 2000;342:605-12.
20 Pradel FG, Limcangco MR, Mullins CD, Bartlett ST. Patients' attitudes about living donor transplantation and living donor nephrectomy. Am J Kidney Dis 2003;41:849-58.
21 Gossmann J, Wilhelm A, Kachel HG, Jordan J, Sann U, Geiger H, et al. Long-term consequences of live kidney donation follow-up in 93% of living kidney donors in a single transplant center. Am J Transplant 2005;5:2417-24.
22 Torffvit O, Kamper AL, Strandgaard S. Tamm-Horsfall protein in urine after uninephrectomy/transplantation in kidney donors and their recipients. Scand J Urol Nephrol 1997;31:555-9.
23 Morgan BR, Ibrahim HN. Long-term outcomes of kidney donors. Curr Opin Nephrol Hypertens 2011;20:605-9.
24 Ibrahim HN, Foley R, Tan L, Rogers T, Bailey RF, Guo H, et al. Long-term consequences of kidney donation. N Engl J Med 2009;360:459-69.
25 Fehrman-Ekholm I, Elinder CG, Stenbeck M, Tyden G, Groth CG. Kidney donors live longer. Transplantation 1997;64:976-8.
26 Gibbons N, Nicol D. The CARI guidelines. Surgical techniques in living donor nephrectomy. Nephrology (Carlton) 2010;15(suppl 1):S88-95.
27 British Kidney Patient Association. 2011. www.britishkidney-pa.co.uk/.
28 Kuss R, Teinturier J, Milliez P. [Some attempts at kidney transplantation in man]. Mem Acad Chir (Paris) 1951;77:755-64.
29 Kayler L, Kang D, Molmenti E, Howard R. Kidney transplant ureteroneocystostomy techniques and complications: review of the literature. Transplant Proc 2010;42:1413-20.
30 Humar A, Matas AJ. Surgical complications after kidney transplantation. Semin Dial 2005;18:505-10.
31 Weikert BC, Blumberg EA. Viral infection after renal transplantation: surveillance and management. Clin J Am Soc Nephrol 2008;3(suppl 2):S76-86.
32 Chadban S. Glomerulonephritis recurrence in the renal graft. J Am Soc Nephrol 2001;12:394-402.
33 Luan FL, Steffick DE, Ojo AO. New-onset diabetes mellitus in kidney transplant recipients discharged on steroid-free immunosuppression. Transplantation 2011;91:334-41.
34 Josephson MA, McKay DB. Considerations in the medical management of pregnancy in transplant recipients. Adv Chronic Kidney Dis 2007;14:156-67.
35 McKay DB, Josephson MA. Pregnancy in recipients of solid organs—effects on mother and child. N Engl J Med 2006;354:1281-93.
36 European best practice guidelines for renal transplantation. Section IV: Long-term management of the transplant recipient. IV.10. Pregnancy in renal transplant recipients. Nephrol Dial Transplant 2002;17(suppl 4):50-5.

Related links

bmj.com
- Get CME points at BMJ Learning

bmj.com/archive
- Diagnosis and management of anal intraepithelial neoplasia and anal cancer (2011;343:d6818)
- Management of deep vein thrombosis and prevention of post-thrombotic syndrome (2011;343:d5916)
- Diagnosis and management of autism in childhood (2011;343:d6238)
- Diagnosis and management of maturity onset diabetes of the young (MODY) (2011;343:d6044)

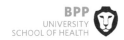

Management of anal fistula

Jonathan Alastair Simpson, specialist registrar in colorectal surgery,
Ayan Banerjea, colorectal consultant,
John Howard Scholefield, professor of surgery

¹Division of Digestive Diseases, Queen's Medical Centre Campus, Nottingham University Hospitals, Nottingham NG7 2UH, UK

Correspondence to: J A Simpson
alastairsimpson@hotmail.com

Cite this as: BMJ 2012;345:e6705

DOI: 10.1136/bmj.e6705

http://www.bmj.com/content/345/bmj.e6705

Anal fistula is part of the spectrum of perianal sepsis. It is a chronic condition that may present de novo or after an acute anorectal abscess. Anal fistula causes a variety of prolonged or intermittent symptoms including pain, discharge, and social embarrassment.

The goals of management are to eradicate the fistula and prevent recurrence while maintaining continence. Simple anal fistula may be easy to treat, but complex cases may require several procedures over months (or years). In some cases, treatment may result in a stoma formation or incontinence, which has a profound effect on the patient's quality of life.

This article aims to provide a pragmatic overview of this often poorly understood condition and enable primary care doctors and other non-specialists to appreciate the common management pathways that their patients might experience.

What is an anal fistula?

A fistula is defined as an abnormal communication between two epithelial surfaces. Anal fistula is a communication between the anorectal canal and the perianal skin that is lined with granulation tissue. It may be useful to consider it as a tunnel during discussions with patients. The fistula may harbour chronic infection, which may discharge continuously or intermittently through the opening on to the skin. Intermittent discharge is usually caused by cyclical accumulation of an abscess with associated discomfort and pain before some relief from discharge, which is followed by further accumulation. In the most severe cases, faecal material may also pass through the tunnel and cause soiling of underwear and skin irritation.

Who gets anal fistula?

The prevalence of anal fistula is 1-2 per 10 000 of the population in European studies,[1] [2] but this is probably an underestimate, with many patients being reluctant to present to medical services. The reported incidence in England is 18.4 per 100 000 per year. Men are twice as likely to be affected, and it most commonly presents in the third, fourth, and fifth decades, with a peak around 40 years of age.

How do anorectal fistulas develop?

Most (~90% in most case series) anal fistulas are idiopathic.[1] [3] Infection of glands in the intersphincteric space of the anal canal is thought to underlie both acute anorectal abscesses and anal fistulas (fig 1)—the "cryptoglandular hypothesis." The exact cause or mechanism of infection has not been fully elucidated, but it spreads through pathways of least resistance, and in so doing creates a track that persists thereafter. Hence, a common presentation is an acute abscess that fails to heal after surgical drainage or recurs at the same site. It is not clear why certain cases of perianal sepsis are limited to abscess formation whereas others are associated with fistula formation. It is widely accepted that adequate surgical drainage is the optimal treatment for acute abscesses and that antibiotics are indicated only for treatment of surrounding cellulitis.[4] A recent review of perianal abscess and fistula quotes a fistula formation rate of 26-37% after perianal abscess.[5]

Microbiological culture of pus from an adequately drained abscess may help to predict fistula formation. Small case series have shown that the abscess is unlikely to recur or develop into a fistula if only skin organisms are grown (0-30% of cases in most studies).[6] [7] When gut organisms are cultured, most studies have shown that 80% or more abscesses have an underlying fistula.

Some cases of anal fistula will be associated with other condition such as Crohn's disease, tuberculosis, hidradenitis suppurativa, and previous surgery or radiotherapy (box). Cancer may present as a fistula or arise within a chronic complex fistula. Fistula arising from anorectal or obstetric trauma may be prevented if the wound is carefully debrided and repaired at the time of injury. Doctors need to be aware of the potential for underlying disease because the management approach will differ depending on the underlying cause.

How are fistulas classified?

Classification and successful management of anal fistula require expert knowledge of anorectal anatomy. A variety of classification systems have been described, but the most useful and widely accepted classification is that described by Parks (fig 2).[8] This classification system is based on the relation between the primary track—the main tunnel that constitutes the fistula—and the sphincter muscles around the anal canal. In simple terms, consider the sphincters as two rings of muscle, with the inner ring termed the internal sphincter and the outer one the external sphincter.

What are the different types of anal fistula?

Low versus high

For the non-specialist, the key distinction is whether the primary track is "low" or "high." In a low fistula the track passes through few or no sphincter muscle fibres and is relatively close to the skin. Examples include superficial fistulas, low intersphincteric fistulas, and low trans-sphincteric fistulas (fig 2). In the absence of complicating factors or underlying conditions these fistulas may be

SOURCES AND SELECTION CRITERIA

We searched PubMed and the Cochrane Library for clinically relevant studies using the search terms anal fistula and perianal sepsis. We consulted guidelines from the National Institute for Health and Clinical Excellence, in addition to both the Association of Surgeons of Great Britain and Ireland and the Association of Coloproctology clinical guidance.

SUMMARY POINTS

- A high index of suspicion of anal fistula is needed when examining patients with a perianal abscess or sepsis
- All fistulas consist of a primary track but may also have secondary extensions
- Complex fistulas need careful assessment and investigation; many months of treatment and several procedures may be needed before resolution
- Some patients are best treated with a seton alone
- Counsel patients who consent to surgery of the anal sphincter about possible post-procedural incontinence

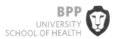

CONDITIONS ASSOCIATED WITH ANAL FISTULA

- Crohn's disease
- Tuberculosis
- Pilonidal disease
- Hidradenits suppurativa
- HIV infection
- Trauma
- Foreign bodies
- Previous surgery (including ileoanal pouch surgery)
- Radiotherapy
- Bridging of an anal fissure
- Lymphogranuloma venereum
- Prescaral dermoid cysts
- Sacrococcygeal teratoma
- Rectal duplication
- Perianal actinomycosis

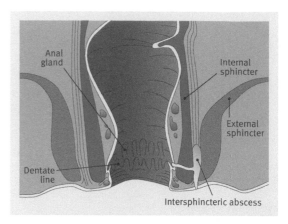

Fig 1 Anatomy of the anal canal and the cryptoglandular hypothesis of the development of an intersphincteric fistula

relatively easy to manage, because laying open and healing by secondary intention (fistulotomy) may pose little threat to continence. However, there is considerable debate among colorectal surgeons as to whether it is appropriate to divide any sphincter muscle at all (see below).

A high fistula describes a track that passes through or above a large amount of muscle; its route may be more complicated and further away from the skin. Examples include high intersphincteric fistulas, high trans-sphincteric fistulas, suprasphincteric fistulas, and extrasphincteric fistulas (fig 2). Laying open of such fistulas would damage considerable amounts of sphincter muscle and result in impaired bowel control. These fistulas are therefore also considered complex.

Simple versus complex

After considering whether a fistula track is high or low, additional complexity arises from the presence of secondary tracks or residual abscess cavities (fig 3). These may be explained to patients as branches or caverns off the main tunnel. Examples of such complexity include secondary tracks and cavities that extend above the levator muscles, supralevator or suprasphincteric extensions, those that extend in an almost circumferential manner around the anal canal—so called horseshoe extensions. Successful management of anal fistula requires that all secondary tracks and extensions are drained and eradicated before or at the same time as attempting definitive treatment of the primary track.

Conditions such as Crohn's disease, previous surgery or radiotherapy, and cancer also make the management of anal fistula more complicated, as does pre-existing impairment of continence. Thus a fistula with a low primary track may also be complex and difficult to treat if secondary tracks are present, specific disease underlies the fistula, or the sphincters have previously been damaged.

How are anal fistulas assessed?

Primary care

Anal fistula should be part of the differential diagnosis in any patient presenting with chronic or recurrent perianal pain, lump, or discharge. Recurrent abscesses or failure of healing at an incision and drainage site often indicates the presence of anal fistula. Ask about previous perianal sepsis, surgery or radiotherapy, trauma (obstetric or otherwise), and associated conditions (see box). Determine the patient's baseline level of continence.

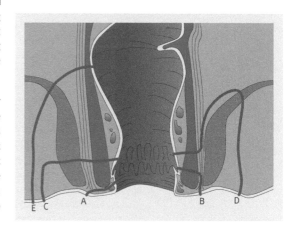

Fig 2 Parks's classification of anal fistula. (A) A superficial fistula track beneath the internal and external anal sphincters. (B) An intersphincteric fistula track between the internal and external anal sphincter muscles in the intersphincteric space. (C) A trans-sphincteric fistula track crossing both the external and internal anal sphincters. (D) A suprasphincteric fistula travels outside the internal and external sphincters over the top of the puborectalis muscle and penetrates the levator muscle before tracking down to the skin. (E) An extrasphincteric fistula tracks outside the external anal sphincter and penetrates the levator muscle into the rectum

Abdominal examination will often be normal but is necessary to exclude obvious intra-abdominal pathology. Document any external openings, tracks, or internal openings. An external opening may appear as a simple pit in the skin or may be obviously discharging, with or without a surrounding rim of raised granulation tissue. Some external openings are within the scar of a previous abscess. Recurrent swelling and pain under such a scar indicate an underlying fistula, even if an obvious opening or frank discharge is not evident. It is conventional to describe external openings by their distance from the anal verge and by their position on a clock face, with the anterior midline as 12 o'clock (fig 3).

Palpation of the perianal area with a lubricated finger may discern a palpable track that feels like a cord-like structure below the skin, indicating that the fistula is more likely to be "low." A digital rectal examination with the tip of the finger in the anal canal may detect indentation or induration, often described as "a grain of rice," associated with the internal opening. Digital examination higher up may also show bogginess or induration associated with chronic sepsis. Such patients should be referred for further assessment and evaluation to a specialist colorectal outpatient clinic.

Secondary care
Assessment
A full history and examination (including proctosigmoidoscopy) are fundamental to assessment. The aim of assessment is to determine the site and number of external and internal openings, the anatomy of primary and secondary tracks in relation to the sphincter muscles, and the exclusion of other conditions (such as Crohn's disease). Careful inspection and examination of the perianal skin and digital rectal examination provide a considerable amount of this information. The position of an external opening also guides the surgeon, because those less than 2-3 cm away from the anal verge are often associated with lower tracks than those further away.[9]

Goodsall's rule, much beloved by surgical examiners, states that external openings posterior to a line drawn from 9 o'clock to 3 o'clock should have a track that follows a course to the posterior midline. External openings anterior to this line should run directly radially to the anal canal. However, this rule is often unreliable in anterior fistulas and those with underlying disease.

The anatomy of the anal fistula can be further characterised by examination under anaesthesia. This allows a more thorough assessment of openings, and tracks may be probed or injected with agents such as hydrogen peroxide to define the anatomy of the fistula more accurately. Make it clear to patients that this procedure is part of their investigation. A simple fistula may be treated definitively at the time of examination, but in complex cases, although the insertion of a seton (see below) may be the first step of management, further investigations and procedures are usually necessary.

Imaging
Numerous non-randomised comparative studies have shown that endoanal ultrasound and magnetic resonance imaging (MRI) improve the characterisation of fistula anatomy and are the most useful imaging techniques in complex cases.[10] Anal ultrasound is cheaper but operator dependent, provides anatomical detail of the tracks and the sphincters, and can be used intraoperatively to give surgeons more information at the time of examination with anaesthesia. Accuracy can be improved by injection of hydrogen peroxide into fistula tracks. However, ultrasound has a limited field of view (about 2 cm from the anal probe) and is poor at evaluating pathology beyond the sphincters (both laterally and above).

MRI is considered the "gold standard" for imaging fistula anatomy. It provides excellent soft tissue resolution in multiple planes without the need for ionising radiation. It is indicated for all recurrent fistulas and primary fistulas that appear to be complex after examination under anaesthesia or endoanal ultrasound. Unfortunately, some patients have implants that preclude MRI or they find the procedure intolerable. In these cases, thin slice spiral computed tomography may be useful and may also be informative if abdominal or pelvic sources of sepsis are suspected; its value is otherwise limited. Similarly, fistulography has been superseded by endoanal ultrasound and MRI, and its role is limited to cases where an extrasphincteric track is suspected. A recent meta-analysis of four studies confirmed that endoanal ultrasound and MRI had similar sensitivity for detecting fistulas (87%), but that MRI had a higher specificity (69% v 43%).[11]

Anal manometry measures pressures within the anal canal and allows objective assessment of sphincter function. It is particularly useful in patients with compromised continence or those at risk, such as patients with previous sphincter surgery or injury.

What are the management options for anal fistulas?
A range of treatment options are available, but none is universally successful or without risk.[12] Key principles for the management of anal fistula are described by the acronym SNAP, which stands for sepsis, nutrition, anatomy, and procedure. Eradication of sepsis is the first step—a fistula will not heal while infection is present. As with wound healing in general, anal fistulas heal poorly in malnourished patients. Fistula openings and therefore the underlying track anatomy are not always clear, and failure to recognise secondary tracks may lead to treatment failure. Selection of the appropriate procedure is key to successful management.

Anal fistulas will not heal without intervention, and failure to treat may lead to progression of the disease process. If left untreated, anal fistulas are at risk of recurrent formation of a perianal abscess interspersed with partial healing of the fistula track. This can become a chronic septic focus with the establishment of a complex fistula network. The consequences for the patient may include pain, bleeding, incontinence, cellulitis, and systemic sepsis.

Seton
A seton is a simple thread placed through the anal fistula track and tied to form a continuous ring between the internal and external openings (figs 4 and 5). The primary application is in high trans-sphincteric fistula, where division of greater than one third of the anal sphincter muscle risks incontinence. Setons maintain patency of the fistula track, allow drainage, and prevent the development of perianal sepsis. The thread is usually a non-absorbable suture or vascular sling. The placement of a draining seton is usually the first step in treating a complex fistula. It reduces inflammation, allowing the establishment of a well formed track and defining the anatomy of the fistula.[13] Secondary treatment will be required to close the track.

A subsequent option for trans-sphincteric fistulas is the use of a cutting seton. This involves regular tightening of the seton to encourage gradual cutting through of the sphincteric muscle with associated inflammation followed by fibrosis. This process aims to resolve the fistula without allowing the muscle to spring apart, thereby maintaining continence. However, high rates of functional disturbance have been reported[14]: a prospective study that examined the use of a slow cutting seton for the treatment of intersphincteric and trans-sphincteric fistulas reported an incontinence rate of 25% at 42 months.[15]

Fistulotomy
Fistulotomy describes division of superficial tissue and thus laying open of a fistula track. It is the most effective method of dealing with a fistula and is the standard treatment for submucosal (low) fistulas because there is no risk to continence and recurrence is low (0-2%).[16] [17] Its use in the treatment of fistulas that involve the sphincter mechanism is controversial, however, because division of muscle risks incontinence. Practice parameters described for the management of perianal abscess and fistula-in-ano in 2005 stated that fistulotomy may be used in the treatment of simple perianal fistulas in

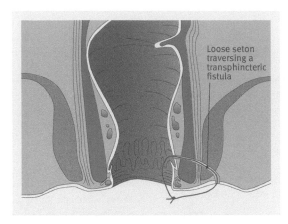

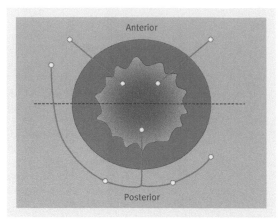

Fig 3 Diagram of the anal canal showing external openings and Goodsall's rule. The rule states that fistulas with an external opening anterior to a plane passing transversely through the centre of the anus will follow a straight radial course to the dentate line. Fistulas with openings posterior to this line will follow a curved course to the posterior midline. Exceptions to this rule are external openings more than 3 cm from the anal verge. These almost always originate as a primary or secondary tract from the posterior midline, consistent with a previous horseshoe abscess

Fig 4 Cross sectional diagram of a loose seton traversing a trans-sphincteric fistula

cryptoglandular disease.[18] A simple fistula was defined as a single non-recurrent track that crossed less than 50% of the external anal sphincter, but not the anterior sphincter in women, in people with perfect continence and no history of Crohn's disease or pelvic radiation.

The amount of sphincter that should be divided during fistulotomy is unclear. Some surgeons prefer not to divide any external sphincter muscle because of the fear of causing incontinence. Several sphincter preserving methods have been developed and are discussed below. However, others argue that persistence with such procedures after failure or recurrence often leads to protracted treatment with multiple procedures and prolonged suffering. Some patients, when counselled appropriately, may prefer to choose a long term loose seton. Others, particularly those who have had a protracted course, may accept the risks of minor soiling or incontinence associated with sphincter division for the almost certain cure that fistulotomy offers.

Sphincter saving methods

Fibrin glue
Fibrin glue is a combination of fibrinogen, thrombin, and calcium in a matrix, which is injected into the fistula track while the patient is under general anaesthesia. It heals the fistula by first inducing clot formation within the track and then encouraging growth of collagen fibres and healthy tissue. The internal and external openings do not need to be closed but there should be no deficiencies in the track when filling it with glue; this raises particular problems in complex fistulas and multiple tracks.

Observational cohort studies and controlled trials report healing rates of 31-85%.[19] Reasons for this wide variation include aspects of trial design such as length of follow-up, heterogeneity of patients, and variable fistula anatomy included in the treatment and control arms. In addition, a review highlights the importance of ensuring that all perianal sepsis has resolved and that stool softeners are used and a sedentary lifestyle is maintained after surgery to minimise dislodgement of the glue.[20]

Infiltration of fibrin glue is a simple, benign, sphincter sparing technique, and in simple tracks most authors conclude that the fistula heals in one to two thirds of

patients treated. This makes it an attractive early option, particularly because failure does not preclude other subsequent treatments.

Fistula plug
The biological fistula plug is manufactured from porcine small intestinal mucosa. It is resistant to infection, does not induce a foreign body reaction, and encourages host cells to populate it and ultimately fill the fistula track.

Insertion of a fistula plug is a sphincter sparing procedure with limited dissection. The plug is pulled through the fistula track and secured in place at the internal opening, then trimmed at the external opening, which is left open for drainage. A recent systematic review of 20 studies found that this technique resulted in fistula closure in 54% of patients, excluding those with Crohn's disease.[21] Further randomised controlled trials are awaited to confirm the efficacy of the fistula plug. One of the largest is the Fistula In Ano Trial (FIAT), which is due to report in 2015 (www.acpgbi.org.uk/members/research/fiat-trial/).

Endorectal advancement flap
Advancement flaps aim to stop the fistula track communicating with the bowel and cover the internal opening with disease-free anorectal wall. The procedure involves dissection of a full or partial thickness flap of the proximal rectal wall, which is then advanced on its pedicled blood supply to cover the previously excised internal opening. Principles for success include adequate flap vascularity and anastomosis of the flap to a site well distal of the previous internal opening. Modifications include curved incisions, rhomboid flaps, anorectal flaps with proximal advancement, and closure or dissection of the remaining fistula track (or both).

Failure or ischaemia of the flap may result in the creation of a much larger defect than previously existed, and dissection in a scarred anorectum risks damage to the underlying sphincter. Consequently, observational cohort studies report widely variable success rates—from 0% to 63%.[22][23] Most surgeons quote a success rate of 30% overall.

LIFT procedure
Ligation of the intersphincteric fistula track (LIFT) was first described in 2007.[24] A skin incision is made between the internal and external anal sphincters; the fistula track is exposed within the intersphincteric space and subsequently ligated and divided. A 94% success rate was initially reported, with no effect on continence.

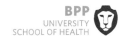

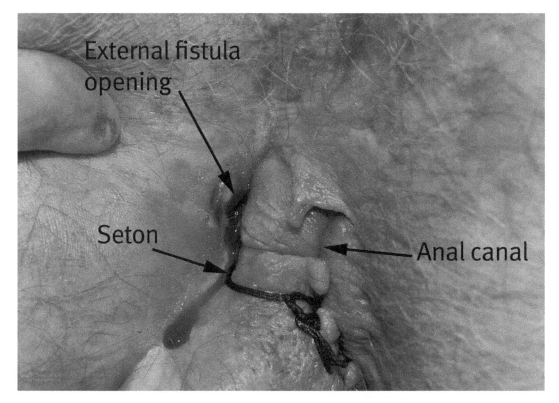

Fig 5 Photograph of a loose seton traversing a trans-sphincteric fistula

A Malaysian research group applied the technique to 45 patients (five with recurrent fistulas); after a median follow-up of nine months the healing rate was 82%.[25] A North American cohort study found a 57% success rate at median follow-up of 20 weeks.[26] The technique is sphincter sparing, inexpensive, and if it fails it does not prohibit other treatment methods. Recent modifications known as the BioLIFT involve placing a biological mesh in the intersphincteric space to act as a barrier to refistulisation. However, a larger area of dissection is needed, and the introduction of foreign material increases the risk of infection.

ADDITIONAL EDUCATIONAL RESOURCES

Resources for healthcare professionals

- Williams JG, Farrands PA, Williams AB, Taylor BA, Lunniss PJ, Sagar PM, et al. The treatment of anal fistula: ACPGBI position statement. *Colorectal Dis* 2007;9(suppl 4):18-50
- American Society of Colon and Rectum Surgeons. Anal fistula/abscess (www.fascrs.org/physicians/education/core_subjects/2009/anal_fistula_abscess/)—Summary of the management of anal fistula from an American perspective

Resources for patients

- NHS choices. Anal fistula (www.nhs.uk/conditions/Anal-fistula/Pages/Introduction.aspx)—Provides general information in lay language
- Crohn's and Colitis UK (www.nacc.org.uk/downloads/factsheets/fistula.pdf)—Crohn's and colitis fistula fact sheet for patients living with anal fistula

---

TIPS FOR NON-SPECIALISTS

- Consider possible underlying causes in a patient with a suspected anal fistula
- When performing a digital rectal examination in patients with perianal abscess or fistula, an internal opening classically feels like palpating a grain of rice
- Microbiology swabs of the affected perianal area may help determine whether the primary bacteria are skin or bowel commensals
- Although antibiotics are not usually effective in treating perianal abscess or infection associated with anal fistula, they are recommended in patients who have associated spreading cellulitis

Stem cells

The use of stem cells is a novel treatment. In a comparative study of 49 patients with cryptoglandular fistulas or Crohn's related fistulas the patient's own adipose tissue was processed and centrifuged to provide adipose derived stem cells. These cells were cultured and injected into the fistula track. A stem cell plus fibrin glue group was compared with a fibrin glue alone group and the healing rate was 71% versus 16%. The recurrence rate was 17.6% in the stem cell group at one year, with no recurrences in the control group.[27] However, this technology is not available in most centres.

Defunctioning

In rare cases where perianal sepsis is difficult to control and multiple tracks exist, the bowel may need to be defunctioned by bringing out the proximal colon as a colostomy. This improves symptoms of perianal leakage and diverts the bowel contents away from the anorectum, thus providing the optimum environment for sepsis resolution. However, the operation involves entering the peritoneal cavity and establishing a stoma. Postoperative problems include bleeding, infection, thrombosis, ileus, leaks, and complications associated with colostomy. Defunctioning is therefore considered only as a last resort in non-healing anal fistula. Once treatment of the anal fistula is complete it is possible to reverse the colostomy and restore intestinal continuity in some patients.Special cases

Crohn's disease

The cumulative incidence of anal fistula in patients with Crohn's disease is 20-25%.[28] [29] Fistulas are often complex and multiple in these patients; this makes the treatment challenging and seriously affects the patient's quality of life. Randomised clinical trials have confirmed the efficacy of the anti-tumour necrosis factor α antibody, infliximab,[30] [31] and this agent should be considered first line treatment.[32] In one multicentre randomised double blind trial, conducted

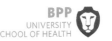

at 45 sites, 306 patients were enrolled to receive infliximab maintenance therapy or a control maintenance therapy. Over the 54 week study, nearly twice as many patients who received infliximab, as compared with placebo, had complete and durable closure of their fistula.[31] Surgical options are considered if medical treatment fails, but because of the poor rate of wound healing in active Crohn's disease, a defunctioning colostomy is a more common strategy.

Tuberculosis

Tuberculosis may be the cause of anal fistula in some cases. The clinical presentation may imitate that of Crohn's disease or cancer, and it is more likely to be the underlying cause in patients with HIV.[33] Tuberculosis should be suspected in patients who fail to respond to standard treatment or who develop recurrent fistulas.[34] Diagnosis is made through the histological finding of granulomatous disease and the positive identification of acid fast bacilli.[35] Antituberculous drugs are the first line treatment.

Contributors: JAS and AB contributed equally to the writing and revision of the manuscript. JHS was responsible for editing and revision.

Patient consent obtained.

Funding: No special funding received.

Competing interests: All authors have completed the ICMJE uniform disclosure form at www.icmje.org/coi_disclosure.pdf (available on request from the corresponding author) and declare: no support from any organisation for the submitted work; no financial relationships with any organisations that might have an interest in the submitted work in the previous three years; no other relationships or activities that could appear to have influenced the submitted work.

Provenance and peer review: Not commissioned; externally peer reviewed.

1   Zanotti C, Martinez-Puente C, Pascual I, Pascual M, Herreros D, García-Olmo D. An assessment of the incidence of fistula-in-ano in four countries of the European Union. *Int J Colorect Dis*2007;22:1459-62.
2   Sainio P. Fistula-in-ano in a defined population. Incidence and epidemiological aspects. *Ann Chir Gynaecol*1984;73:219-24.
3   Sileri P, Cadeddu F, D'Ugo S, Franceschilli L, Del Vecchio Blanco G, De Luca E, et al. Surgery for fistula-in-ano in a specialist colorectal unit: a critical appraisal. *BMC Gastroenterol*2011;11:120.
4   Meislin HW, McGehee MD, Rosen P. Management and microbiology of cutaneous abscesses. *JACEP*1978;7:186-91.
5   Malik AI, Nelson RL, Tou S. Incision and drainage of perianal abscess with or without treatment of anal fistula. *Cochrane Database Syst Rev*2010;7:CD006827.
6   Grace RH, Harper IA, Thompson RG. Anorectal sepsis: microbiology in relation to fistula-in-ano. *Br J Surg*1982;69:401-3.
7   Toyonaga T, Matsushima M, Tanaka Y, Shimojima Y, Matsumura N, Kannyama H, et al. Microbiological analysis and endoanal ultrasonography for diagnosis of anal fistula in acute anorectal sepsis. *Int J Colorectal Dis*2007;22:209-13.
8   Parks AG, Gordon PH, Hardcastle JD. A classification of fistula-in-ano. *Br J Surg*1976;63:1-12.
9   Becker A, Koltun L, Sayfan J. Simple clinical examination predicts complexity of perianal fistula. *Colorectal Dis*2006;8:601-4.
10   Halligan S, Stoker J. Imaging of fistula in ano. *Radiology*2006;239:18-33.
11   Siddiqui MR, Ashrafian H, Tozer P, Daulatzai N, Burling D, Hart A, et al. A diagnostic accuracy meta-analysis of endoanal ultrasound and MRI for perianal fistula assessment. *Dis Colon Rectum*2012;55:576-85.
12   Jacob TJ, Perakath B, Keighley MR. Surgical intervention for anorectal fistula. *Cochrane Database Syst Rev*2010;5:CD006319.
13   Faucheron JL, Saint-Marc O, Guibert L, Parc R. Long-term seton drainage for high anal fistulas in Crohn's disease—a sphincter-saving operation? *Dis Colon Rectum*1996;39:208-11.
14   Christensen A, Nilas L, Christiansen J. Treatment of transsphincteric anal fistulas by the seton technique. *Dis Colon Rectum*1986;29:454-5.
15   Hammond TM, Knowles CH, Porrett T, Lunniss PJ. The snug seton: short and medium term results of slow fistulotomy for idiopathic anal fistulae. *Colorectal Dis*2006;8:328-37.
16   Tyler KM, Aarons CB, Sentovich SM. Successful sphincter-sparing surgery for all anal fistulas. *Dis Colon Rectum*2007;50:1535-9.
17   Atkin GK, Martins J, Tozer P, Ranchod P, Phillips RK. For many high anal fistulas, lay open is still a good option. *Tech Coloproctol*2011;15:143-50.
18   Whiteford MH, Kilkenny J 3rd, Hyman N, Buie WD, Cohen J, Orsay C, et al. Practice parameters for the treatment of perianal abscess and fistula-in-ano (revised). *Dis Colon Rectum*2005;48:1337-42.
19   Sentovich SM. Fibrin glue for all anal fistulas. *J Gastrointest Surg*2001;5:158-61.
20   Shawki S, Wexner SD. Idiopathic fistula-in-ano. *World J Gastroenterol*2011;17:3277-85.
21   O'Riordan JM, Datta I, Johnston C, Baxter NN. A systematic review of the anal fistula plug for patients with Crohn's and non-Crohn's related fistula-in-ano. *Dis Colon Rectum*2012;55:351-8.
22   Ortiz H, Marzo J. Endorectal flap advancement repair and fistulectomy for high trans-sphincteric and suprasphincteric fistulas. *Br J Surg*2000;87:1680-3.
23   Van der Hagen SJ, Baeten CG, Soeters PB, van Gemert WG. Long-term outcome following mucosal advancement flap for high perianal fistulas and fistulotomy for low perianal fistulas: recurrent perianal fistulas: failure of treatment or recurrent patient disease? *Int J Colorectal Dis*2006;21:784-90.
24   Rojanasakul A, Pattanaarun J, Sahakitrungruang C, Tantiphlachiva K. Total anal sphincter saving technique for fistula-in-ano; the ligation of intersphincteric fistula tract. *J Med Assoc Thai*2007;90:581-6.
25   Shanwani A, Nor AM, Amri N. Ligation of the intersphincteric fistula tract (LIFT): a sphincter-saving technique for fistula-in-ano. *Dis Colon Rectum*2010;53:39-42.
26   Bleier JI, Moloo H, Goldberg SM. Ligation of the intersphincteric fistula tract: an effective new technique for complex fistulas. *Dis Colon Rectum*2010;53:43-6.
27   Garcia-Olmo D, Herreros D, Pascual I, Pascual JA, Del-Valle E, Zorrilla J, et al. Expanded adipose-derived stem cells for the treatment of complex perianal fistula: a phase II clinical trial. *Dis Colon Rectum*2009;52:79-86.
28   Hellers G, Bergstrand O, Ewerth S, Holmstrom B. Occurrence and outcome after primary treatment of anal fistulae in Crohn's disease. *Gut*1980;21:525-7.
29   Tang LY, Rawsthorne P, Bernstein CN. Are perineal and luminal fistulas associated in Crohn's disease? A population-based study. *Clin Gastroenterol Hepatol*2006;4:1130-4.
30   Sands BE, Blank MA, Diamond RH, Barrett JP, Van Deventer SJ. Maintenance infliximab does not result in increased abscess development in fistulizing Crohn's disease: results from the ACCENT II study. *Aliment Pharmacol Ther*2006;23:1127-36.
31   Sands BE, Anderson FH, Bernstein CN, Chey WY, Feagan BG, Fedorak RN, et al. Infliximab maintenance therapy for fistulizing Crohn's disease. *N Engl J Med*2004;350:876-85.
32   Taxonera C, Schwartz DA, Garcia-Olmo D. Emerging treatments for complex perianal fistula in Crohn's disease. *World J Gastroenterol*2009;15:4263-72.
33   Donoghue HD, Holton J. Intestinal tuberculosis. *Curr Opin Infect Dis*2009;22:490-6.
34   Bokhari I, Shah SS, Inamullah, Mehmood Z, Ali SU, Khan A. Tubercular fistula-in-ano. *J Coll Physicians Surg Pak*2008;18:401-3.
35   Wijekoon NS, Samarasekera DN. The value of routine histopathological analysis in patients with fistula in-ano. *Colorectal Dis*2010;12:94-6.

Related links

bmj.com/archive
Previous articles in this series
- Plantar fasciitis (2012;345:e6603)
- Cardiopulmonary resuscitation (2012;345:e6122)
- Weight faltering and failure to thrive in infancy and early childhood (2012;345:e5931)
- Preimplantation genetic testing (2012;345:e5908)
- Early fluid resuscitation in severe trauma (2012;345:e5752)

bmj.com
- Get CME credits for this article

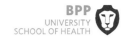

Management of faecal incontinence in adults

Mukhtar Ahmad, specialist registrar, general surgery[1],
Iain J D McCallum, teaching and research fellow[2],
Mark Mercer-Jones, consultant surgeon[1]

[1]Queen Elizabeth Hospital, Gateshead NE9 6SX

[2]North Tyneside General Hospital, North Shields NE29 8NH

Correspondence to: mark.mercer-jones@ghnt.nhs.uk

Cite this as: BMJ 2010;340:c2964

DOI: 10.1136/bmj.e7183

http://www.bmj.com/content/345/bmj.e7183

Faecal incontinence is the involuntary loss of stool or flatus. It is a distressing condition that can have a substantially negative effect on quality of life.[1][2] According to a systematic review it may affect 11-15% of the population.[3] The estimated cost of absorbent products (such as pads) is around £94m (€112m; $138m) per annum in the United Kingdom.[4] Because faecal incontinence is a heterogeneous problem that ranges from minor faecal soiling to incapacitating urge or passive faecal incontinence and embarrassment may prevent patients from seeking help, estimates of prevalence may not be accurate. Incontinence is a common reason for admission to residential care even though in many cases simple measures are available in primary care that could enable people to remain at home. We review evidence on causes, diagnosis, and management of faecal incontinence in adults and summarise the findings of systematic reviews and guidelines where possible.

Who is affected by faecal incontinence?

An epidemiological survey showed a rising incidence with advancing age and the highest prevalence in elderly people in long term care, with no sex difference in adults aged over 40.[5] The higher reported prevalence of faecal incontinence in younger women is probably the result of childbirth related injuries, and a prospective study showed that the greatest risk follows the first vaginal delivery.[6]

How does faecal incontinence present?

Two main patterns of presentation exist. Urge faecal incontinence occurs when the patient senses the need to defecate but is unable to control or resist the urge. Passive incontinence occurs without warning. Some patients have faecal soiling without frank incontinence. We mention this here because the initial assessment of this group is similar to that for faecal incontinence with the addition of assessing the patient's perianal hygiene routine. Management is similar to that for passive faecal incontinence.

How is continence normally maintained?

The anal canal is surrounded by two layers of muscle, the involuntary internal anal sphincter and the external anal sphincter, which is under voluntary control. The integrity of the anal sphincters is important for maintaining continence, but pelvic floor muscles, anal cushions (three distinct pads of vascular tissue that help maintain continence), nervous control of the anal canal and pelvic floor, the consistency of faeces, and a compliant non-diseased rectal reservoir all play a role. A complex interplay of these factors maintains faecal continence and problems with any of them can lead to incontinence (fig 1).

What are the causes of faecal incontinence?

Faecal incontinence is a symptom rather than a diagnosis. It is a multifactorial condition that usually results from a combination of specific causes, often in the context of physical or cognitive decline in older age. The causes are classified below according to pathophysiology.

Diarrhoea and constipation

The consistency of faeces is an important factor in maintaining continence. Urge incontinence may occur in any patient with larger than average stool volume or loose stools delivered to the rectum. This includes patients with inflammatory bowel disease or irritable bowel disease and patients taking certain drugs (box 1). Patients with faecal impaction may have "overflow diarrhoea," and this is most common in nursing home residents.

Problems with the anal sphincter

After childbirth

A large cohort study of 8774 women found the incidence of faecal incontinence after vaginal delivery to be 29% at three to six months postpartum. Incontinence is particularly common after the use of forceps, in women with a high body mass index, and after prolonged labour.[8] Eighty five per cent of women with recognised third degree tears have residual sphincter damage, and over half of this group have ongoing symptoms despite primary repair at the time of delivery.[9]

Surgery

Incontinence may result from any procedure that damages the anal sphincters. It may be inevitable after complex anal fistula surgery, for example, or occur unexpectedly—for example, after haemorrhoidectomy or surgery for chronic anal fissure or rectal cancer. Evidence from a cohort study suggests that the incidence of iatrogenic damage is reducing with advances in surgical techniques.[w1]

Degeneration of the internal anal sphincter

In the absence of structural damage, primary isolated degeneration of the smooth muscle of the internal anal sphincter may cause passive leakage of stool.[10] It is most common in middle age and affects men and women. In a recently published case series, 9% of patients attending a faecal incontinence clinic had faecal soiling with no obvious cause. The exact incidence of internal anal sphincter degeneration is difficult to determine because of the heterogeneity in its description and because it is one of the "causes" of idiopathic faecal soiling.[w2]

SOURCES AND SELECTION CRITERIA

We searched PubMed, National Institute for Health and Clinical Excellence guidelines, Embase, and the Cochrane library using the search terms faecal/fecal incontinence. We retrieved potentially useful studies and critically evaluated them for inclusion.

SUMMARY POINTS

- Faecal incontinence is common and socially debilitating
- Most cases of faecal incontinence can be managed in the community by non-specialists
- The aetiology is multifactorial and treatment must be individually tailored
- Often the condition cannot be "cured" but its effects mitigated to improve patients' lives
- When conservative methods fail referral to a specialist is indicated

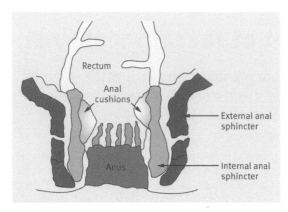

Section through the anal canal showing the anal sphincters and anal cushions

Neurological disease

A prevalence study reported that 50% of patients with multiple sclerosis had faecal incontinence.[11] Patients with diabetes and autonomic neuropathy may also have incontinence. A controlled study showed that rectal sensation is impaired in patients with diabetes who also have faecal incontinence compared with those without.[w3] Autonomic neuropathy is thought to impair the reflex that enables a person to distinguish between solid, liquid, and gaseous rectal contents. Pudendal neuropathy causes neurogenic incontinence and reduced external anal sphincter function.

Congenital disorders

Patients with spina bifida commonly report incontinence or faecal soiling. Surgery for congenital disorders such as anal atresia or Hirschsprung's disease may lead to incontinence. One study of 60 patients with this disease found that about 50% had severe soiling.[w4]

Other conditions

Rectal prolapse, which results from a combination of factors including weakness or degeneration of the pelvic floor muscles and anal sphincters, may lead to incontinence. Prolapsing internal haemorrhoids may also cause faecal soiling by interfering with closure of the anal canal.

Idiopathic incontinence

Some patients with faecal incontinence have normal anal sphincters on endoanal ultrasound, normal rectal compliance, intact sensation, and no evidence of neuropathy.

BOX 1 DRUGS THAT CAN EXACERBATE FAECAL INCONTINENCE[7]

Drugs that alter sphincter tone
- Nitrates, calcium channel antagonists, β blockers, sildenafil, selective serotonin reuptake inhibitors

Broad spectrum antibiotics (multiple mechanisms)
- Cephalosporins, penicillins, macrolides

Topical anal drugs
- Glyceryl trinitrate ointment, diltiazem gel, bethanechol cream, botulinum A toxin

Drugs causing profuse loose stools
- Laxatives, metformin, orlistat, selective serotonin reuptake inhibitors, antacids containing magnesium, digoxin

Constipating drugs
- Loperamide, opioids, tricyclic antidepressants, antacids containing aluminium, codeine

Tranquillisers or hypnotics (reduce alertness)
- Benzodiazepines, tricyclic antidepressants, selective serotonin reuptake inhibitors, antipsychotics

---

Specific aetiologies are yet to be fully defined. Atrophy of the anal cushions (which contribute to 10-15% of the resting pressure of the anal canal) is one possibility.[12] Rectoanal intussusception has been found in patients with otherwise normal investigations,[13] and its correction by laparoscopic ventral rectopexy produced encouraging results in one short term prospective study.[14]

How do I assess a patient with faecal incontinence in primary care?

Most patients will never undergo formal testing of anorectal function and can be managed in primary care. Recent guidelines commissioned by the National Institute for Health and Clinical Excellence (NICE) found no studies that examined the initial assessment of faecal incontinence, so NICE provided guidelines based on expert consensus.[7] Initial history underpins an accurate diagnosis and is summarised in box 2. The most important factor is an accurate assessment of the effect of incontinence on a patient's lifestyle. This allows benchmarks to be set for judging the success of interventions.

Examination should focus on causes suspected from the history. NICE guidelines recommend a minimum of a general examination, digital anorectal examination, and assessment of cognitive function.[7] The first two examinations are aimed at identifying or ruling out some of the conditions discussed above. Specific conditions that will need to be identified and treated before the empirical treatment of faecal incontinence can begin are: colitis, other causes of diarrhoea, faecal loading, suspected colorectal cancer, rectal prolapse, acute sphincter injury, and central disc prolapse.[7]

Scoring systems have been devised to assess the severity of faecal incontinence. The most widely used one is the Wexner or Cleveland Clinic system (table).[15] Its original description has been modified to give a simple, practical and reproducible tool with good concurrence between patients' scores and doctors' scores.[15] One cross sectional study of 154 patients showed that those with more severe incontinence had poorer quality of life.[w5] However, larger studies of patients with incontinence have not found clear associations between quality of life scores and severity, so both should be assessed to judge the effect of interventions properly.[w6] Box 4 gives advice on when to refer patients to a specialist.

What investigations may be carried out in secondary care?

Investigations in secondary care depend on the suspected aetiology. They may include flexible sigmoidoscopy, defecating proctography, endoanal ultrasound examination, magnetic resonance imaging, anorectal manometry, rectal compliance and distension sensitivity, pudendal nerve latency, and electromyography. Evidence to support the use of any specific single investigation or combination is limited.[7] Endoscopy is warranted if colorectal cancer is suspected.

What non-surgical treatments are currently available?

Treatment depends on the underlying structural and functional abnormalities, as well as the severity of symptoms and their effects on quality of life. Many patients will have had the problem for years, and they may have been subject to social stigmatisation as well as anxiety or depression. Treatment options can be divided broadly into conservative non-surgical interventions and surgical procedures. Most cases can be managed successfully in primary care. NICE

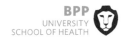

guidelines recommend patient centred management.[7] Most interventions will not "cure" faecal incontinence but will reduce its effect on the patient's life.

Diet and fluids

Some patients find that eating stimulates the gastrocolic reflex—increased colonic motility in response to distension of the stomach after a meal—with resulting urgency. If this is the case, changing the timing of meals and their size may help. Box 3 lists foods that can exacerbate faecal incontinence.[7] Fibre supplementation has been used as strategy to bulk stools, and a study of 336 women who were overweight and had urinary incontinence found that low dietary fibre intake was an independent risk factor for faecal incontinence.[w7] One small, underpowered, randomised controlled trial (n=26) found that fibre supplements of gum arabic or psyllium reduced the proportion of incontinent stools.[w8] Another trial combined either fibre supplements or a low residue diet with loperamide in a crossover design. It found that both groups improved, but neither fibre supplementation nor low residue diet was superior. The response varied greatly within each group, probably because of differing causes of incontinence; this led the authors to conclude that dietary strategies should be individually tailored.[16]

Drugs

Box 1 lists the drugs that are known to exacerbate faecal incontinence.[7] A Cochrane review examined the effectiveness of drugs used to treat faecal incontinence—the antidiarrhoeals—loperamide, codeine phosphate, and co-phenotrope (diphenoxylate and atropine).[17] These drugs are usually prescribed in the order stated above (according to the severity of their side effects). The review concluded that there was evidence to support the use of titrated antidiarrhoeals for faecal incontinence and that side effects were common.[17]

Mechanical options

A recent Cochrane review examined the use of anal plugs for faecal incontinence. Only two small trials had examined the use of plugs versus no treatment, and studies were prone to high levels of dropout (36%). Although plugs were useful and effective in some patients, they were unacceptable to many.[18]

A Cochrane review and a Health Technology Assessment (HTA) report have examined the usefulness and cost effectiveness of absorbent products such as pads. Both found that preference varied considerably, depending on sex, location (nursing home or community), level of independence, and severity of incontinence.[4][19] The HTA report concluded that allowing users (patients or carers) to choose within a budget would probably be most cost effective.[4]

Biofeedback and pelvic floor exercises

Biofeedback is a technique that allows cognitive and mechanical re-training of the complex muscular systems needed to maintain continence and defecation.[w9] Positive case series have led to support for the use of biofeedback as a primary intervention,[20] but the evidence is prone to publication bias and the large placebo effect often noted in functional gastrointestinal disorders. A recent Cochrane review examined the use of biofeedback and any form of pelvic floor or anal exercises to treat incontinence.[21] The review was limited by heterogeneity of aetiology, specific treatment strategies, and outcome measures between studies, however, as well as limitations in trial design and size. It concluded that there was no evidence from the limited randomised controlled trials available to support the use of biofeedback therapy.[21]

Rectal irrigation

Rectal irrigation has been used to prevent incontinence on the assumption that a patient cannot be incontinent if the rectum is kept empty. One prospective trial found improved continence scores in all 18 patients treated with irrigation.[w10] Long term results in 348 patients with constipation or incontinence treated with rectal irrigation showed success in 47% of patients at 21 months. Anal insufficiency, low rectal volume at urge to defecate, and low maximal rectal capacity were the conditions most likely to improve with this treatment.[22]

What are the surgical options?

Surgical procedures are aimed at correcting obvious mechanical defects or occasionally augmenting functionally deficient but structurally intact sphincters.

Anal bulking

There are three distinct elevations within the anal canal formed by collections of blood vessels. These anal "cushions" are thought to play an important role in maintaining passive faecal continence. Anal bulking refers to the intra-anal injection of synthetic agents to correct asymmetry of the anal canal that may result from atrophy of the anal cushions. A recent Cochrane review found only four randomised controlled trials of variable quality and concluded that there was no robust evidence but a trend towards improvement in the short term.[23] Case series have shown that anal bulking is a safe treatment and can reduce the severity of faecal incontinence.[24][25] Careful selection of patients is crucial because only those with mild to moderate faecal incontinence are likely to benefit.

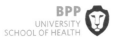

Sacral nerve stimulation

A Cochrane review concluded that sacral nerve stimulation can improve continence in some people with faecal incontinence.[26] If conservative measures fail, sacral nerve stimulation offers an effective yet minimally invasive approach in patients with weak but mostly intact anal sphincters and rectal function. Electrodes are inserted in the lower back and attached to a pulse generator. The exact mechanism of action is poorly understood, but the pulses of electricity produced stimulate the sacral nerve roots and are thought to modulate the neural control of the anal sphincters and possibly enhance rectal sensation. A temporary electrode is placed initially, and if symptoms improve by 50% or more, a permanent implant is inserted. It is an expensive procedure but cost analysis shows it to be cost effective compared with colostomy or dynamic graciloplasty.[w11]

BOX 3 FOOD AND DRINK THAT MAY EXACERBATE FAECAL INCONTINENCE IN PATIENTS WITH LOOSE STOOLS[7]

Fruit and vegetables
- Rhubarb, figs, prunes, and plums (all contain a natural laxative). Beans, pulses, cabbages, and sprouts

Spices
- Such as chilli

Artificial sweeteners
- Found in sugar free or diabetic products

Alcohol
- Especially stout, beers, and ales

Lactose
- Some patients may have a degree of lactase deficiency, although they may be able to tolerate small quantities of milk and yoghurt

Caffeine
- Can loosen stool in susceptible patients

Vitamin and mineral supplements
- Excessive doses of vitamin C, magnesium, phosphorus, or calcium can increase faecal incontinence

Olestra fat substitute
- Can cause loose stools

BOX 4 WHEN DO I REFER TO A SPECIALIST?
- Referral to a specialist is indicated when simple conservative measures fail[7]
- Some special cases should prompt early referral:
- Sphincter injury
- Trauma
- Recent change in bowel pattern
- Previous surgery for incontinence

---

faecal incontinence symptom severity scoring system[15]*

Event	Never	Rarely (<1/month)	Sometimes (<1/week, ≥1/ month)	Usually <1/day, ≥1/week	Always ≥1/day
Solid leakage	0	1	2	3	4
Liquid leakage	0	1	2	3	4
Gas leakage	0	1	2	3	4
Use of pads	0	2	2	2	2
Use of constipating agents	0	2	2	2	2
Altered lifestyle	0	1	2	3	4

Numerical scores are given for how often in the past month the patient experienced an event, although a flat score of 2 is given for use of pads and use of constipating agents.

Sphincter repair

Anterior overlapping sphincteroplasty is the treatment of choice in patients with external sphincter defects, although the success of sacral nerve stimulation in these patients has called it into question. The procedure involves dissecting the external anal sphincter from surrounding structures to allow an overlapping repair to be performed using sutures. A recently published case series showed good long term outcome in 60% of patients, although outcome was worse in patients who were older than 50 years at the time of surgery.[27]

Randomised trials have compared different surgical techniques but failed to show superiority of one technique.[w12 w13] A Cochrane review found not enough evidence from trials to judge whether surgery is better than non-surgical management.[28] This is probably because the wide range of procedures available and the varied aetiology of incontinence in the trial subjects hinder standardisation.

Sphincter replacement

Artificial sphincters

A small randomised trial showed that all patients who had an artificial sphincter implanted improved more than those who had only supportive treatment. The same trial reported significant morbidity associated with the implants, however.[29]

Graciloplasty

This technique transposes the gracilis muscle so that it encircles the anus and provides a neosphincter. Electrodes are then implanted in the muscle and connected to a neurostimulator, which the patient can use to control the sphincter. A systematic review found that this was better at restoring continence than colostomy, although complication rates were higher.[30]

Antegrade colonic enema

Antegrade colonic enema refers to antegrade irrigation of the colon via an appendicostomy, caecostomy, or tapered ileostomy. It reduces the frequency of incontinence by intermittently cleansing the colon. The procedure can be carried out laparoscopically. A recent retrospective study of 80 patients showed favourable long term results across the spectrum of surgical procedures performed.[31] It should be considered before resorting to colostomy.

Diversion stoma

When all measures to achieve continence fail a diversion stoma (usually a colostomy) remains the only way to restore continence and dignity. The patient should be assessed thoroughly and all non-surgical and surgical options should be considered by a specialist team. If the decision is to create a stoma, stoma specialists should be involved early in the process so that the patient can make an informed decision after the potential risks and long term consequences have been explained.

Which patients are challenging?

Those with severe cognitive impairment

It is important to determine whether there is any behavioural reason for faecal incontinence.[7] If behavioural causes are identified, specific interventions can be planned to resolve them, and the input of multiple specialties will be required. Physical measures are usually needed to augment psychotherapeutic or behavioural interventions.

Competing interests: All authors have completed the Unified Competing Interest form at www.icmje.org/coi_disclosure.pdf (available on request from the corresponding author) and declare: (1) No financial support for the submitted work; (2) No relationships with companies that might have an interest in the submitted work in the previous three years; (3) No spouses, partners, or children with financial relationships that may be relevant to the submitted work; and (4) No non-financial interests that may be relevant to the submitted work.

Provenance and peer review: Not commissioned; externally peer reviewed.

Patient consent obtained.

MA and IJDM contributed equally to the manuscript and should be considered joint first authors.

 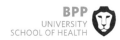

ADDITIONAL EDUCATIONAL RESOURCES

Resources for healthcare professionals

- National Institute for Health and Clinical Excellence (www.nice.org.uk/CG49)—In addition to the full guideline, a quick reference guide includes key points in the management of faecal incontinence
- Cochrane Library (www.thecochranelibrary.com/view/0/browse.html?cat=ccochgastrfaecalincontinence)—This website contains 12 systematic reviews on all aspects of management of faecal incontinence
- Gallas S, Michot F, Faucheron JL, Meurette G, Lehur PA, Barth X, et al. Predictive factors for successful sacral nerve stimulation in the treatment of faecal incontinence: results of trial stimulation in 200 patients. *Colorectal Dis* 2010; online 10 March

Resources for patients

- UpToDate (www.uptodate.com/patients/content/topic.do?topicKey=~foab4wp/xXlpnf)—Patient version of this useful online information
- US National Library of Medicine and the National Institutes of Health (www.nlm.nih.gov/medlineplus/bowelincontinence.html)—Provides a simple overview of the topic and links to relevant journal articles
- American College of gastroenterology (http://www.gi.org/patients/gihealth/fi.asp)—Useful question and answer format on causes and management options

A PATIENT'S PERSPECTIVE

Living with faecal incontinence is debilitating and demoralising, but if you can overcome your immense personal distress help is available.

My story began 18 years ago after childbirth. My bowel control changed—severe urgency would give me minutes or less to find a toilet, and leakage with flatus happened frequently. I said nothing. I tried to manage as best I could, wearing pads all the time. I work as a midwife and was struggling to do my job properly and to continue to live an active life because of this problem.

Two years ago rectal bleeding made me go to my general practitioner; I managed to blurt out my "other" problems and was referred to a consultant.

The journey was tough; the tests needed for diagnosis were distressing in themselves. After a ventral rectopexy and insertion of a permanent sacral nerve stimulation implant my bowel control has improved immensely. The implant isn't without its drawbacks; I feel a permanent pulsing through my buttock which can be uncomfortable.

However, I feel that this is a small price to pay for the immense relief from my condition and the subsequent growth in my self esteem and confidence. My life has changed dramatically and I feel that I belong to the human race again.

Those with neuromuscular disease

For patients with neuromuscular disease, try to maximise their understanding of how the underlying disease has altered bowel function. In addition to dietary modification, rectal evacuants (enemas or suppositories) and oral laxatives help establish a predictable pattern of bowel evacuation. Digital anorectal stimulation may be beneficial for people with spinal cord injuries or other neurogenic bowel disorders. Manual removal of faeces may be necessary when faecal impaction occurs. Rectal irrigation might help to prevent incontinence by clearing out faeces. Unfortunately, these measures are time consuming and may impose further restrictions on an already challenged life. Surgical options including stoma may be considered if conservative measures fail or become too burdensome.

Nursing home residents with faecal impaction

A treatment strategy for this group aims at producing a tailor made plan for each patient that reduces the chances of recurrence. The plan will include a combination of interventions such as laxatives, rectal evacuants, and dietary modification. Some people require the regular use of rectal evacuants to produce planned evacuations.

1. Chelvanayagam S, Norton C. Quality of life with faecal continence problems. (Role of patient focus groups in developing a quality of life measure for faecal incontinence. *Nurs Times*2000;96(31 suppl):15-7.
2. Collings S, Norton C. Women's experiences of faecal incontinence: a study. *Br J Community Nurs*2004;9:520-3.
3. Macmillan AK, Merrie AE, Marshall RJ, Parry BR. The prevalence of faecal incontinence in community-dwelling adults: a systematic review of the literature. *Dis Colon Rectum*2004;47:1341-9.
4. Fader M, Cottenden A, Getliffe K, Gage H, Clarke-O'Neill S, Jamieson K, et al. Absorbent products for urinary/faecal incontinence: a comparative evaluation of key product designs. *Health Technol Assess*2008;12(29):iii-iv, ix-185.
5. Perry S, Shaw C, McGrother C, Matthews RJ, Assassa RP, Dallosso H, et al. Prevalence of faecal incontinence in adults aged 40 years or more living in the community. *Gut*2002;50:480-4.
6. Fynes M, Donnelly V, Behan M, O'Connell PR, O'Herlihy C. Effect of second vaginal delivery on anorectal physiology and faecal continence: a prospective study. *Lancet*1999;354:983-6.
7. National Institute for Health and Clinical Excellence. Faecal incontinence: the management of faecal incontinence in adults. CG49. 2007. www.nice.org.uk/CG49.
8. Guise JM, Morris C, Osterweil P, Li H, Rosenberg D, Greenlick M. Incidence of faecal incontinence after childbirth. *Obstet Gynelcol*2007;109:281-8.
9. Kamm MA. Obstetric damage and faecal incontinence. *Lancet*1994;344:730-3.
10. Vaizey CJ, Kamm MA, Bartram CI. Primary degeneration of the internal anal sphincter as a cause of passive faecal incontinence. *Lancet*1997;349:612-5.
11. Hinds JP, Eidelman BH, Wald A. Prevalence of bowel dysfunction in multiple sclerosis. A population survey. *Gastroenterology*1990;98:1538-42.
12. Thekkinkattil DK, Dunham RJ, O'Herlihy S, Finan PJ, Sagar PM, Burke DA. Measurement of anal cushions in idiopathic faecal incontinence. *Br J Surg*2009;96:680-4.
13. Collinson R, Cunningham C, D'Costa H, Lindsey I. Rectal intussusception and unexplained faecal incontinence: findings of a proctographic study. *Colorectal Dis*2009;11:77-83.
14. Collinson N, Wijffels N, Cunningham C, Lindsey I. Laparoscopic ventral rectopexy for internal rectal prolapse: short-term functional results. *Colorectal Dis*2010;12:97-104.
15. Rockwood TH, Church JM, Fleshman JW, Kane RL, Mavrantonis C, Thorson AG, et al. Patient and surgeon ranking of the severity of symptoms associated with faecal incontinence: the faecal incontinence severity index. *Dis Colon Rectum*1999;42:1525-32.
16. Lauti M, Scott D, Thompson-Fawcett MW. Fibre supplementation in addition to loperamide for faecal incontinence in adults: a randomized trial. *Colorectal Dis*2008;10:553-62.
17. Cheetam MJ, Brazzelli M, Norton CC, Glazener CMA, Drug treatment for faecal incontinence in adults. *Cochrane Database Syst Rev*2002;3:CD002116.
18. Deutekom M, Dobben AC. Plugs for containing faecal incontinence. *Cochrane Database Syst Rev*2005;3:CD005086.
19. Fader M, Cottenden AM, Getliffe K. Absorbent products for moderate-heavy urinary and/or faecal incontinence in women and men. *Cochrane Database Syst Rev* 2008;4:CD007408.
20. Norton C, Kamm MA. Anal sphincter biofeedback and pelvic floor exercises for faecal incontinence in adults—a systematic review. *Aliment Pharmacol Therapeut*2001;15:1147-54.
21. Norton CC, Cody JD, Hosker G. Biofeedback and/or sphincter exercises for the treatment of faecal incontinence in adults. *Cochrane Database Syst Rev* 2009;1:CD002111.
22. Christensen P, Krogh K, Buntzen S, Payandeh F, Laurberg S. Long-term outcome and safety of transanal irrigation for constipation and faecal incontinence. *Dis Colon Rectum*2009;52:286-92.
23. Maeda Y, Laurberg S, Norton C. Perianal injectable bulking agents as treatment for faecal incontinence in adults. *Cochrane Database Syst Rev* 2010;5:CD007959.
24. Altomare DF, La Torre F, Rinaldi M, Binda GA, Pescatori M. Carbon-coated microbeads anal injection in outpatient treatment of minor faecal incontinence. *Dis Colon Rectum*2008;51:432-5.
25. Bartlett L, Ho YH. PTQ anal implants for the treatment of faecal incontinence. *Br J Surg*2009;96:1468-75.

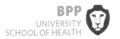

26 Mowatt G, Glazener CMA, Jarrett M. Sacral nerve stimulation for faecal incontinence and constipation in adults. *Cochrane Database Syst Rev* 2007;3:CD004464.

27 Oom DM, Gosselink MP, Schouten WR. Anterior sphincteroplasty for faecal incontinence: a single centre experience in the era of sacral neuromodulation. *Dis Colon Rectum*2009;52:1681-7.

28 Brown SR, Nelson RL. Surgery for faecal incontinence in adults. *Cochrane Database Syst Rev* 2007;2:CD001757.

29 O'Brien PE, Dixon JB, Skinner S, Laurie C, Khera A, Fonda D. A prospective randomized controlled clinical trial of placement of the artificial bowel sphincter (Acticon neosphincter) for the control of faecal incontinence. *Dis Colon Rectum*2004;47:1852-60.

30 Chapman AE, Geerdes B, Hewett P, Young J, Eyers T, Kiroff G, et al. Systematic review of dynamic graciloplasty in the treatment of faecal incontinence. *Br J Surg*2002;89:138-53.

31 Worsøe J, Christensen P, Krogh K, Buntzen S, Laurberg S. Long-term results of antegrade colonic enema in adult patients: assessment of functional results. *Dis Colon Rectum*2007;50:1023-31.

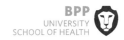

Diagnosis and management of anal intraepithelial neoplasia and anal cancer

J A D Simpson, academic surgical registrar, J H Scholefield, professor of surgery

[1]Division of Gastrointestinal Surgery, Queens Medical Centre Campus, Nottingham University Hospital, Nottingham NG7 2UH, UK

Correspondence to: J A Simpson
alastairsimpson@hotmail.com

Cite this as: BMJ 2011;343:d6818

DOI: 10.1136/bmj.d6818

http://www.bmj.com/content/343/bmj.d6818

Anal cancer accounts for about 4% of large bowel malignancies, but data from the Surveillance Epidemiology and End Results programme show a considerable rise in incidence since 1975[1] from 0.8 to 1.7 per 100 000. The World Health Organization recently estimated that between 350 and 500 new cases of anal squamous cell carcinoma are detected each year in England and Wales.[2]

Observational studies have shown that individuals with genital human papillomavirus (HPV) infection and those who are immunosuppressed, including HIV positive patients, are at increased risk of developing anal cancer.[3] [4] A history of cervical or vulval HPV infection and premalignant changes also increases the risk of developing anal cancer, with a reported incidence rate ratio of between 3.97 and 31.09, dependent on age at diagnosis, compared with controls.[5] General practitioners and practice nurses who screen women as part of national programmes for detecting cervical malignancy should be aware of the association between HPV infection and anal cancer.

The majority of anal cancers are of squamous cell origin and 80% are preceded by relatively innocuous skin changes. Early identification is important because anal cancer can often be prevented or treated with conservative management strategies, whereas late presentation often necessitates radical surgery associated with substantial morbidity. We discuss causes, diagnosis, and management of anal cancer, focusing particularly on recent changes in management strategies. We draw on the findings of systematic reviews and cite recognised guidelines where possible.

Who is most at risk?

Observational evidence from the UK has shown that in the past three decades, the greatest increase in incidence of anal cancer has occurred in women.[6] [7] Figure 1 illustrates this trend as seen in south east England from the late 1800s

through to 1964. The average age for diagnosis in both men and women is 57 years.

Population based case-control studies from Denmark and Sweden[w1] showed that anal cancer is associated with HPV infection in 90% of patients,[1] and a large case-control study found positive associations between incidence of anal cancer and various health and lifestyle factors.[8] This study identified cigarette smoking as a substantial risk factor in both men and women (relative risks 9.4 and 7.7, respectively, compared with non-smoking controls);[8] 28% of patients with anal cancer gave a history of genital warts as a result of HPV infection, compared with only 1-2% of controls, and a history of receptive anal intercourse in men increased the relative risk of developing anal cancer by 33 times compared with controls with colon cancer. HIV infection in men who have sex with men was associated with approximately double the risk of developing anal cancer compared with men who have sex with men who were HIV negative.[8] [9]

How do patients with anal cancer present?

Common presenting symptoms include anal pain, bleeding, discharge, pruritus, and ulceration (fig 2). If the anal sphincters are infiltrated by tumour patients may report faecal incontinence and tenesmus. Locally advanced disease may present with perianal infection and fistula formation. It is important to identify palpable inguinal lymphadenopathy at presentation because worse outcomes, higher local failure, and decreased survival have been reported if nodal spread has occurred.[10] Radiological assessment is required to detect distant metastases. Although metastases are not common, occurring in less than 10% of patients with anal cancer, the ACT 1 trial indicated that 40% of this patient subgroup died as a consequence of metastatic spread.[11] Invasive anal cancer is occasionally an unexpected finding after excision of anal tags or haemorrhoids.

Red flag symptoms that should raise suspicion of anal cancer and for which a patient must be promptly referred for investigation are perianal bleeding, a palpable anal mass, and perianal ulceration.

Understanding anal anatomy

Definitions of anal anatomy are not consistent and surgeons, radiologists, and pathologists differ in how they classify structures. The following description is a pragmatic definition taken from the 2011 position statement for management of anal cancer from the Association of Coloproctology of Great Britain and Ireland[12] and relates directly to figure 3.

The anus can be divided into the anal canal and the anal margin; the former is 3.5-4 cm long in men and shorter in women. The anal canal begins where the rectum enters the puborectalis sling at the apex of the anal sphincter complex, and ends with the squamous mucosa blending with the perianal skin, which roughly coincides with the palpable intersphincteric groove. Immediately proximal to the dentate line, a narrow zone of transitional mucosa is

SOURCES AND SELECTION CRITERIA

We searched PubMed for clinically relevant studies, and the Cochrane library, using the search terms anal cancer and anal intraepithelial neoplasia. We consulted the National Institute for Health and Clinical Excellence guidelines and the Association of Coloproctology position statements.

SUMMARY POINTS

- Human papillomavirus infection increases an individual's risk of developing squamous cell carcinoma of the anus; cigarette smoking, high number of previous sexual partners, and previous pre-cancerous lesions of the cervix or vulva (in women) are also associated with increased risk

- Although anal cancer is not an AIDS defining cancer, its incidence is increased in HIV positive individuals and in those who are immunosuppressed

- Anal intraepithelial neoplasia usually precedes development of invasive squamous anal carcinoma and can present in various forms.

- The management of anal cancer has changed in recent years; chemo-irradiation rather than surgery is the first choice treatment for most lesions.

- Surgery may be the primary treatment modality for small perianal lesions which can be locally excised, but is now usually reserved for tumours that fail to respond to chemo-irradiation or for recurrent disease.

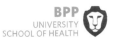

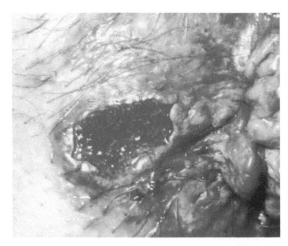

Fig 2 Perianal ulceration, typical of invasive anal cancer, often associated with symptoms of bleeding, pain, and pruritus.

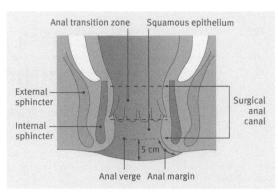

Fig 3 Cross sectional anatomy of the anal canal. Adapted from Renehan et al[12]

variably present—the anal transition zone. Distal to this, the mucosa consists of squamous epithelium devoid of hairs and glands. The anal margin extends distal to the anal verge (the junction of the hair bearing skin) to a 5 cm circumferential area from it. Lymphatic drainage of the anal canal depends on location: below the dentate line drainage is to the inguinal group of nodes; above, lymph drains to the mesorectal, lateral pelvic and inferior mesenteric nodes.[12]

What is anal intraepithelial neoplasia and how do I recognise it?

Anal intraepithelial neoplasia usually precedes the development of invasive squamous anal carcinoma. It can involve both the perianal skin and anal canal. A population based, case-control study has shown that anal intraepithelial neoplasia is strongly associated with HPV infection.[3] It can present as part of a multifocal disease process involving any or all sites of anogenital cancer.[13] There are aetiological and clinical parallels between anal intraepithelial neoplasia, vulval intraepithelial neoplasia, and cervical intraepithelial neoplasia. A recent Association of Coloproctology Position statement suggests that the progression of anal intraepithelial neoplasia to invasive anal cancer more closely resembles the natural history of vulval intraepithelial neoplasia, with expected malignant transformation in about 10% of immunocompetent patients over five years.[14]

Patients may present with pruritus or anal discharge. Suspicious lesions may be raised, scaly, white plaques, erythematous, pigmented, fissured, or eczematous (fig 4).[15] Anal intraepithelial neoplasia is present in 28-35% of excised anal condylomata.[16w2]

How are suspicious lesions investigated?

Evaluation in primary care

Ask the patient about risk factors for anal cancer. Obtaining a careful medical history (including asking about chronic diseases) will help to evaluate a patient's fitness for any future surgery and other treatment. Age over 75 years is associated with reduced tolerance to chemoradiotherapy and increased risk of local disease relapse.[17][18] In view of the association with HPV it is also prudent for a thorough sexual history to be taken.

Although anal cancer is not an AIDS defining cancer (meaning that diagnosis of anal cancer does not indicate the conversion of HIV to AIDS), it is 30 times more common in HIV positive individuals. Therefore HIV status should be considered, and for known HIV positive patients it is sensible to obtain up to date results for viral load and CD4 count.[12]

Patients who describe perianal symptoms consistent with anal intraepithelial neoplasia or anal cancer require examination of the perineum, digital rectal examination, and examination of the inguinal area for palpable nodes. Consider vaginal examination in women because of the multifocal nature of the disease, specifically with a view to identifying lesions on the vulval skin or vaginal mucosa. Suspicious lesions may suggest the presence of vulval intraepithelial neoplasia and should trigger referral to a gynaecological specialist.

Note any changes in pigmentation of the perianal region, as well as ulceration and the presence of skin tags or condylomata. As part of the digital rectal examination it is important to document any palpable mass lesion, if possible indicating the distance from the anal verge at which the mass is felt and the proportion of the anal circumference that it occupies. Inspect the glove for blood from the anal canal.

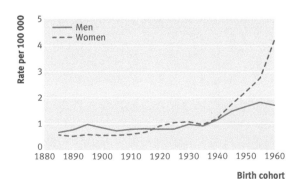

Fig 1 Age standardised rates of anal cancer by birth cohort. Adapted from Robinson et al (Br J Cancer 2009)[7]

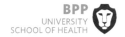

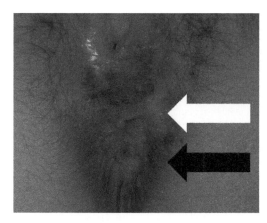

Fig 4 Perianal pigmented anal intraepithelial neoplasia III lesion (black arrow) and associated white plaque (white arrow)

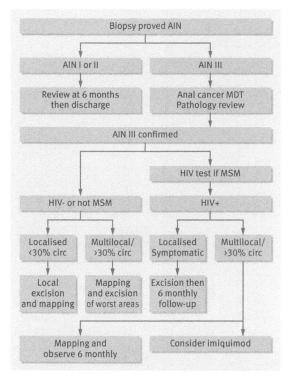

Fig 5 Treatment algorithm for the management of anal intraepithelial neoplasia (AIN).[14] MDT=multidisciplinary team. MSM=men who have sex with men. % circ=percentage of the circumference of the perianal skin/anal canal occupied by lesion

Before referral to a specialist it is helpful to request a full blood count, serum urea and electrolytes, and, in HIV positive patients, an assessment of current CD4 status.

Diagnosing anal intraepithelial neoplasia

Diagnosis of anal intraepithelial neoplasia requires primary care practitioners to maintain a high index of suspicion particularly in patients with known risk factors who present with new symptoms. For a definitive diagnosis a biopsy of the suspicious area is needed. This will normally be performed by a specialist following referral.

Referral of patients with suspected anal cancer

Guidelines from the UK National Institute of Health and Clinical Excellence recommend that patients presenting with bleeding from the anus that has lasted longer than six weeks, a palpable mass on rectal examination, or anaemia without a known cause should be referred for urgent investigation for cancer. Pragmatically this means that they will be included in the two week wait rule and receive a diagnostic investigation within 14 days of referral, because urgent consultation with a specialist has been recognised as a priority.

Investigations undertaken in specialist care

After referral to a specialist, the patient is likely to undergo biopsy of the suspect lesion in order to establish a histological diagnosis. Biopsy often takes place as part of a formal examination under anaesthesia, which can also provide information about the size of the lesion and involvement of adjacent structures, and may be supplemented by sigmoidoscopy.

Imaging is used to inform tumour staging. Distant metastatic spread can be determined by computed tomography of the thorax, abdomen, and pelvis. Magnetic resonance imaging of the pelvis allows assessment of tumour size and local invasion and the involvement of local lymph nodes. Endoanal ultrasound provides a 360° image of the anal canal and is useful for assessing tumour depth, particularly if there is concern that the anal sphincters may be involved. It is useful for assessing local response to treatment but is limited by its restricted field of view and may miss lymph nodes in the mesorectum.

How is anal intraepithelial neoplasia treated?

The priorities of managing anal intraepithelial neoplasia are to minimise symptoms and prevent the development of anal cancer. A number of different strategies can be employed to achieve these end points.

Observation only

Conservative management derives from a combination of single centre studies that have shown low rates of malignant transformation in immunocompetent patients with anal intraepithelial neoplasia[19w3] and high recurrence rates after aggressive surgery. Recurrences after surgery are thought to occur because of the inability to completely eradicate local HPV. Therefore patients with low grade anal dysplasia are followed up every six to 12 months.[w4]

Chemoradiotherapy

No supporting evidence has been established for the use of chemoradiotherapy in anal intraepithelial neoplasia, but anecdotal reports have described success in vulval intraepithelial neoplasia. However the use of radiotherapy in particular may lead to the development of anal stenosis.

Surgery

Local excision of small lesions preserves tissue histology, which can help to guide future management. Local excision is suitable for lesions that cover less than a third of the anal circumference. Before excision the surgeon will usually perform anal mapping to determine the extent of the disease. Mapping involves taking eight to 12 biopsies from around the anal margin and canal. It is useful to record the procedure on an operative mapping sheet or with digital photography.

Brown et al performed preoperative mapping and local excision on 34 patients with high grade anal intraepithelial neoplasia. On review 56% had margin involvement and 63% recurred within 12 months.[w5] No patient developed carcinoma but five developed anal stenosis or faecal incontinence.

Wide local excision has also been considered for larger anal lesions, but these techniques present an even greater

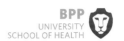

risk of postoperative complications and are probably overly aggressive for a disease process in which the natural history is still not fully understood. If the worst areas are excised then the remaining lesions can be managed expectantly.

Immunomodulation therapy

Imiquimod is a nucleoside analogue of the imidazoquinoline family and has pro-inflammatory, anti-tumour, and anti-viral activity. It is prescribed as a 5% cream, and applied topically it can induce regression of anal intraepithelial neoplasia and eradication of HPV. A double blind randomised controlled trial showed sustained regression of high grade intraepithelial neoplasia in 61% of patients, with a median follow-up of 36 months.[w6] In a separate review of cohort studies and case reports, imiquimod was associated with a complete regression in 48% of anal intraepithelial neoplasia lesions and a partial response in 34%. This was associated with a recurrence rate of 36% over 11-39 months of follow-up.[w7] Most studies of imiquimod have assessed its use in HIV positive populations with short follow-up, and the drug has rarely been compared with other treatment strategies. Despite the relative success of this treatment, caution should be used when extrapolating this evidence to other populations of patients with anal intraepithelial neoplasia.

HPV immunotherapy

Vaccination against HPV was first approved in the United States in 2006. The evidence for its use in preventing cervical intraepithelial neoplasia and cervical malignancies as part of a population based immunisation programme is well established.[w8] The quadrivalent vaccine has also shown efficacy against anogenital warts in phase II/III trials. However, clarification of some uncertainties—notably vaccine efficacy in men and HIV infected individuals, and the feasibility to offer vaccination programmes to both sexes—is required to establish the benefits of HPV vaccines for the prevention of malignant and premalignant anal lesions.

Photodynamic therapy

Case reports and small uncontrolled trials have supported the use of photodynamic therapy in anal intraepithelial neoplasia.[w9] However this type of therapy is painful and often requires multiple treatments.[w10] Larger series with long term follow up are required before it could be recommended as standard therapy.

Ablation

Goldstone et al[w11] retrospectively reviewed 75 cases of high grade anal intraepithelial neoplasia in which patients had received infrared coagulator ablative therapy. They quoted the probability of success as 81% after a single treatment, rising with repeated treatment and with no evidence of serious complications. However, the follow-up period was limited (one to two years) and the outcomes were not as good if the patient was HIV positive before treatment. Other reviews point to a high recurrence rate and substantial postoperative pain, also questioning the ability of ablation

---

> **WHO HISTOLOGICAL CLASSIFICATION OF TUMOURS OF THE ANAL CANAL**
>
> **Epithelial tumours**
> - Intraepithelial neoplasia (dysplasia)
> - Squamous or transitional epithelium
> - Glandular
> - Paget disease
>
> **Carcinoma**
> - Squamous cell carcinoma
> - Adenocarcinoma
> - Mucinous adenocarcinoma
> - Small cell carcinoma
> - Undifferentiated carcinoma
> - Others
> - Carcinoid tumour
>
> **Malignant melanomaNon-epithelial tumours**
> *Adapted from Salmo et al[21]*

to clear HPV.[14] Ablative therapies can include laser ablation, cryotherapy, and electrocautery, but none of these provide histology, which can be useful when planning a patient's long term management.

Anal intraepithelial neoplasia is a complex disease process, the natural history of which remains unclear. Low grade dysplasia (anal intraepithelial neoplasia I and II) represents a much more indolent disease than high grade dysplasia (anal intraepithelial neoplasia III). Progression of disease and therefore associated treatment is more aggressive in HIV positive populations. With this in mind we have reproduced the treatment algorithm from the 2011 Association of Coloproctology guidelines (fig 5).[14]

How is anal cancer classified and staged?

The current WHO classification of anal tumours (box) categorises by histological tissue types. Squamous cell carcinoma is the most common type of anal cancer, seen in 80-85% of patients.[w12] Adenocarcinoma of the anus is less common, constituting 5-18% of cases.[20] Other malignancies are very rare.

Squamous cell carcinoma of the anal canal can be graded histologically, but neither the histological type nor the degree of differentiation seem to influence prognosis strongly.[22] Other authors have used anal cancer databases to perform multivariate analysis and establish factors that influence prognosis, which include the patient's sex, tumour stage, node involvement, and response to radiotherapy or combined treatment.[23 24 25]After confirmation of the diagnosis of anal cancer, tumour staging is needed. Anal cancers are staged in accordance with the American Joint Committee on Cancer/tumour node metastasis (TNM) classification. Staging provides prognostic significance based on five year survival (table).

How is anal cancer managed?

Anal cancer is a rare malignancy that requires care at specialist referral centres where diagnostic and treatment decisions can be referred to a single multidisciplinary team. This team ensures that treatment decisions are made involving experienced specialists from surgical, radiological, oncological, and gynaecological divisions. Given that 10% or less of patients with anal cancer have metastases at presentation, the mainstay of treatment is usually local control.

Five year survival for anal cancer on the basis of stage at diagnosis[26]

Tumour stage	5 year survival (%)
I	69.5
II	61.8
IIIA	45.6
IIIB	39.6
IV	15.3

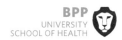

Non-surgical treatment

An important change in the recommended approach for treating anal cancer over the past two decades has been that chemoradiotherapy is now the first choice treatment for invasive anal cancer, with surgery reserved for salvage of local recurrence. The reasons for loss of enthusiasm for surgery as first line therapy included the high associated morbidity and frequent recurrence rates, presumably because although surgical resection removed the malignant tissue it could not eradicate the underlying HPV infection.

Six randomised trials of non-surgical treatment have been reviewed in the Association of Coloproctology position statement on anal cancer,[27] which supports the use of combination chemoradiotherapy including 5-fluorouracil and mitomycin C, but also acknowledges that conclusions are based on a cohort of 1628 patients spread across trials with heterogeneous methodology.

Patients who receive chemoradiotherapy may lose fertility and may need a colostomy either before or after treatment. Pelvic radiotherapy can lead to faecal incontinence and the development of rectovaginal fistula. These complications may reduce a patient's quality of life and patients should be counselled about them when treatment is discussed.

Surgical treatment

Well differentiated anal margin tumours less than 2 cm in diameter (T1 No) or occupying less than half the anal circumference can initially be treated by local excision, which provides definitive treatment if all resection margins are clear.[28w13]

Currently the main role for surgery in anal cancer is for "salvage treatment" after failure of chemoradiotherapy. A retrospective review showed that disease relapse is most likely within the first three years and rare after five years.[29]

Renehan and O'Dwyer recently reviewed the management of local disease relapse after treatment for anal cancer.[30] Following examination of 13 studies that had reported oncological outcomes after salvage surgery for relapsed anal cancer they concluded that salvage surgery with abdominoperineal excision offers the only opportunity for cure in these patients. The excision margins for anal cancer surgery are wider than for rectal cancer and therefore perineal reconstruction and the assistance of urological, plastic, and gynaecological surgeons may be required. There are a number of reasons for the wider margins: firstly, to take account of local spread, the perineal skin resection is wider; secondly, the lateral oncological margin for salvage surgery is the level of the ischial tuberosity; thirdly, owing to the preoperative fibrosing effects of radiotherapy, a wide excision margin may be needed to ensure a well vascularised skin edge; and finally, involvement of adjacent pelvic organs is common.

The most frequent operation performed for anal cancer that has failed to respond to chemoradiotherapy is an abdominoperineal resection with perineal reconstruction. This operation involves the removal of the anal canal and rectum and the formation of a permanent stoma, usually sited on the left lower quadrant of the abdomen. Outcomes for this type of surgery have only been described in small, retrospective, single centre studies with heterogeneous methodology, but the results suggest a five year survival between 30% and 69%.[29w14-w18]

Factors that have been associated with decreased survival include positive lymph nodes at presentation, increased tumour size, advanced age of the patient, comorbidities, and positive resection margins (that is, when pathology shows the tumour extending to the margin of resection, suggesting incomplete excision). Debate continues over whether the presence of persistent or recurrent disease as the reason for surgery has a true effect on survival.[w14-w18]

Perineal reconstruction refers to the use of local and distant tissue flaps or commercial material to fill the defect left after excision. This type of wound repair involves a risk of postoperative complications, with infection and breakdown reported in 35% to 72% of cases.[w15 w16 w18]

Rare anal tumours

Although true anal adenocarcinomas do occur, adenocarcinoma of the anal canal is more commonly a very low rectal cancer that has spread distally. True adenocarcinomas probably originate from the anal glands and then spread outwards to involve the anal sphincter. This is a very rare tumour that is sensitive to chemoradiotherapy.[w19 w20]

Malignant melanoma accounts for 1% of malignant anal canal tumours. In presentation, they may mimic a thrombosed haemorrhoid. Anal melanoma is an aggressive disease with early infiltration and distant spread resulting in poor overall prognosis. It is not sensitive to chemotherapy or radiotherapy. Review of 85 patients treated at a single centre showed a median survival of 19 months.[w21] A recent systematic review compared abdominoperineal resection of the rectum with wide local excision and found no distinct survival advantage for either procedure.[w22] As chances of cure are minimal, radical surgery should not be considered as a primary treatment, but local excision may provide useful palliation.

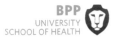
Contributors: JADS was responsible article concept, design, drafting and revision. JHS was responsible for revising the article critically and final approval of the published version.

Competing interests: All authors have completed the ICMJE uniform disclosure form at www.icmje.org/coi_disclosure.pdf (available on request from the corresponding author) and declare: no support from any organisation for the submitted work; no financial relationships with any organisations that might have an interest in the submitted work in the previous three years; no other relationships or activities that could appear to have influenced the submitted work.

Provenance and peer review: Not commissioned, externally peer reviewed.

1 Parkin DM. The global health burden of infection-associated cancers in the year 2002. Int J Cancer2006;118:3030-44.

2 WHO/ICO Information Centre on HPV and Cervical Cancer (HPV Information Centre). Human Papillomavirus and Related Cancers in United Kingdom. Summary Report. 2010. http://apps.who.int/hpvcentre/statistics/dynamic/ico/country_pdf/GBR.pdf?CFID=27804&CFTOKEN=18959369.

3 Daling JR, Madeleine MM, Johnson LG, Schwartz SM, Shera KA, Wurscher MA, et al. Human papillomavirus, smoking, and sexual practices in the etiology of anal cancer. Cancer2004;101:270-80.

4 Critchlow CW, Hawes SE, Kuypers JM, Goldbaum GM, Holmes KK, Surawicz CM, et al. Effect of HIV infection on the natural history of anal human papillomavirus infection. Aids1998;12:1177-84.

5 Edgren G, Sparen P. Risk of anogenital cancer after diagnosis of cervical intraepithelial neoplasia: a prospective population-based study. Lancet Oncol2007;8:311-6.

6 Brewster DH, Bhatti LA. Increasing incidence of squamous cell carcinoma of the anus in Scotland, 1975-2002. Br J Cancer2006;95:87-90.

7 Robinson D, Coupland V, Moller H. An analysis of temporal and generational trends in the incidence of anal and other HPV-related cancers in Southeast England. Br J Cancer2009;100:527-31.

8 Daling JR, Weiss NS, Hislop TG, Maden C, Coates RJ, Sherman KJ, et al. Sexual practices, sexually transmitted diseases, and the incidence of anal cancer. N Engl J Med1987;317:973-7.

9 Patel P, Hanson DL, Sullivan PS, Novak RM, Moorman AC, Tong TC, et al. Incidence of types of cancer among HIV-infected persons compared with the general population in the United States, 1992-2003. Ann Intern Med2008;148:728-36.

10 Bartelink H, Roelofsen F, Eschwege F, Rougier P, Bosset JF, Gonzalez DG, et al. Concomitant radiotherapy and chemotherapy is superior to radiotherapy alone in the treatment of locally advanced anal cancer: results of a phase III randomized trial of the European Organization for Research and Treatment of Cancer Radiotherapy and Gastrointestinal Cooperative Groups. J Clin Oncol1997;15:2040-9.

11 UKCCCR Anal Cancer Trial Working Party, UK Co-ordinating Committee on Cancer Research. Epidermoid anal cancer: results from the UKCCCR randomised trial of radiotherapy alone versus radiotherapy, 5-fluorouracil, and mitomycin. Lancet1996;348:1049-54.

12 Renehan AG, O'Dwyer ST. Initial management through the anal cancer multidisciplinary team meeting. Colorectal Dis 2011;13(suppl 1):21-8.

13 Carter JJ, Madeleine MM, Shera K, Schwartz SM, Cushing-Haugen KL, Wipf GC, et al. Human papillomavirus 16 and 18 L1 serology compared across anogenital cancer sites. Cancer Res2001;61:1934-40.

14 Scholefield JH, Harris D, Radcliffe A. Guidelines for management of anal intraepithelial neoplasia. Colorectal Dis2011;13(suppl 1):3-10.

15 Zbar AP, Fenger C, Efron J, Beer-Gabel M, Wexner SD. The pathology and molecular biology of anal intraepithelial neoplasia: comparisons with cervical and vulvar intraepithelial carcinoma. Int J Colorectal Dis2002;17:203-15.

16 Carter PS, de Ruiter A, Whatrup C, Katz DR, Ewings P, Mindel A, et al. Human immunodeficiency virus infection and genital warts as risk factors for anal intraepithelial neoplasia in homosexual men. Br J Surg1995;82:473-4.

17 Chauveinc L, Buthaud X, Falcou MC, Mosseri V, De la Rochefordiere A, Pierga JY, et al. Anal canal cancer treatment: practical limitations of routine prescription of concurrent chemotherapy and radiotherapy. Br J Cancer2003;89:2057-61.

18 Renehan AG, Saunders MP, Schofield PF, O'Dwyer ST. Patterns of local disease failure and outcome after salvage surgery in patients with anal cancer. Br J Surg2005;92:605-14.

19 Scholefield JH, Castle MT, Watson NF. Malignant transformation of high-grade anal intraepithelial neoplasia. Br J Surg2005;92:1133-6.

20 Licitra L, Spinazze S, Doci R, Evans TR, Tanum G, Ducreux M. Cancer of the anal region. Crit Rev Oncol Hematol2002;43:77-92.

21 Salmo E, Haboubi N. Anal cancer: pathology, staging and evidence-based minimum data set. Colorectal Dis 2011;13(suppl 1):11-20.

22 Hill J, Meadows H, Haboubi N, Talbot IC, Northover JM. Pathological staging of epidermoid anal carcinoma for the new era. Colorectal Dis2003;5:206-13.

23 Scott NA, Beart RW, Jr., Weiland LH, Cha SS, Lieber MM. Carcinoma of the anal canal and flow cytometric DNA analysis. Br J Cancer1989;60:56-8.

24 Peiffert D, Bey P, Pernot M, Hoffstetter S, Marchal C, Beckendorf V, et al. Conservative treatment by irradiation of epidermoid carcinomas of the anal margin. Int J Radiat Oncol Biol Phys1997;39:57-66.

25 Ajani JA, Winter KA, Gunderson LL, Pedersen J, Benson AB, 3rd, Thomas CR Jr, et al. Prognostic factors derived from a prospective database dictate clinical biology of anal cancer: the intergroup trial (RTOG 98-11). Cancer2010;116:4007-13.

26 Edge SB, American Joint Committee on Cancer. AJCC cancer staging manual. 7th ed. Springer, 2009.

27 Kronfli M, Glynne-Jones R. Chemoradiotherapy in anal cancer. Colorectal Dis 2011;13(suppl 1):33-8.

28 Glynne-Jones R, Northover JM, Cervantes A. Anal cancer: ESMO Clinical Practice Guidelines for diagnosis, treatment and follow-up. Ann Oncol2010;21(suppl 5):v87-92.

29 Pocard M, Tiret E, Nugent K, Dehni N, Parc R. Results of salvage abdominoperineal resection for anal cancer after radiotherapy. Dis Colon Rectum 1998;41:1488-93.

30 Renehan AG, O'Dwyer ST. Management of local disease relapse. Colorectal Dis2011;13(suppl 1):44-52.

Related links

bmj.com/archive
Previous articles in this series
- Management of deep vein thrombosis and prevention of post-thrombotic syndrome (2011;343:d5916)
- Diagnosis and management of autism in childhood (2011;343:d6238)
- Diagnosis and management of maturity onset diabetes of the young (MODY) (2011;343:d6044)
- Actinomycosis (2011;343:d6099)
- Managing perioperative risk in patients undergoing elective non-cardiac surgery (2011;343:d5759)

bmj.com
- Get CME points at BMJ Learning

More titles in The BMJ Clinical Review Series

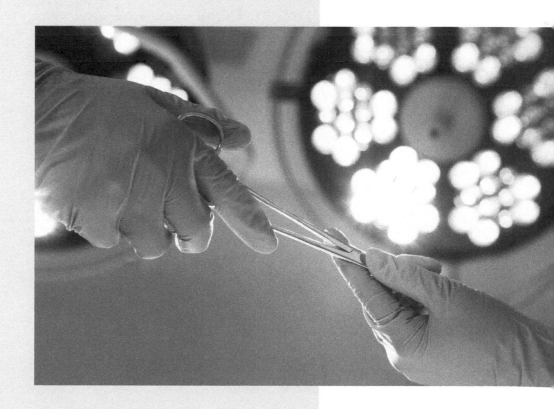

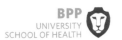
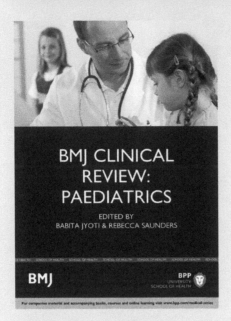
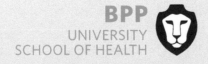

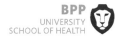
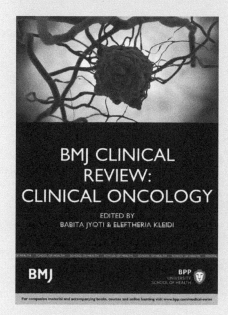
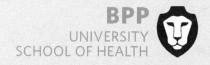

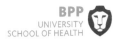

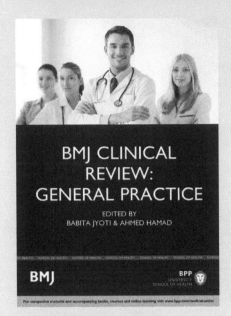
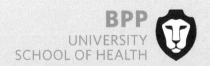

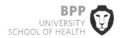
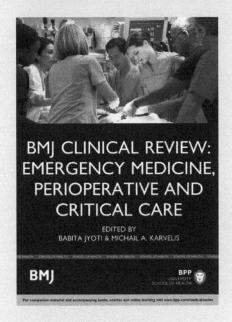
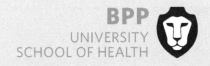

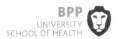

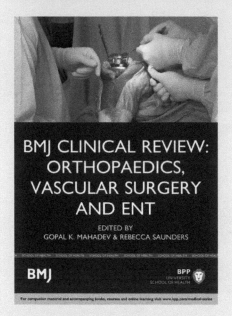
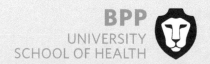

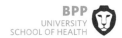
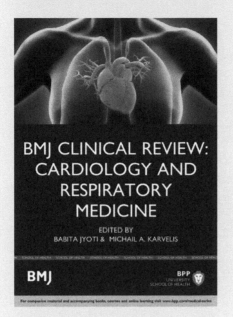
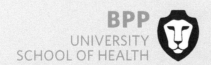

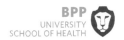
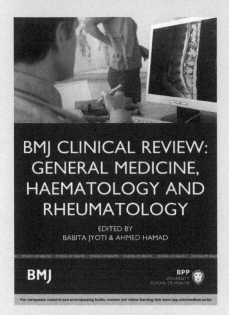
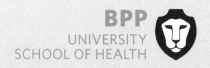

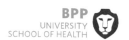

More titles in The Progressing your Medical Career Series

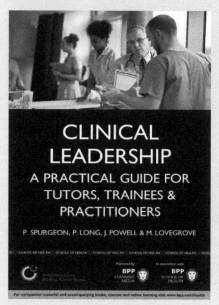

CLINICAL LEADERSHIP
A PRACTICAL GUIDE FOR TUTORS, TRAINEES & PRACTITIONERS

P. SPURGEON, P. LONG, J. POWELL & M. LOVEGROVE

£24.99

June 2015

Paperback

978-1-472727-83-1

Are you a healthcare professional or student who wishes to acquire and develop your leadership and management skills? Do you recognise the role and influence of strong leadership and management in modern healthcare?

Clinical leadership is something in which all healthcare professionals can participate in, in terms of driving forward high quality care for their patients. In this up-to-date guide, the authors take you through the latest leadership and management thinking, and how this links in with the Clinical Leadership Competency Framework. As well as influencing undergraduate curricula this framework forms the basis of the leadership component of the curricula for all healthcare specialties, so a practical knowledge of it is essential for all healthcare professionals in training.

Using case studies and practical exercises to provide a strong work-based emphasis, this practical guide will enable you to build on your existing experiences to develop your leadership and management skills, and to develop strategies and approaches to improving care for your patients.

This book addresses:

- Why strong leadership and management are crucial to delivering high quality care;
- The theory and evidence behind the Clinical Leadership Competency Framework;
- The practical aspects of leadership learning in a wide range of clinical environments
- How clinical professionals and trainers can best facilitate leadership learning for their trainees and students within the clinical work-place.

Whether you are a student just starting out on your career, or an established healthcare professional wishing to develop yourself as a clinical leader, this practical, easy-to-use guide will give you the techniques and knowledge you require to excel.

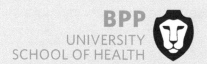

BPP
UNIVERSITY
SCHOOL OF HEALTH

www.bpp.com/medical-series

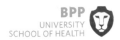
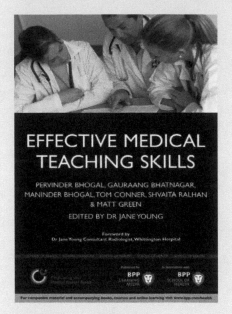
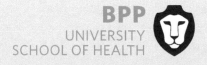

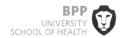
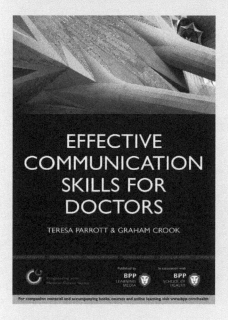

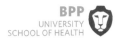

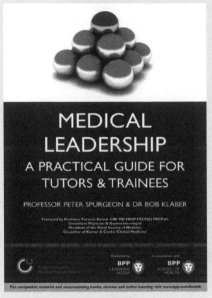
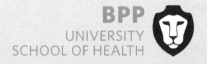

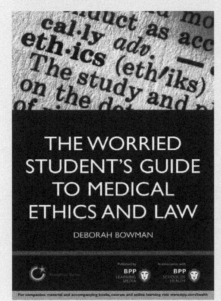
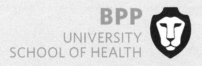

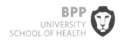
More Titles in The Progressing Your Medical Career Series

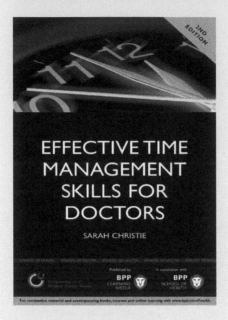

EFFECTIVE TIME MANAGEMENT SKILLS FOR DOCTORS

SARAH CHRISTIE

£19.99

October 2011

Paperback

978-1-906839-08-6

Do you find it difficult to achieve a work-life balance? Would you like to know how you can become more effective with the time you have?

With the introduction of the European Working Time Directive, which will severely limit the hours in the working week, it is more important than ever that doctors improve their personal effectiveness and time management skills. This interactive book will enable you to focus on what activities are needlessly taking up your time and what steps you can take to manage your time better.

By taking the time to read through, complete the exercises and follow the advice contained within this book you will begin to:

- Understand where your time is being needlessly wasted

- Discover how to be more assertive and learn how to say 'No'

- Set yourself priorities and stick to them

- Learn how to complete tasks more efficiently

- Plan better so you can spend more time doing the things you enjoy

In recent years, with the introduction of the NHS Plan and Lord Darzi's commitment to improve the quality of healthcare provision, there is a need for doctors to become more effective within their working environment. This book will offer you the chance to regain some clarity on how you actually spend your time and give you the impetus to ensure you achieve the tasks and goals which are important to you.

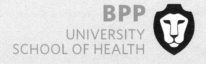

BPP
UNIVERSITY
SCHOOL OF HEALTH

www.bpp.com/medical-series

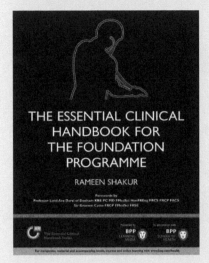
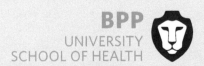

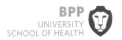
More titles in The Essential Clinical Handbook Series

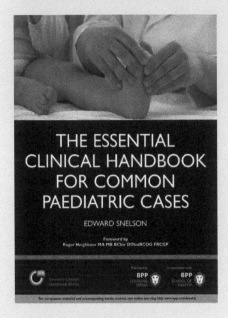

THE ESSENTIAL
CLINICAL HANDBOOK
FOR COMMON
PAEDIATRIC CASES

EDWARD SNELSON

Foreword by
Roger Neighbour MA MB BChir DObstRCOG FRCGP

September 2011

Paperback

978-1-445379-60-9

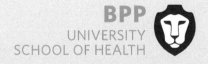

BPP
UNIVERSITY
SCHOOL OF HEALTH

Not sure what to do when faced with a crying baby and demanding parent on the ward? Would you like a definitive guide on how to manage commonly encountered paediatric cases?

This clear and concise clinical handbook has been written to help healthcare professionals approach the initial assessment and management of paediatric cases commonly encountered by Junior Doctors, GPs, GP Specialty Trainee's and allied healthcare professionals. The children who make paediatrics so fun, can also make it more than a little daunting for even the most confident person. This insightful guide has been written based on the author's extensive experience within both a General Practice and hospital setting.

Intended as a practical guide to common paediatric problems it will increase confidence and satisfaction in managing these conditions. Each chapter provides a clear structure for investigating potential paediatric illnesses including clinical and non-clinical advice covering: background, how to assess, pitfalls to avoid, FAQs and what to tell parents. This helpful guide provides :

- A problem/symptom based approach to common paediatric conditions

- As essential guide for any doctor assessing children on the front line

- Provides easy-to-follow and step-by-step guidance on how to approach different paediatric conditions

- Useful both as a textbook and a quick reference guide when needed on the ward

This engaging and easy to use guide will provide you with the knowledge, skills and confidence required to effectively diagnose and manage commonly encountered paediatric cases both within a primary and secondary care setting.

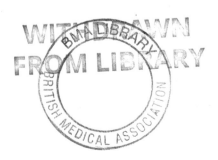